# Health Promotion Programs

## From Theory to Practice

### CARL I. FERTMAN
### DIANE D. ALLENSWORTH

#### EDITORS

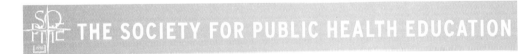

THE SOCIETY FOR PUBLIC HEALTH EDUCATION

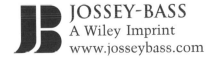

JOSSEY-BASS
A Wiley Imprint
www.josseybass.com

Published by Jossey-Bass
A Wiley Imprint
989 Market Street, San Francisco, CA 94103-1741—www.josseybass.com

Jossey-Bass books and products are available through most bookstores. To contact Jossey-Bass directly call our Customer Care Department within the U.S. at 800-956-7739, outside the U.S. at 317-572-3986, or fax 317-572-4002.

Jossey-Bass also publishes its books in a variety of electronic formats. Some content that appears in print may not be available in electronic books.

**Library of Congress Cataloging-in-Publication Data**
Health promotion programs: from theory to practice/Carl I. Fertman, Diane D. Allensworth, editors.
　　p.;　cm.
　　Includes bibliographical references and index.
　　ISBN 978-0-470-24155-4 (pbk.)
　　　1. Health promotion.　I. Fertman, Carl I., date.　II. Allensworth, Diane DeMuth.
　　[DNLM: 1. Health Promotion—United States.　2. Health Education—United States.
WA 590 H4396 2010]
　　RA427.8.H5255 2010
　　613—dc22

2009054080

Printed in the United States of America
FIRST EDITION
*PB Printing*　　　　10 9 8 7 6 5 4

# CONTENTS

## PART TWO: PLANNING HEALTH PROMOTION PROGRAMS

## PART THREE: IMPLEMENTING HEALTH PROMOTION PROGRAMS

7. **Advocacy**   181

Regina A. Galer-Unti, Kelly Bishop Alley, Regina McCoy Pulliam

8. **Communicating Health Information Effectively**   203

Neyal J. Ammary-Risch, Allison Zambon, Kelli McCormack Brown

9. **Developing and Increasing Program Funding**   233

Carl I. Fertman, Karen A. Spiller, Angela D. Mickalide

# PART FOUR: EVALUATING AND SUSTAINING HEALTH PROMOTION PROGRAMS

10. **Evaluating and Improving a Health Promotion Program**   259

Daniel Perales, Andy Fourney, Barbara MkNelly, Edward Mamary

## PART FIVE: HEALTH PROMOTION PROGRAMS IN DIVERSE SETTINGS

# FIGURES, TABLES, AND EXHIBITS

## Figures

## Tables

# Exhibits

# PREFACE

**The need for health promotion programs** is all around us. Workers in hospitals, factories, businesses, schools, colleges, day care centers, government offices, churches, health clinics, community centers, and local health departments are all thinking about how to improve the lives and productivity of people where they live, work, and play. And if you are working or planning to work in health education, public health, medicine, nursing, or any other health-related field, you're probably going to be involved with a health promotion program at some time. In the process, you'll use your clinical and professional expertise as well as academic training to develop and implement a plan to improve the health status of individuals and populations as well as reduce the risk of persons becoming ill or help restore their health. You'll most likely be part of a team that is organizing a health promotion program. At first, the concept of a program to improve or promote the health of people may sound a little intimidating. Ultimately, it becomes clear that although the idea of a health promotion program is appealing and seems worthwhile, turning the idea into reality demands work and expertise. In other words, it is easy to say that something should be done or needs to be done. It is very different to know how to design and implement a program to actually achieve a specific health outcome or an improvement in the overall health status of a specific population. It is a complex process.

Undergraduate and graduate programs that prepare professionals to work in public health, health education, and health promotion and wellness have been flourishing in the United States and throughout the world for more than half a century. Thousands of students graduate every year with a baccalaureate or advanced degree in health promotion and get jobs in schools, colleges, businesses, health care facilities, community organizations, and government.

As the premier organization of professionals trained and working in health education and health promotion, leaders of the Society for Public Health Education (SOPHE) recognized the need for a book to help advance the field at the undergraduate level. Escalating rates of chronic disease, soaring health care costs, increasing diversity of the U.S. population, as well as aging of the current health education workforce, all call for training a new generation of health promoters. The SOPHE board of trustees, executive director, and members offer this book, which combines the theoretical and practice base of the field with a step-by-step practical section on how to develop, implement, and evaluate health promotion programs. SOPHE hopes that this book, read in its entirety or in part, will help not only undergraduate students who choose to major or minor in health education, health promotion, community health, public health, or health-related fields (for example, environmental health, physical activity, allied health, nursing, or medicine) but also professionals already working who want to acquire the technical knowledge and skills to develop successful health promotion programs. Acquiring the competencies to effectively plan, implement, and evaluate health promotion programs can improve health outcomes, promote behavioral and social change, and contribute to eliminating health disparities. This book offers a concise summary of the many years of research in the fields of health education and health promotion, along with the expertise of many SOPHE members working in diverse contemporary settings and programs. The book also reflects SOPHE's mission and its commitment to professional preparation and continuing education for the purpose of improving the quantity and quality of the lives of individuals and communities.

We are enormously grateful to the many SOPHE members who wrote this book. Their expertise in many fields, including health education, public health, sociology, anthropology, psychology, nursing, medicine, physical education, nutrition, allied health, and many others, have been braided into this health promotion anthology. They have shared the foundations of the field as well as their own practical experiences in health promotion planning. May this book help teach, guide, inspire, catalyze, and transform students and professionals in their quest to develop successful health promotion programs that address the health challenges of both today and tomorrow.

## ABOUT THIS BOOK

Opportunities to prevent disease and to promote health are abundant. Promoting health helps people to lead socially and economically productive lives. The goal of the book is to provide a comprehensive introduction to health promotion programs by combining the theory and practice with a hands-on guide to program planning, implementation, and evaluation. One of the fundamental premises of this book is the importance of using an approach based in both research and practice to guide and inform planning, implementation, and evaluation of health promotion programs. A secondary goal of this book is to review the widespread opportunities to implement health promotion programs in schools, communities, workplaces, and health care organizations. This text addresses the needs of students and professionals who are pursuing careers in health education as well as nursing, medicine, public health, and allied health.

Since 1950, SOPHE has been a leading organization in the field of health promotion. This book reflects its commitment to responding to the needs of its members, future members, and the broader field by delivering quality products and services. Principles of integrity, accountability, and transparency guided the book's development. Every step in the writing process was shared and discussed among members. Teamwork, collaboration, and diversity were cornerstones for the writing teams for each chapter. It is not always easy to write about something you do every day. It is challenging to write down your thoughts and let others read and comment on them. With respect and care, the process encouraged innovation and creativity that made the book better for readers and the subsequent programs that they will develop.

## WHO SHOULD READ THIS BOOK

This book is aimed at three audiences. The first audience is individuals pursuing an undergraduate major or minor in health education, health promotion, community health, public health, or health-related fields such as environmental health, physical activity and education, allied health, nursing, or medicine. The second audience is young and mid-career practitioners, practicing managers, researchers, and instructors who for the first time are responsible for teaching, designing, or leading health promotion programs. The third audience is colleagues and professionals not trained in the health fields but working in settings where health promotion programs are increasingly prevalent and might be under their supervision (for example, school superintendents and principals, human resource directors working in business and health care, college deans of student affairs, faculty members, board members of nonprofit organizations, community members, and employers and staff members in businesses and health care organizations).

## OVERVIEW OF THE CONTENTS

The book is divided into five parts. Part One presents the foundations of health promotion programs: what health and health promotion are, the history of health promotion, sites of health promotion programs, and the key people (stakeholders) involved in programs. Highlighted and explored are the two guiding forces in planning, implementing, and evaluating health promotion programs. The first is eliminating health disparities. The second is use of health theories and models.

Parts Two (planning), Three (implementation), and Four (evaluation) provide a step-by-step guide to planning, implementing, and evaluating a health promotion program. Each chapter covers specific phases of health promotion program planning, implementation, and evaluation. Practical tips and specific examples aim to facilitate readers' understanding of the phases as well as to build technical skills in designing and leading evidence-based health promotion programs.

Part Five presents health promotion programs across four settings: schools (elementary to college), health care organizations, workplaces, and communities. Each chapter presents keys for effective site-specific programs to promote health.

At the beginning of each chapter, a set of Learning Objectives provides a framework and guide to the chapter topics. The key terms at the end of each chapter can be used as a reference while reading this book as well as a way to recap key definitions in planning, implementation, and evaluation of health promotion programs. At the end of the text, all the key terms are listed and defined in a glossary.

Practical examples throughout this book reinforce the need for health promotion programs to be based on in-depth understanding of the intended audiences' perceptions, beliefs, attitudes, behaviors, and barriers to change as well as the cultural, social, and environmental context in which people live. By referring to current theories and models of health promotion, this book also reinforces the need for health promotion practitioners to base their programs on theories, models, and approaches that guide and inform health promotion program design, implementation, and evaluation.

Each chapter ends with practice and discussion questions that help the reader to reflect upon as well as utilize key terms. Finally, all chapters are interconnected but are also designed to stand alone and provide a comprehensive overview of the topic they cover.

## FEATURES

- Learning objectives
- Practice and discussion questions
- Lists of key terms
- Glossary of key terms

## EDITORS' NOTE

As editors, we hope that we contribute to preventing disease and promoting health. We believe that understanding the theory and practice of health promotion program planning, implementation, and evaluation will allow more individuals and groups to enjoy the benefits of good health and will encourage more schools, workplaces, health care organizations, and communities to be designated as health-promoting sites. We are grateful to the SOPHE members who have authored chapters in this text and admire their commitment and dedication to making a difference in the health outcomes of the individuals, communities, groups, and organizations they serve.

We appreciate the opportunity that the SOPHE board of trustees, executive director, staff, and members provided to us to plan and edit this text. SOPHE provides leadership and works to contribute to the health of all people and the elimination of disparities through advances in health promotion theory and research, excellence in professional preparation and practice, and advocacy for public policies conducive to health. SOPHE and its members advocate and support the work of thousands of professionals who are committed to improving people's health where they live, work, worship, or play. We hope that this book helps advance these goals and helps guide and inspire a healthier world.

## ACKNOWLEDGMENTS

*Health Promotion Programs: From Theory to Practice* is a team effort. We acknowledge and thank Andrew Pasternack, editor, and Seth Schwartz, associate editor, at Jossey-Bass for their support. We thank the chapter authors as well as their supporting organizations and families. We also recognize the staff of the Maximizing Adolescent Potentials Program in the Department of Health and Physical Activity, School of Education, University of Pittsburgh, for their support and effort on behalf of the text. We thank Dr. John Jakicic, chair of the Department of Health and Physical Activity, for his support, and we thank the Allegheny Department of Human Services staff for their support and insights.

In addition, we appreciate and acknowledge the hundreds of SOPHE members and the SOPHE staff and board members who work to promote people's health worldwide. Thank you.

*February 2010*                                                    Carl I. Fertman
                                                                   *Pittsburgh, Pennsylvania*

                                                                   Diane D. Allensworth
                                                                   *Atlanta, Georgia*

# THE CONTRIBUTORS

## EDITORS

**Carl I. Fertman**
Associate Professor
Executive Director, Maximizing Adolescent
Potentials Program (MAPS)
Department of Health and Physical Activity
School of Education
University of Pittsburgh

**Diane D. Allensworth**
Professor Emeritus
College of Education
Kent State University

## CHAPTER AUTHORS

**Kelly Bishop Alley**
Health Education Specialist
Centers for Disease Control and Prevention

**Neyal J. Ammary-Risch**
Deputy Director, National Eye Health Education Program
National Eye Institute
National Institutes of Health

**M. Elaine Auld**
Chief Executive Officer
Society for Public Health Education

**Jean M. Breny Bontempi**
Associate Professor
Department of Public Health
Southern Connecticut State University

**Kelli McCormack Brown**
Professor and Associate Dean for Academic Affairs
Department of Health Education and Behavior
University of Florida

**Frances D. Butterfoss**
President, Coalitions Work
Professor
Department of Pediatrics
Eastern Virginia Medical School

**Huey-Shys Chen**
Associate Professor
School of Nursing
University of Medicine and Dentistry of New Jersey

**W. William Chen**
Professor
Department of Health Education and Behavior
University of Florida

**Sara L. Cole**
Adjunct Faculty
University of Central Oklahoma

**Katherine Crosson**
Associate Director
Center for Quality Improvement and Patient Safety
Agency for Healthcare Research and Quality

**Joseph A. Dake**
Associate Professor
Department of Health and Rehabilitative Services
College of Health Science and Human Service
University of Toledo

**Michael C. Fagen**
Clinical Assistant Professor
Community Health Sciences
School of Public Health
University of Illinois at Chicago

**Andy Fourney**
Evaluation Specialist
Public Health Institute
California Department of Public Health

**Regina A. Galer-Unti**
Faculty Member
Walden University

**Cezanne Garcia**
Senior Program and Resource Specialist
Institute for Family-Centered Care

**Melissa Grim**
Assistant Professor
Department of Exercise, Sport, and Health Education
Radford University

**Jim Grizzell**
Health Educator
California State Polytechnic University

**Tyra Gross**
Support Coordinator
Easter Seals Louisiana

**Michael T. Hatcher**
Chief, Environmental Medicine and Education Services Branch
Division of Toxicology and Environmental Medicine Agency for Toxic
Substances and Disease Registry
Centers for Disease Control and Prevention

**Leonard Jack Jr.**
Associate Dean for Research; Director, Center for Minority Health, Health
Disparities, Research and Education; Endowed Chair of Minority Health
Disparities; and Professor, Division of Clinical and Administrative Services
College of Pharmacy
Xavier University of Louisiana

**Camara Phyllis Jones**
Research Director on Social Determinants of Health and Equity
Emerging Investigations and Analytic Methods Branch
Division of Adult and Community Health
National Center for Chronic Disease Prevention and Health Promotion
Coordinating Center for Health Promotion
Centers for Disease Control and Prevention

**Laura Linnan**
Associate Professor
Department of Human Behavior and Education
Gilling School of Global Public Health
University of North Carolina at Chapel Hill

**Sara Lynch**
Student
Health Sciences Center
School of Public Health
Louisiana State University

**Edward Mamary**
Professor
Department of Health Science
San José State University

**Francisco Soto Mas**
Associate Professor of Health Education
Translational Hispanic Health Research Initiative
University of Texas at El Paso

**Carlen McLin**
Associate Professor
Department of Public Health
Dillard University

**Angela D. Mickalide**
Director of Education and Outreach
Home Safety Council

**Barbara MkNelly**
Research Scientist
Public Health Institute
California Department of Public Health

**Kimberly L. Peabody**
Assistant Professor
Health Sciences Department
James Madison University

**Daniel Perales**
Professor
Department of Health Science
San José State University

**James H. Price**
Professor
Department of Health and Rehabilitative Services
College of Health Science and Human Service
University of Toledo

**Regina McCoy Pulliam**
Associate Professor
University of North Carolina–Greensboro

**Kathleen M. Roe**
Professor
Department of Health Science
San José State University

**Jiunn-Jye Sheu**
Assistant Professor
Department of Health Education and Behavior
University of Florida

**David A. Sleet**
Associate Director for Science
Division of Unintentional Injury Prevention
Centers for Disease Control and Prevention

**Karen A. Spiller**
Manager, Jump Up & Go Program
Blue Cross Blue Shield of Massachusetts

**Marlene K. Tappe**
Associate Professor
Department of Health Science
Minnesota State University, Mankato

**Louise Villejo**
Director
Patient Education Department
M. D. Anderson Cancer Center
The University of Texas

**Britney Ward**
Assistant Director of Health Planning
Hospital Council of Northwest Ohio

**Jennifer Wieland**
Associate Transportation Planner
Seattle Department of Transportation

**Allison Zambon**
Health Communications Specialist
NOVA Research Company

## SOPHE

**The Society for Public Health Education** (SOPHE) is a nonprofit professional organization founded in 1950. SOPHE's mission is to provide global leadership to the profession of health education and health promotion and to promote the health of society through advances in health education theory and research, excellence in professional preparation and practice, advocacy for public policies conducive to health, and the achievement of health equity for all. SOPHE is the only independent professional organization devoted exclusively to health education and health promotion.

SOPHE's membership extends health education principles and practices to many settings, including schools; universities; medical and health care settings; work sites; voluntary health agencies; international organizations; and federal, state, and local governments.

Contact SOPHE at 10 G Street N.W., Suite 605, Washington, DC 20002-4242; telephone: (202) 408-9804; Web site: www.sophe.org.

For my wife, Barbara Murock, promoter of love,
family, health, and biking
—*Carl I. Fertman*


To my best friend, colleague, and husband, John,
who encouraged and supported my dreams
—*Diane D. Allensworth*

# PART ONE

# FOUNDATIONS OF HEALTH PROMOTION PROGRAMS

# CHAPTER ONE

# WHAT ARE HEALTH PROMOTION PROGRAMS?

CARL I. FERTMAN

DIANE D. ALLENSWORTH

M. ELAINE AULD

## LEARNING OBJECTIVES

- Define *health* and *health promotion*, and describe the role of health promotion in fostering good health and quality of life

- Summarize the key historical developments in health promotion over the last century

- Describe the national public-private initiative for health promotion

- Compare and contrast health education and health promotion

- Describe the nature and advantages of each health promotion program setting

- Identify health promotion program stakeholders, including the role each can play in fostering the development or continuation of health promotion programming

HEALTH PROMOTION PROGRAMS can improve physical, psychological, educational, and work outcomes for individuals and help control or reduce overall health care costs by emphasizing prevention of health problems, promoting healthy lifestyles, improving patient compliance, and facilitating access to health services and care. Health promotion programs play a role in creating healthier individuals, families, communities, workplaces, and organizations. They contribute to an environment that promotes and supports the health of individuals and the overall public. Health promotion programs take advantage of the pivotal position of their setting (for example, schools, workplaces, health care organizations, or communities) to reach children, teenagers, adults, and families with the knowledge and skills they need to make informed decisions about their health. This chapter sets the stage for discussing how to plan, implement, and evaluate health promotion programs.

## HEALTH, HEALTH PROMOTION, AND HEALTH PROMOTION PROGRAMS

The World Health Organization (1947) defined health as "a state of complete physical, mental and social well-being, and not merely the absence of disease or infirmity." While most of us can identify when we are sick or have some infirmity, identifying the characteristics of complete physical, mental, and social well-being is often a bit more difficult. What does complete physical, mental, and social well-being look like? How will we know when or if we arrive at that state? If it is achieved, does it mean that we will not succumb to any disease, from the common cold to cancer?

In 1986, the first International Conference of Health Promotion, held in Ottawa, Canada, issued the *Ottawa Charter for Health Promotion*, which defined health in a broader perspective: "health has been considered less as an abstract state and more as a means to an end which can be expressed in functional terms as a resource which permits people to lead an individually, socially, and economically productive life" (World Health Organization, 1986). Accordingly, health in this view is a resource for everyday life, not the object of living. It is a positive concept emphasizing social and personal resources as well as physical capabilities.

Arnold and Breen (2006) identified the characteristics of health not only as well-being but also as a balanced state, growth, functionality, wholeness, transcendence, and empowerment and as a resource. Perhaps the view of health as a balanced state between the individual (host), agents (such as bacteria, viruses, and toxins), and the environment is one of the most familiar. Most individuals can readily understand that occasionally the host-agent interaction becomes unbalanced and the host (the individual) no longer is able to ward off the agent (for example, when bacteria overcome a person's natural defenses, making the individual sick). When needed, the interventions of a health specialist may restore balance (for example, by providing drugs to help the individual's natural defenses fight against the foreign agents or bacteria). But as will be explained before the end of this chapter, it is now the host-environment interactions that, we are learning through emerging research, are making us ill in ways that we previously were not aware of. Environmental factors are ascending as a focus of interest, and interventions to address host-environment interactions are increasingly being employed to address the prevention of chronic and infectious diseases as well as injuries and developmental disorders in order to ensure balance and prevent disease in specific populations.

Clearly, good health doesn't just happen; it's more than just luck. Although being born with good genes and having access to health care are important, they do not provide a guaranteed ticket to wellness. The food we eat, levels of physical activity, exposure to tobacco smoke, social interactions, the environment in which we live, and many other factors ultimately influence our health or lack thereof. The health of individuals as well as the health of our communities reflects the unique combination of biological, psychological, social, intellectual, and spiritual components as well as the cultural, economic, and political environment in which we live. Exploration of the interaction that occurs between individuals and their environment in regard to health has been a hallmark in the progress of nations in promoting and improving the health of individuals and the community at large. This ecological perspective on health emphasizes the interaction between and interdependence of factors within and across levels of a health problem. The ecological perspective highlights people's interaction with their physical and sociocultural environments. McLeroy, Bibeau, Steckler, and Glanz (1988) identified three levels of influence for health-related behaviors and conditions: (1) the intrapersonal or individual level, (2) the interpersonal level, and (3) the population level. The population level encompasses three types of factors: institutional or organizational factors, social capital factors, and public policy factors (see Table 1.1).

The ecological health perspective helps to locate intervention points for promoting health by identifying multiple levels of influence on individuals' behavior and recognizing that individual behavior both shapes and is shaped by the environment. Using the ecological perspective as a point of reference, health promotion is viewed as planned change of health-related lifestyles and life conditions through a variety of individual, interpersonal, and population-level changes.

TABLE 1.1    Ecological Health Perspective: Levels
of Influence

| Concept | Definition |
|---------|-----------|
| **Intrapersonal level** | Individual characteristics that influence behavior, such as knowledge, attitudes, beliefs, and personality traits |
| **Interpersonal level** | Interpersonal processes and primary groups, including family, friends, and peers, that provide social identity, support, and role definition |
| **Population level** | |
| Institutional factors | Rules, regulations, policies, and informal structures that may constrain or promote recommended behaviors |
| Social capital factors | Social networks and norms or standards that may be formal or informal among individuals, groups, or organizations |
| Public policy factors | Local, state, and federal policies and laws that regulate or support healthy actions and practices for prevention, early detection, control, and management of disease |

*Source*: Adapted from McLeroy, Bibeau, Steckler, and Glanz, 1988.

Health promotion programs provide planned, organized, and structured activities and events over time that focus on helping individuals make informed decisions about their health. In addition, health promotion programs promote policy, environmental, regulatory, organizational, and legislative changes at various levels of government and organizations. These two complementary types of interventions are designed to achieve specific objectives that will improve the health of individuals as well as, potentially, all individuals at a site. Health promotion programs are now designed to take advantage of the pivotal position of their setting within schools, workplaces, health care organizations, or communities to reach children, adults, and families by combining interventions in an integrated, systemic manner.

This focus on planned change in health promotion can be applied among individuals in varied settings and at any stage in the natural history of an illness or health problem. Using a framework proposed by Leavell and Clark (1965), health promotion programs can help prevent new cases or incidents of a health problem (for example, preventing falls among the elderly, smoking and drug abuse among middle school and high school students, or risky drinking among college students).

These are programs that take action prior to the onset of a health problem to intercept its causation or to modify its course before people are involved. This level of health promotion is called *primary prevention*. Health promotion programs can interrupt problematic behaviors among those who are engaged in unhealthy decision making and perhaps showing early signs of disease or disability. This type of health promotion is called *secondary prevention*. Examples of this type of health promotion program include smoking cessation programs for tobacco users and physical activity and nutrition programs for overweight and sedentary individuals. Health promotion programs can improve the life of individuals with chronic illness (*tertiary prevention*). Examples are programs that work to improve the quality of life for cancer survivors or individuals with HIV/AIDS. Health promotion programs are a bridge between medicine and health and are part of an ongoing dialogue about how to improve the health and well-being of individuals across settings. Here are some examples of strategies for primary, secondary, and tertiary prevention applied in health promotion and disease prevention.

- Primary health promotion and disease prevention strategies include
  - Identifying and strengthening protective ecological conditions that are conducive to health
  - Identifying and reducing various health risks
- Secondary health promotion and disease prevention strategies address low-risk factors and high protective factors through
  - Identifying, adopting, and reinforcing specific protective behaviors
  - Early detection and reduction of existing health problems
- Tertiary health promotion and disease prevention strategies include
  - Improving the quality of life of individuals affected by health problems
  - Avoiding deterioration, reducing complications from specific disorders, and preventing relapse into risky behaviors

Health promotion programs are designed to work with a priority population (in the past called a target population)—a defined group of individuals who share some common characteristics related to the health concern being addressed. Programs are planned, implemented, and evaluated for their priority population. The foundation of any successful program lies in gathering information about a priority population's health concerns, needs, and desires. Also, engaging the schools, workplaces, health care organizations, and communities where people live and work as partners in the process of promoting health is most effective.

Finally, health promotion programs are also concerned with prevention of the root causes of poor health and lack of well-being resulting from discrimination, racism, or environmental assaults—in other words, the social determinants of health. Addressing root causes of health problems is often linked to the concept of social justice. Social justice is the belief that every individual and group is entitled to fair and equal rights and equal participation in social, educational, and economic opportunities. Health promotion programs have a role in increasing understanding of oppression and inequality and taking action to overcome them and to improve the quality of life for everyone.

## HISTORICAL CONTEXT FOR HEALTH PROMOTION

Kickbush and Payne (2003) identified three major revolutionary steps in the quest to promote healthy individuals and healthy communities. The first step, which focused on addressing sanitary conditions and infectious diseases, occurred in the mid-nineteenth century. The second step was a shift in community health practices that occurred in 1974 with the release of the Lalonde report, which identified evidence that an unhealthy lifestyle contributed more to premature illness and death than lack of health care access (Lalonde, 1974). This report set the stage for health promotion efforts. The third and current revolutionary step in promoting health for everyone challenges us to identify the various combinations of forces that influence the health of a population.

In the mid-nineteenth century, John Snow, a physician in London, traced the source of cholera in a community to the source of water for that community. By removing the pump handle on the community's water supply, he prevented the agent (cholera bacteria) from invading community members (hosts). This discovery not only led to the development of the modern science of epidemiology but also helped governments recognize the need to address infectious diseases. Initially, governmental efforts focused only on preventing the spread of infectious diseases across borders by implementing quarantine regulations (Fidler, 2003), but ultimately, additional ordinances and regulations governing sanitation and urban infrastructure were instituted at the community level. As an outgrowth of the New Deal in the United States, water and sewer systems were constructed across the nation. By the 1940s, the regulatory focus had expanded to include dairy and meat sanitation, control of venereal disease, and promotion of prenatal care and childhood vaccinations (Perdue, Gostin, & Stone, 2003).

As environmental supports for addressing infectious diseases were initiated (for example, potable water and vaccinations), deaths from infectious diseases were reduced. Compared with people who lived a century ago, most people in our nation and around the world are living longer and have a better quality of life—and better health. While new infectious diseases (HIV/AIDS, bird flu, MRSA) emerged at the end of the twentieth century and continue to demand the attention of health workers, the emphasis of health promotion shifted in the last quarter of the twentieth century to focus on the prevention and treatment of chronic diseases and injury, which were the leading causes of illness and death. This change was stimulated, in part, by the Lalonde report, which observed in 1974 that health was determined more by lifestyle than by human biology or genetics, environmental toxins, or access to appropriate health care. It was estimated that one's lifestyle—specifically, those health risk behaviors chosen by individuals—could account for up to 50 percent of premature illness and death. Substituting healthy behaviors, such as avoiding tobacco use, choosing a diet that was not high in fat or calories, and engaging in regular physical activity, for high-risk behaviors (tobacco use, poor diet, and a sedentary lifestyle) could prevent the development of various chronic diseases, including heart disease, diabetes, and cancer (Breslow, 1999). By emphasizing the importance of one's lifestyle to the ultimate manifestations of disease, a shift in the understanding of disease causation occurred, making health status the responsibility not only of the physician, who ensures health with curative treatments, but also of the individual, whose choice of lifestyle plays an important role in preventing disease.

The Lalonde report set the stage for the third and current revolution in promoting health by laying the groundwork for the World Health Organization meeting in which the *Ottawa Charter for Health Promotion* (World Health Organization, 1986) was developed. This pivotal report was a milestone in international recognition of the value of health promotion. The report outlined five specific strategies (actions) for health promotion:

- Develop healthy public policy.
- Develop personal skills.
- Strengthen community action.
- Create supportive environments.
- Reorient health services.

In the United States, the Lalonde report formed the foundation for *Healthy People: The Surgeon General's Report on Health Promotion and Disease Prevention* (U.S. Department of Health and Human Services, 1979), which set national goals for reducing premature deaths. *Healthy People* is discussed in the next chapter section.

In 1997, the *Jakarta Declaration on Leading Health Promotion into the 21st Century* (World Health Organization, 1997) added to and refined the strategies of the *Ottawa Charter* by articulating the following priorities:

- Promote social responsibility for health.
- Increase investment for health developments in all sectors.

- Consolidate and expand partnerships for health.
- Increase community capacity and empower individuals.
- Secure an infrastructure for health promotion.

The *Jakarta Declaration* gave new prominence to the concept of the health setting as the place or social context in which people engage in daily activities in which environmental, organizational, and personal factors interact to affect health and well-being. No longer were health programs the sole province of the community or school. Various settings were to be used to promote health by reaching people who work in them, by allowing people to gain access to health services, and through the interaction of different settings. Most prominently, workplaces and health care organizations as well as schools and communities were now seen as sites for action in health promotion (World Health Organization, 1998).

Much has happened as part of the current revolution in health promotion. Many of the topics and concepts that have been advanced are discussed in this text. These include partnerships for health, health outcomes, risk factors, advocacy, health indicators, health status and health communications, and poverty and equity. The breadth of the work is represented in the Canadian Centre for Health Promotion's quality of life model, which conceptualizes health promotion as aligned with a quality life (Table 1.2). Although the model has its roots in the developmental disability sector, its concepts are valid for other individuals and populations. The definition of *quality of life* is the degree to which an individual can enjoy his or her life. The model's definition of quality of life is based on nine life sectors that are grouped in three major themes: being, belonging, and becoming (Raeburn & Rootman, 2007).

Today, health promotion is a specialized area in the health fields that involves the planned change of health-related lifestyles and life conditions through a variety of individual and environmental changes. Figure 1.1 illustrates the dynamic interaction between strategies aimed at the individual and strategies targeting the entire population. In actuality, the distinction is somewhat artificial in that individuals constitute the population. Nonetheless, certain health promotion strategies are needed to effect changes in knowledge and skill so that population-based or environmental strategies can be enacted. Although there is no question that regulatory and legislative actions generate the quickest behavioral changes within a population, these actions are the most difficult to enact and cannot be achieved without support from enough individuals who understand the value and health benefits of these actions and are willing to contact their legislators to urge support for the legislative actions under consideration.

TABLE 1.2 Quality of Life Model from the Centre for
Health Promotion

| | |
|---|---|
| *Being*<br>Physical Being | *Who one is*<br>• Physical health<br>• Personal hygiene<br>• Nutrition<br>• Exercise<br>• Grooming and clothing<br>• General physical appearance |
| Psychological Being | • Psychological health and adjustment<br>• Cognitions<br>• Feelings<br>• Self-esteem, self-concept, and self-control |
| Spiritual Being | • Personal values<br>• Personal standard of conduct<br>• Spiritual beliefs |
| *Belonging*<br>Physical Belonging | *Connections with one's environment*<br>• Home<br>• Workplace<br>• School<br>• Neighborhood, community |
| Social Belonging | • Family<br>• Friends<br>• Co-workers<br>• Neighborhood, community |
| Community Belonging | • Adequate income<br>• Health and social services<br>• Employment<br>• Educational programs<br>• Recreational programs<br>• Community events and activities |
| *Becoming*<br>Practical Becoming | *Achieving personal goals, hopes, and aspirations*<br>• Domestic activities<br>• Paid work<br>• School or volunteer activities<br>• Meeting health and social needs |
| Leisure Becoming | • Activities that promote recreation and stress reduction |
| Growth Becoming | • Activities that promote improvement of knowledge and skills<br>• Adapting to change |

*Source*: Adapted from University of Toronto, Centre for Health Promotion, Quality of Life Research Unit. (n.d.).

FIGURE 1.1   Health Promotion Interactions

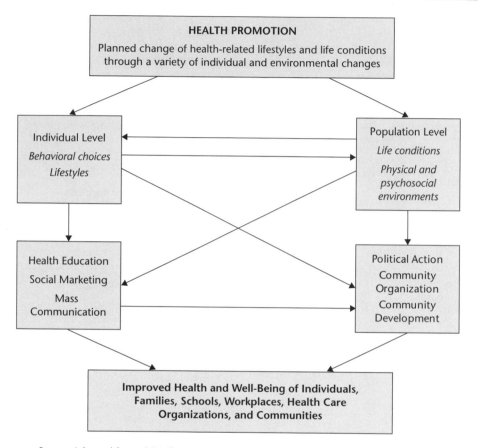

Source: Adapted from O'Neill & Stirling, 2007.

## HEALTHY PEOPLE: A NATIONAL PUBLIC-PRIVATE PARTNERSHIP TO PROMOTE HEALTH

In the United States, the Lalonde report formed the foundation for *Healthy People: The Surgeon General's Report on Health Promotion and Disease Prevention* (U.S. Department of Health and Human Services, 1979), which provided national goals for reducing premature deaths. This report was followed by *Promoting Health/Preventing Disease: Objectives for the Nation* in 1980 (U.S. Department of Health and Human Services, 1980), which set forth 226 targeted health objectives for the nation to achieve over the next ten years. At that time, this report was unique in that it was developed through a broad consultation process that included both public and private health professionals—government scientists as well as health practitioners and academics—at the national, state, and local levels. This initiative asked states and local communities to use the report to focus and guide their health promotion efforts as well as to track and monitor their progress. Every decade since 1980, the U.S. Department of Health and Human Services has reinstituted the same public-private process and released an updated version of *Healthy People* that provides the overarching goals and objectives that will guide and direct the health promotion actions of federal agencies; local and state health departments; and practitioners, academics, and health workers at all levels of government.

The mission of the 2020 Healthy People initiative (The Secretary's Advisory Committee on National Health Promotion and Disease Prevention Objectives for 2020, 2009) is to

- Identify nationwide health improvement priorities.
- Increase public awareness and understanding of the determinants of health, disease, and disability and the opportunities for progress.
- Provide measurable objectives and goals that are applicable at the national, state, and local levels.
- Engage multiple sectors to take actions to strengthen policies and improve practices that are driven by the best available evidence and knowledge.
- Identify critical research, evaluation, and data collection needs.

The vision for the 2020 initiative is a society in which all people live long, healthy lives. The specific goals for the decade leading up to 2020 are to

- Eliminate preventable disease, disability, injury, and premature death.
- Achieve health equity, eliminate disparities, and improve the health of all groups.
- Create social and physical environments that promote good health for all.
- Promote healthy development and healthy behaviors across every stage of life.

One value of the Healthy People initiative in the planning, implementation, and evaluation of health promotion programs is access to national data and resources. Because the initiative addresses such a broad range of health and disease topics, health promotion program staff can usually find objectives that are similar to those they are planning to address. Using Healthy People information allows program staff to compare their program data with national data and to use resources that have been generated nationally in order to achieve the national objectives.

Like its predecessors, Healthy People 2020 reflects continuing efforts on the part of national and various other health promotion program sites (see Figure 1.2). It will help set programming initiatives by federal public health agencies, as well as provide a framework for state and local public health departments to address risk factors, diseases, and disorders and also the determinants of health that affect the health of individuals across health settings. Furthermore, many other national nongovernmental health and educational organizations, philanthropies, and public and private universities will consult the Healthy People 2020 objectives when setting the direction for their respective health promotion programs. This decade's initiative also aims to engage nontraditional sectors such as businesses, faith-based organizations, state and local elected officials, policy organizations, health care organizations, and all others whose actions have significant health consequences. Health promotion is not just an activity for public health workers but an endeavor that requires the collaboration of traditional and nontraditional partners, particularly because understanding of the root factors of disease has

**FIGURE 1.2    Action Model to Achieve the Overarching
Goals of Healthy People 2020**

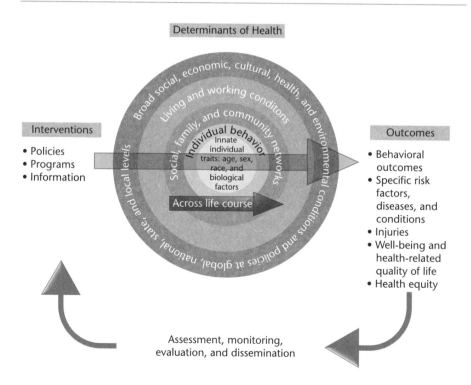

expanded to include the social determinants of health (The Secretary's Advisory Committee on National Health Promotion and Disease Prevention Objectives for 2020, 2009).

## HEALTH EDUCATION AND HEALTH PROMOTION

Health promotion has its roots in health education (Chen, 2001). In the United States, health education has been in existence for more than a century. The first academic programs trained health educators to work in schools, but the role of health educators working within communities became increasingly popular in the 1940s and 1950s. Health education promotes a variety of learning experiences to facilitate voluntary action that is conducive to health (Green, Kreuter, Deeds, & Partridge, 1980). These educational experiences facilitate gaining new knowledge, adjusting attitudes, and acquiring and practicing new skills and behaviors that could change health status. The educational strategies are delivered through individual (one-to-one) or group instruction or interactive electronic media in order to promote changes in individuals, groups of individuals, or the general population. Mass communication strategies that might be used include public service announcements, webinars, social marketing techniques, and other new strategies from text messaging to blogging.

Health education as a discipline has a distinct body of knowledge, a code of ethics, a skill-based set of competencies, a rigorous system of quality assurance, and a system for credentialing health education professionals (Livingood & Auld, 2001). Approximately 250 professional preparation programs offer degrees in health education at the baccalaureate, master's, or doctoral levels. Health education was one of the first disciplines to engage in rigorous, scientific role delineation, a process that resulted in verified competencies for health education practice. The distinct occupation of health educator is recognized and tracked by the U.S. Department of Labor, which estimated that there were some 62,000 health educators in the workforce in 2006 (U.S. Department of Labor, Bureau of Labor Statistics, 2008). When health educators working in schools and businesses are added, the number is even greater. According to the Bureau of Labor Statistics, employment of health educators is expected to grow by 26 percent between 2006 and 2016, which is greater than the average growth for all occupations. "Growth will result from the rising cost of health care and the increased recognition of the need for qualified health educators" (U.S. Department of Labor, Bureau of Labor Statistics, 2008).

*Health promotion* has been defined as the combination of two levels of action: (1) health education and (2) environmental actions to support the conditions for healthy living (Green & Kreuter, 1999). Environmental actions target populations in organizations as well as in the larger community. Such environmental strategies and interventions include political, economic, social, organizational, regulatory, and legislative changes that can improve the health groups of individuals (see Table 1.3). As noted earlier, the priorities for health promotion programs identified by the World Health Organization (1997) were promoting social responsibility for health, the empowerment of individuals, and an increase in community capacity, which requires consolidating and expanding partnerships for health within the community, securing an infrastructure for health promotion, and increasing investments for health developments in all sectors. Health promotion uses complementary strategies at both personal and population levels (see Table 1.3). In the past, *health education* was used as a term to encompass the wider range of environmental actions. These methods are now encompassed in the term *health promotion*, and a narrower definition of health education is used to emphasize the distinction.

In 2008, the Galway Consensus Conference promoted global exchange and understanding in regard to domains of core competency in the professional preparation and practice of health promotion and health education specialists. The conference was designed to provide a forum for discussion among key leaders in order to identify the domains of core competency necessary to build capacity for health promotion, as well as systems that can ensure quality in education, training, and practice. Developing a shared vision for workforce capacity building and a set of standards is a critical foundation for subsequent strategic plans of action, which can be developed by many stakeholders and partners.

In the Galway Consensus Conference Statement, the terms *health promotion* and *health education* are often used interchangeably; however, depending on the

**TABLE 1.3   Components of Health Promotion Programs**

| Health Education to Improve | Environmental Actions to Promote |
|---|---|
| Health knowledge | • Advocacy |
| Health attitudes | • Environmental change |
| Health skills | • Legislation |
| Health behaviors | • Policy mandates, regulations |
| Health indicators | • Resource development |
| Health status | • Social support |
|  | • Financial support |
|  | • Community development |
|  | • Organizational development |

country or context, these terms can have different meanings. In this text, the term *health promotion* is defined as it is in the *Ottawa Charter*: "the process of enabling people to increase control over their health and its determinants, and thereby improve their health" (World Health Organization, 1986). Thus, health promotion is considered vital in contributing to the public's health. Health promotion and health education orchestrate a wide range of complementary actions at individual, community, and societal levels. The Galway Consensus Conference Statement underscores the idea that although health promotion is now established as a recognized field in many parts of the world, it is only emerging in others where the political will and resources to support capacity for health promotion are scarce and thus undermine its development. Health promotion occurs at many levels, is unique in the ways that it can contribute to society, and is characterized by a unique set of competencies and skills that involve integrating interdisciplinary theories and approaches (Allegrante et al., 2009).

Health promotion is guided by a set of core values and principles. These values and principles form the habits of mind that provide a common basis for the practice of health promotion and include the ecological perspective on health, which takes into account the cultural, economic, and social determinants of health; a commitment to equity, civil society, and social justice; a respect for cultural diversity and sensitivity; a dedication to sustainable development; and a participatory approach to engaging the population in identifying needs, setting priorities, and planning, implementing, and evaluating practical and feasible health promotion solutions to address needs.

The Galway Consensus Conference Statement focuses primarily on the domains of core competencies. The competencies required to engage in the practice of health promotion fall into the eight domains listed here. The domains represent key skill areas for effective health promotion program planning, implementation, and evaluation (Allegrante et al., 2009). All the areas are discussed in this text.

1. Catalyzing change—Enabling change and empowering individuals and communities to improve their health.
2. Leadership—Providing strategic direction for developing healthy public policy, mobilizing and managing resources for health promotion, and building capacity.
3. Assessment—Conducting assessment of needs and assets in communities and systems that leads to the identification and analysis of the behavioral, cultural, social, environmental, and organizational determinants that promote or compromise health.

4. Planning—Developing measurable goals and objectives in response to assessment of needs and assets, and identifying strategies that are based on knowledge derived from theory, evidence, and practice.

5. Implementation—Carrying out effective and efficient, culturally sensitive, and ethical strategies to ensure the greatest possible improvements in health, including management of human and material resources.

6. Evaluation—Determining the effectiveness of health promotion programs and policies. This includes utilizing appropriate evaluation and research methods to support program improvements, sustainability, and dissemination.

7. Advocacy—Advocating with and on behalf of individuals and communities to improve their health and well-being and building their capacity for undertaking actions that can both improve health and strengthen community assets.

8. Partnerships—Working collaboratively across disciplines, sectors, and partners to enhance the impact and sustainability of health promotion programs and policies.

## SETTINGS FOR HEALTH PROMOTION PROGRAMS

Earlier in this chapter, we discussed the impact of the *Jakarta Declaration* in giving prominence to the concept of the health setting as the place or social context in which people engage in daily activities and in which environmental, organizational, and personal factors interact to affect health and well-being. Health is promoted through interactions with people who work in various settings, through people's use of settings to gain access to health services, and through the interaction of different settings. Most prominently, workplaces and health care organizations as well as schools and communities are now sites for health promotion (World Health Organization, 1998), and this text focuses on these four settings for health promotion programs. Health promotion programs are planned, implemented, and evaluated for specific sites, reflecting the unique characteristics of the environment as well as the individuals at the site.

### Schools

*Schools* are pivotal to the growth and development of healthy children, adolescents, and young adults. School settings include child care; preschool; kindergarten; elementary, middle, and high schools; two-year and four-year colleges; universities; and vocational-technical programs. Young people spend large portions of their lives in schools. Increasingly, postsecondary institutions are sites where one can find nontraditional students (for example, adults seeking a career change or retired individuals seeking enrichment). The correlation between learning and health has been documented. Graduation from high school is associated with an increase in average life span of six to nine years (Wong, Shapiro, Boscardin, & Ettner, 2002). It has been noted that as a nation, we could save an annual amount of more than $17 billion in Medicaid and expenditures for health care for the uninsured if all students were to graduate (Alliance for Excellent Education, 2006).

## Workplaces

*Workplaces* are anywhere that people are employed—business and industry (small, large, and multinational) as well as governmental offices (local, state, and federal). Employers have found that it makes financial sense to encourage and support employees' healthy practices. Employers, both on their own initiative and because of federal regulations administered by the Occupational Safety and Health Administration, have been active in creating safe and drug-free workplaces. As employers become aware that behaviors such as smoking, lack of physical activity, and poor nutritional habits adversely affect the health and productivity of their employees, they are providing their employees with a variety of work site–based health promotion programs. These programs have been shown to improve employee health, increase productivity, and yield a significant return on investment for employers (O'Donnell, 2002; National Institute for Occupational Safety and Health, 2009).

## Health Care Organizations

*Health care organizations* provide services and treatment to reduce the impact and burden of illness, injury, and disability and to improve the health and functioning of individuals. Health care practitioners work with individuals in community hospitals, specialty hospitals, community health centers, physician offices, clinics, rehabilitation centers, skilled nursing and long-term care facilities, and home health and other health-related entities. Traditionally, these sites are thought of as being part of the health care industry, which is one of the largest industries in the United States and provides 13.5 million jobs. The U.S. Department of Labor reports that eight of the twenty occupations projected to grow the fastest are in health care. More new wage and salary jobs—about 27 percent, or 3.6 million—will be created between 2004 and 2014 in health care. The roughly 545,000 establishments that make up the health care industry vary greatly in size, staffing patterns, and organizational structures. About 76 percent of health care establishments are offices of physicians, dentists, or other health practitioners. Although hospitals constitute only 2 percent of all health care establishments, they employ 40 percent of all health care workers. While health promotion programs might seem out of place in a treatment facility, in fact, much work is done in such facilities to reduce the negative consequences associated with disease.

## Communities

*Communities* are usually defined as places where people live—for example, neighborhoods, towns, villages, cities, and suburbs. However, communities are more than physical settings. They are also groups of people who come together for a common purpose. The people do not need to live near each other. People are members of many different communities at the same time (families, cultural and racial groups, faith organizations, sports team fans, hobby enthusiasts, motorcycle riders, hunger awareness groups, environmental organizations, animal rights groups, and so on). These community groups often have their own physical locations (for example, community recreation centers; golf, swimming, and tennis clubs; temples, churches, and mosques; or parks). These affinity groups all exist within communities, as part of communities, and at the same time, they are their own community. Health promotion programs frequently seek out people both in the physical environment of the neighborhood where they live and within the affinity groups that they form and call their community.

Within a community, the local health department and community health organizations work to improve health, prolong life, and improve the quality of life among all populations within the community. Local and state health departments are part of the government's efforts to support healthy lifestyles and create supportive environments for health by addressing such issues as sanitation, disease surveillance, environmental risks (for example, lead or asbestos poisoning) and ecological risks (for example, destruction of the ozone layer or air and water pollution). The staff at a local health department includes a wide variety of professionals who are responsible for promoting health in the community: public health physicians, nurses, public health educators, community health workers, epidemiologists, sanitarians, and biostatisticians.

Community health organizations have their roots in local community members' health concerns, issues, and problems. These organizations work at the grassroots level, frequently operating a range of health promotion programs that target community members. In this text, the term *community health organization* is synonymous with the terms *community agency, program, initiative, human services*, and *project*. Some community health organizations do not choose to use these terms in their names, deciding to use a name that reflects whom they serve, the health issue they address, or their mission—for example, the American Cancer Society, Caring Place, Compass Mark, Youth Center, Maximizing Adolescent Potentials, Bright Beginnings, Strength and Courage, Healthy Hearts, or Drug Free Youth. Regardless of their names, the common bond for community health organizations is their shared health focus.

## STAKEHOLDERS IN HEALTH PROMOTION PROGRAMS

In beginning to plan, implement, and evaluate a health promotion program, the first step is to know who the stakeholders are in regard to the health issue under consideration. Stakeholders are the people and organizations that have an interest in the health of a specific group or population of people. Stakeholders are people or organizations that have a legitimate interest (a stake) in what kind of health promotion program is implemented. First and foremost are the program participants, also called the *priority population* (for example, students, employees, community members, patients). The program is for their benefit and works to address their health concerns and problems. Although the authors of this book believe that the audience of any health promotion initiative should be regarded as the primary stakeholders, the term *stakeholders* traditionally has referred to other stakeholder groups that also have an interest in a program—for example, top civic, business, or health leaders in the community. The term *stakeholders* may also be used to describe the sponsoring organization's executives, administrators, and supervisors; funding agencies; or government officials. In other words, stakeholders in a health promotion program are people who are directly or indirectly involved in the program.

In the case of a business implementing a health promotion program for employees, stakeholders would include the employees, supervisors, and owners. Other stakeholders might include funders, employees' family members, customers, or health care providers, including health insurance providers. Stakeholder groups often have similar interests in the program but may have different goals; for example, employees and supervisors both want employees to be healthy and productive. However, one group might want time off during the work day for physical activity and exercise, while the other might prefer that employees exercise before or after work.

### Involving Stakeholders

Involving the stakeholders in a health promotion program is essential for its success. Involvement creates value and meaning for the stakeholders—for example, enlisting stakeholders to assist in identifying a program's approaches and strategies in order to ensure congruence with stakeholders' values and beliefs will strengthen stakeholders' commitment to the program. Different stakeholders have different roles. Some stakeholders might help to define what is addressed in a program by sharing their personal health needs and concerns (a process called *needs assessment*, which is discussed in Chapter Four). Other stakeholders might offer services and activities in conjunction with the program (service collaborators). Stakeholders might serve as members of a program's advisory board or as program champions or advocates, roles that are often essential in creating successful health promotion programs.

## Advisory Boards

Most health promotion programs form some type of advisory board or advisory group (also sometimes called a *team*, *task force*, *planning committee*, *coalition*, or *ad hoc committee*) to provide program support, guidance, and oversight. These groups look different across settings. Some are formal, with bylaws, regular meeting schedules, member responsibilities, and budgets. Others are informal, perhaps without any meetings but acting instead as a loose network of individuals who will offer advice and information when called upon by program staff.

Advisory boards play important roles at different points of planning, implementing, and evaluating a program. For example, during planning, advisory board members are involved with determining program priorities as part of the needs assessment, developing program goals and objectives, and selecting program interventions (Chapters Four and Five). During implementation, they might participate in the initial program offering, program participant recruitment, material development, advocacy, and grant writing (Chapters Six, Seven, Eight, and Nine). During evaluation they often review reports and give feedback on how best to disseminate and use the evaluation results and findings (Chapters Ten and Eleven).

Who serves as a member of an advisory group? People with a genuine interest in the setting or program and who communicate well with others. Likewise, it is important to have a diverse group of individuals and organizations represented. Always consider the gender, ethnic, socioeconomic, language, and racial composition of the setting, organization, and community when selecting your membership. In addition, things like geographical boundaries, program representation, and community profile are key factors in the selection process.

For health promotion programs that are based at the site of an organization (for example, at a school or work site), advisory group members typically represent management, supervisors, and individuals involved with the work of the organization (for example, teachers, counselors, clerical staff, or production workers) as well as human resource staff members, medical directors, board members, or representatives of groups such as unions. Some people participate as part of their job responsibilities (for example, a human resource director or a medical director), while others serve because of personal interest. Look for individuals with experience in serving on advisory boards. Avoid personal friends and individuals with a personal agenda. Finally, try to balance the committee with individuals who bring a wide range of interests, skills, and backgrounds to the group.

Frequently, groups in the community will join together to form coalitions that plan and support health promotion programs. Community coalitions might draw on the broad range of agencies and service providers in a community to address a health concern such as underage drinking, violence, teenage pregnancy, or tobacco use. The advisory team for such a community initiative would reflect the diverse groups of the coalition.

Bringing stakeholders together can sometimes be a frustrating task. Some stakeholders may be competitors for resources and attention in the community, so they may have difficulty with trusting one another. Such turf issues or professional or cultural differences may cause communication problems, unrealistic expectations of the committee, or concerns about loss of autonomy—all potential problems. A neutral person with group facilitation skills can often help forge a successful partnership, especially if the partners see a benefit in collaborative participation.

## Champions and Advocates

Health promotion programs often have champions whose advocacy provides leadership and passion for the program. The champion typically knows the setting, the health problems, and the individuals, families, and communities affected by the health problem. In the process of planning, implementing, and evaluating a program, champions provide insight into how the organization operates, who will be supportive, and potential challenges to implementing a health promotion program. They know the history of the health problem and what has worked before in solving it as well as what has not worked. (Frequently, champions are also called *key informants* because they know this important or key information about an organization.) Champions are the people who have initiated the effort to start the program, identify the health problem, or try to solve the problem (often volunteering their time and energy). They fight for resources, funding, and space for the program's operations. Building a trusting and honest relationship with program champions, advocates, and key informants builds the foundation for the work of planning, implementing, and evaluating a health promotion program.

## SUMMARY

Health promotion programs are the product of deliberate effort and work by many people and organizations to address a health concern in a community, school, health care organization, or workplace. And even though individuals across these sites may share broad categories of health concerns focused on diseases and human behavior, each setting is unique. Effective health promotion programs reflect the individual needs of a priority population as well as their political, social, ethnic, economic, religious, and cultural backgrounds.

Health promotion programs represent an evolution that has passed through three revolutionary steps in the quest to promote health. Today, health promotion programs use both health education and environmental actions to promote good health and quality of life for all. The Healthy People initiative is a public-private partnership that allows local health promotion programs to link their health promotion programming with national data and information.

The Galway Consensus Conference identified core competencies for planning, implementing, and evaluating health promotion programs. Health promotion programs involve stakeholders, advisory boards, champions, and advocates in program planning, implementation, and evaluation in order to ensure effective programming.

## FOR PRACTICE AND DISCUSSION

1. What preliminary ideas did you have about the definition and role of health promotion programs prior to reading this chapter? How do these compare with what you have learned in this chapter?

2. The concepts of health and health promotion have evolved from a narrow focus on physical, mental, and social well-being to a broader conceptualization involving a person's quality of life: the degree to which an individual can enjoy his or her life. Use the Quality of Life Model from the Centre for Health Promotion presented in the chapter to discuss the quality of your, your parents' or guardians', and grandparents' quality of life. How are they similar and how do they differ?

3. Visit the Healthy People 2020 Web site (http://www.healthypeople.gov/HP2020). Pick a chapter and explore the objectives. As you explore the chapter think of your school and how you might use the Healthy People 2020 information for a specific objective to build a case for implementing a health

promotion program to address the identified health concern on your campus. Prepare a brief (250-word) statement to use to support your argument for a program.

4. Much of this text is about the eight core competencies defined in the Galway Consensus Statement. What more do you want to know about each competency? What questions do you have about the competencies? As you progress through this book, try to think of additional competencies you believe may be important and define why they are important.

5. What do you think it would be like to work in a health promotion program? This chapter talks about health promotion programs in four different settings—schools, workplaces, health care organizations, and communities. Which setting would be of most interest for you in regard to working in a health promotion program? What is attractive about this setting and the people in the setting? Who would be the stakeholders in this setting?

## KEY TERMS

Advisory boards

Champion

Communities

Core competencies

Ecological health perspective

Galway Consensus Conference Statement

Health

Health care organizations

Health education

Health promotion

Health promotion programs

Health status

Healthy People 2020

Interpersonal level

Intrapersonal level

*Jakarta Declaration*

Key informant

Lalonde report

*Ottawa Charter*

Population level

Primary health promotion

Primary prevention

Priority population

Quality of life

Schools

Secondary health promotion

Secondary prevention

Settings

Stakeholders

Tertiary health promotion

Tertiary prevention

Workplaces

World Health Organization

## REFERENCES

Allegrante, J. P., Barry, M. M., Airhihenbuwa, C. O., Auld, M. E., Collins, J. L., Lamarre, M. C., et al. (2009). Domains of core competency, standards and quality assurance for building global capacity in health promotion: The Galway Consensus Conference Statement. *Health Education & Behavior, 36*(3), 476–482.

Alliance for Excellent Education. (2006, November). *Healthier and wealthier: Decreasing health care costs by increasing educational attainment.* Retrieved May 5, 2008, from http://www.all4ed.org/publication_material/healthier_wealthier.

Arnold, J., & Breen, L. J. (2006). Images of health. In M. O'Neill, S. Dupéré, A. Pederson, & I. Rootman (Eds.), *Health promotion in Canada* (2nd ed., pp. 3–20). Toronto: Canadian Scholars' Press.

Breslow, L. (1999). From disease prevention to health promotion. *Journal of the American Medical Association, 281*(11), 1030–1033.

Chen, W. (2001). The relationship between health education and health promotion: A personal perspective. *American Journal of Health Education, 32*(6), 369–370.

Fidler, D. P. (2003). SARS: Political pathology of the first post-Westphalian pathogen. *Journal of Law, Medicine and Ethics, 31*(4), 485–505.

Green, L., & Kreuter, M. (1999). *Health promotion planning: An educational and ecological approach* (3rd ed.). Mountain View, CA: Mayfield.

Green, L. W., Kreuter, M. W., Deeds, S. G., & Partridge, K. B. (1980). *Health promotion planning: A diagnostic approach.* Palo Alto, CA.: Mayfield.

Kickbush, I., & Payne, L. (2003). Twenty-first century health promotion: The public health revolution meets the wellness revolution. *Health Promotion International, 18*(4), 275–278.

Lalonde, M. (1974). *A new perspective on the health of Canadians.* Ottawa: Health and Welfare Canada.

Leavell, H. R., & Clark, E. G. (1965). *Preventive medicine for the doctor in his community* (3rd ed.). New York: McGraw-Hill.

Livingood, W. C., & Auld, M. E. (2001). The credentialing of population-based health professions: Lessons learned from health education certification. *Journal of Public Health Management and Practice, 7,* 38–45.

McLeroy, K. R., Bibeau, D., Steckler, A., & Glanz, K. (1988). An ecological perspective on health promotion programs. *Health Education Quarterly, 15,* 351–377.

National Institute for Occupational Safety and Health. (2009). *Delivering on the nation's investment in worker safety and health.* Washington, DC: Author. Retrieved October 14, 2009, from http://www.cdc.gov/niosh/docs/2009-144/pdfs/2009-144.pdf.

O'Donnell, M. (2002). *Health promotion in the workplace.* Florence, KY: Delmar Cengage Learning.

O'Neill, M., Pederson, A., Dupéré, S., & Rootman, I. (Eds.). (2007). *Health promotion in Canada: Critical perspectives* (2nd ed.). Toronto: Canadian Scholars' Press.

O'Neill, M., & Stirling, A. (2007). The promotion of health or health promotion? In M. O'Neill, S. Dupéré, A. Pederson, & I. Rootman (Eds.), *Health promotion in Canada* (2nd ed., pp. 32–45). Toronto: Canadian Scholars' Press.

Perdue, W. C., Gostin, L. O., & Stone L. A. (2003). Public health and the built environment: Historical, empirical and theoretical foundations for an expanded role. *Journal of Law, Medicine and Ethics, 31*(4), 557–566.

Raeburn, J., & Rootman, I. (2007). A new appraisal of the concept of health. In M. O'Neill, S. Dupéré, A. Pederson, & I. Rootman (Eds.), *Health promotion in Canada* (2nd ed., pp. 19–31). Toronto: Canadian Scholars' Press.

The Secretary's Advisory Committee on National Health Promotion and Disease Prevention Objectives for 2020. (2009, October 27). *Phase I report: Recommendations for the framework and format of Healthy People 2020.* Retrieved October 27, 2009, from http://www.healthypeople.gov/hp2020/Objectives/fwiFramework.aspx.

University of Toronto, Centre for Health Promotion, Quality of Life Research Unit. (n.d.). *The quality of life model.* Retrieved October 13, 2009, from http://www.Utoronto.ca/qol/concepts.htm.

U.S. Department of Health and Human Services. (1979). Healthy people: The surgeon general's report on health promotion and disease prevention. Washington, DC: Author.

U.S. Department of Health and Human Services (1980). *Promoting health/preventing disease: Objectives for the nation.* Washington, DC: Author.

U.S. Department of Labor, Bureau of Labor Statistics. (2008). *Occupational outlook handbook, 2008–09 edition.* Retrieved April 22, 2009, from http://www.bls.gov/oco/ocos063.htm.

Wong, M., Shapiro, M., Boscardin, W., & Ettner, S. (2002). Contribution of major diseases to disparities in mortality. *New England Journal of Medicine, 347,* 1585–1592.

World Health Organization. (1947). Constitution of the World Health Organization. *Chronicle of the World Health Organization, 1*(1–2), 29–43.

World Health Organization. (1986). *The Ottawa charter for health promotion.* Ottawa: Canadian Public Health Association.

World Health Organization. (1997, July 21–25). *Jakarta declaration on leading health promotion into the 21st century.* Fourth International Conference on Health Promotion: New Players for a New Era— Leading Health Promotion into the 21st Century, Jakarta, Indonesia.

World Health Organization. (1998). *Health promotion glossary.* Retrieved July 20, 2009, from http://www.who.int/hpr/NPH/docs/hp_glossary_en.pdf.

# CHAPTER TWO

# HEALTH PROMOTION PROGRAMS DESIGNED TO ELIMINATE HEALTH DISPARITIES

FRANCISCO SOTO MAS

DIANE D. ALLENSWORTH

CAMARA PHYLLIS JONES

## LEARNING OBJECTIVES

- Define *health disparities* and explain their relevance to planning, implementing, and evaluating a health promotion program

- Describe each of the four major categories for racial and ethnic disparities (societal, environmental, individual and behavioral, and medical)

- Discuss the term *race* as it relates to the distribution of health risks and opportunities in society

- Discuss four strategies health promotion programs can use to reduce health disparities

**E**FFECTIVE HEALTH PROMOTION PROGRAMS are a reflection of the program participants and sites for which the programs are designed, implemented, and evaluated. Every site and group of individuals is different. These differences are most often related to economic status, race and ethnicity, gender, education, disability, geographic location, or sexual orientation. Although genes, behavior, and medical care play a role in how well we feel and how long we live, the social conditions in which we are born, live, and work have the most significant impact on health and longevity. Living in poverty is one of the major conditions associated with poorer health status as well as lack of access to health care. Because more minority individuals live in poverty, they also experience more deficits in health status as well as health care. As a consequence, minority and ethnic groups suffer disproportionately from diseases and conditions that otherwise could be prevented. If health promotion programs are to be effective, then fundamental to their planning, implementation, and evaluation is knowing, identifying, and addressing health disparities among the individuals served by the programs. Elimination of health disparities constitutes an absolute priority in increasing life expectancy and improving quality of life in the United States. Thus, eliminating health disparities is essential in planning, implementing, and evaluating health promotion programs across all settings.

## POPULATION GROUPS AND HEALTH DISPARITIES

The foundation of any health promotion program is matching the program to people's health needs. Critical to making the match is recognizing that health status and health care vary among individuals and groups of people. Disparities (differences) in health status and health care can be identified by gender, income, education, disability, geographic location, sexual orientation, and race or ethnicity.

### Gender

It is obvious that some differences in health between men and women are biological, such as incidence and prevalence of cervical and prostate cancer. However, other differences are more difficult to explain. For instance, the reason why women live longer than men has not fully been explained. In 2005, life expectancy at birth for women in the United States was 80.4 years, and only 75.2 years for men (Miniño, Heron, Murphy, & Kochanek, 2007). Similarly, it has not been scientifically explained why women are at greater risk for Alzheimer's disease than men or why they are twice as likely to be affected by major depression (McBride & Bagby, 2006; Mirowsky & Ross, 1995).

## Income and Education

In the United States, disparities in income and education levels have been associated with differences in the occurrence of many conditions associated with ill health, including heart disease, diabetes, obesity, elevated level of lead in the blood, and low birth weight. National data also indicate that income inequality has increased over the past four decades (Iceland, 2003; Kim & Sakamoto, 2008; Subramanian & Kawachi, 2006; Wheeler, 2005). There are evident demographic differences in poverty by race and ethnicity (see Table 2.1). Similarly, educational attainment differs by race and ethnicity (see Figure 2.1).

## Disability

The Americans with Disability Act (ADA) of 1990 prohibits discrimination against people with disabilities in employment, transportation, public accommodation, communications, and governmental activities. ADA's nondiscrimination standards apply to people who have a physical or mental impairment that substantially limits one or more major life activities.

The last U.S. census, conducted in the year 2000, estimated that nearly 50 million civilian non-institutionalized Americans have a long-lasting disabling condition or impairment. Of those, between 20 and 28 million were women and nearly 17 million were ethnic and racial minorities (Waldrop & Stern, 2003). U.S. Census estimates from 2005 show that 54.5 million people have a disability and 35 million have a severe disability and that 20.1 percent of females reported having a disability, contrasted with only 17.3 percent of men (Brault, 2008).

TABLE 2.1   People Below Poverty Level, by Race, 2006
(numbers in thousands)

| Population | Total | Below Poverty Level | |
|---|---|---|---|
| | | Number | Percentage |
| All races | 296,450 | 36,460 | 12.3 |
| White, not Hispanic | 196,049 | 16,013 | 8.2 |
| Black | 37,306 | 9,048 | 24.3 |
| Asian | 13,177 | 1,353 | 10.3 |
| Hispanic or Latino (any race) | 44,784 | 9,243 | 20.6 |
| Other | 5,134 | 803 | 15.6 |

*Note:* Poverty thresholds in 2006: one person: $10,294; two people: $13,167; four people: $20,614.
*Source:* U.S. Census Bureau, 2007.

FIGURE 2.1   Educational Attainment in U.S. Population Aged
Twenty-Five and Over, by Race, Hispanic Origin,
and Age (percentages)

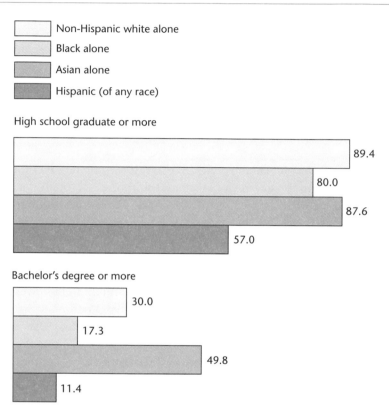

☐ Non-Hispanic white alone

☐ Black alone

☐ Asian alone

☐ Hispanic (of any race)

High school graduate or more

89.4
80.0
87.6
57.0

Bachelor's degree or more

30.0
17.3
49.8
11.4

*Source*: U.S. Census Bureau, 2003.

Data indicate that people with disabilities face barriers that limit their access to routine preventive care and are more likely to report anxiety, pain, sleeplessness, and depression (U.S. Department of Health and Human Services, 2000; Kroll, Jones, Kehn, & Neri, 2006; Wilson, Armstrong, Furrie, & Walcot, 2009). Data also indicate that health professionals may need to make additional efforts to reach out to this population group. For instance, in 2003, the smoking rate among people with disabilities was 31 percent compared with 20 percent among people without disabilities, and 53 percent reported lack of leisure physical activity or being sedentary compared with 34 percent among people without disabilities. In regard to health outcomes, in 2002, 37 percent had high blood pressure compared with 29 percent of adults without disabilities, and 42 percent were affected by obesity compared with 28 percent of adults without disabilities (U.S. Department of Health and Human Services, 2005). People with disabilities who are women and those who are minorities experience additional social and environmental barriers that make them more vulnerable to certain health conditions. For instance, disabled women are more likely to suffer from pain, fatigue, osteoporosis, obesity, and depression (Centers for Disease Control and Prevention, 2006). Disabled minorities are often said to be in double jeopardy because they have two characteristics, being disabled and being from a minority group, that place them at greater risk for health disparities (Jones & Sinclair, 2008; Zawaiza, Walker, Ball, & McQueen, 2003).

## Geographic Location

The place where we are born, grow up, and live has a strong influence on our health status. For example, international studies have found that geography has an important and independent influence on infant mortality and child malnutrition rates. Even in the United States, differences in physical and social environments are apparent and may account for 20 to 25 percent of the variations in illness and death (Satcher & Higginbotham, 2008). In comparison with white children, Hispanic and African American children are more likely to live in communities near toxic waste sites. Further, African Americans are more likely to live in communities that are less likely to have parks, green spaces, walking or biking trails, swimming pools, beaches, or commercial outlets for physical activity such as physical fitness facilities, sports clubs, dance facilities, and golf courses (Robert Wood Johnson Foundation, 2009). Furthermore, those living in very poor neighborhoods often lack supermarkets with fresh produce.

Climate and weather also have a significant impact on human life. Extreme temperatures can cause potentially fatal illnesses such as heat stroke or hypothermia, and excess mortality from heart and respiratory diseases. Natural disasters such as heavy rains, floods, and hurricanes also negatively affect health. According to the World Health Organization (2007), approximately 600,000 deaths occurred worldwide as a result of weather-related natural disasters in the 1990s. Recent studies have suggested that noise constitutes a serious health problem, and at many work sites and in many cities, hazardous noise exposure is considered an increasingly pressing public health problem. Prolonged or excessive exposure to noise can cause hypertension and ischemic heart disease, adversely affect performance, increase aggressive behavior, and lead to accidents (Fyhri & Klæboe, 2009; World Health Organization, 2001).

Rural areas may also contribute to health disparities in the United States. According to the U.S. Census Bureau, nearly 50 million Americans live in rural areas, defined by the Census Bureau as areas comprising open country and settlements with fewer than 2,500 residents. These areas contain only 17 percent of the U.S. population but constitute 80 percent of the land territory (U.S. Department of Agriculture, 2008). The health disparities experienced by minorities in general may be more significant in rural areas due to poverty, transportation problems, lack of public health infrastructure, and limited availability of providers and health care facilities. Immigrants residing in rural communities may face additional cultural and linguistic barriers to health education and medical care. Some studies have found that minorities in rural areas appear to be further disadvantaged in regard to cancer screening and management, cardiovascular disease, and diabetes. This disparity may be due to the fact that people living in rural areas are less likely to use preventive screening services, exercise regularly, or wear seat belts. Lack of health insurance and lack of timely access to emergency services are also significant problems in rural communities (Cristancho, Garces, Peters, & Mueller, 2008; Slifkin, Goldsmith, & Ricketts, 2000; Wong & Regan, 2009). The Office of Rural Health Policy, established in 1987 as part of the Health Resources and Services Administration, promotes better health care service in rural America and informs and advises the U.S. Department of Health and Human Services on issues pertaining to health care services in rural areas (http://www.ruralhealth.hrsa.gov).

## Sexual Orientation

Gay, lesbian, bisexual, and transgender (GLBT) people constitute a segment of our population with particular health concerns, including substance abuse, depression, suicide, and sexually transmitted infections such as HIV/AIDS. Some studies have found higher rates of smoking, obesity, alcohol abuse, and stress among lesbians in comparison with heterosexual women (Gay and Lesbian Medical Association, 2001). The Institute of Medicine has identified pap smear screening and cervical dysplasia among lesbians as two health issues in need of policy development and increased patient education (Grindel, McGehee, Patsdaughter, & Roberts, 2006; Henderson, 2009; Marrazzo, 2004; Mravcak, 2006). Mental health is also of particular relevance among young gays. Gay male adolescents are two to three times more likely than their peers to attempt suicide (U.S. Department of Health and Human Services, 2000; Eisenberg & Resnick, 2006; King et al., 2008). Prejudice and lack of social acceptance contribute to violence and personal safety among GLBT people.

## Race and Ethnicity

Health disparities are well documented in U.S. minority populations such as African Americans, Hispanics, American Indians, Alaska Natives, Asians, Native

Hawaiians, and Pacific Islanders. It is important to keep in mind that the health disparities observed in these groups compared with the white majority population cannot be explained by biological and genetic characteristics or even by socio-economic factors alone.

Differences related to race and ethnicity have become a major focus of the national debate on health disparities. This is partly due to the fact that the U.S. minority population grew to more than 100 million in 2007. Minorities account for one-third of the total population. By 2050, it is projected that they will account for more than half of the U.S. population (see Figure 2.2). This projection is significant, given that compared with non-Hispanic whites, racial and ethnic minorities are in general more likely to be poor or near poor, less likely to have a high school education, and often experience poorer access to care and lower quality of preventive, primary, and specialty care (Agency for Healthcare Research and Quality, 2005).

According to the Office of Minority Health in the U.S. Department of Health and Human Services, the death rate for African Americans is higher than that of whites for heart disease, stroke, cancer, asthma, influenza and pneumonia, diabetes, HIV/AIDS, and homicide. Hispanics in general have higher rates of obesity than non-Hispanic whites. Some Hispanic subgroups present even more alarming disparities in comparison with non-Hispanic whites: the rate of low birth weight for Puerto Ricans is 50 percent higher, and they also suffer disproportionately from asthma, HIV/AIDS, and infant mortality; Mexican Americans suffer disproportionately from diabetes. American Indians and Alaska Natives have an infant death rate almost double the rate for Caucasians; they are twice as likely as Caucasians to have diabetes and also have disproportionately high death rates from unintentional injuries and suicide. Tuberculosis is ten times more common among Asians and five times more common among Native Hawaiian/Pacific Islanders compared with the white population.

*Healthy People 2010* (U.S. Department of Health and Human Services, 2000) identified six focus areas in which racial and ethnic minorities experience serious disparities in health access and outcomes:

- **Cancer screening and management:** African American women are more than twice as likely to die of cervical cancer as are white women and are more likely to die of breast cancer than are women of any other racial or ethnic group.
- **Cardiovascular disease:** Heart disease and stroke are the leading causes of death for all racial and ethnic groups in the United States. In 2000, death rates from diseases of the heart were 29 percent higher and death rates from stroke were 40 percent higher among African American adults than among white adults.

FIGURE 2.2   Projected Population of the United States in
2010 and 2050, by Race and Ethnicity (in millions)

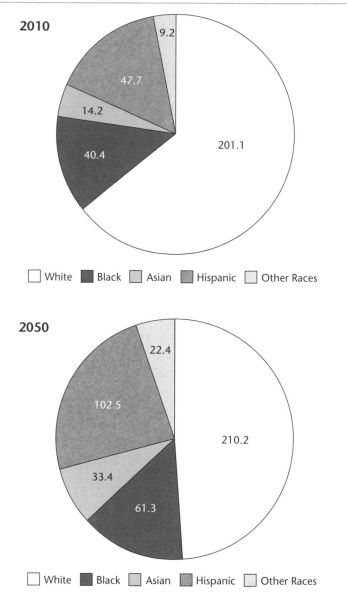

- **Diabetes:** In 2000, American Indians and Alaska Natives were 2.6 times
  more likely than non-Hispanic whites to have diagnosed diabetes; African
  Americans were 2.0 times more likely and Hispanics were 1.9 times more
  likely to have diabetes.

- **HIV infection/AIDS:** Although African Americans and Hispanics represented only 26 percent of the U.S. population in 2001, they accounted for 66 percent of adult AIDS cases and 82 percent of pediatric AIDS cases reported in the first half of that year.

- **Immunizations:** In 2001, Hispanics and African Americans aged sixty-five and older were less likely than non-Hispanic whites to report having received influenza and pneumococcal vaccines.

- **Infant mortality:** African American, American Indian, and Puerto Rican infants have higher death rates than white infants. In 2000, the black-to-white ratio in infant mortality was 2.5 (up from 2.4 in 1998). This widening disparity between black and white infants is a trend that has persisted over the last two decades.

## UNDERSTANDING RACIAL AND ETHNIC DIFFERENCES IN HEALTH

The causes for racial and ethnic disparities have been divided into four major categories (Prevention Institute, 2006): *societal factors*, which include poverty, racism, economics, health illiteracy, limited education, and educational inequality; *environmental factors*, including poor and unsafe physical and social environments, viral and microbial agents, exposure to toxins, inadequate access to nutritious food and exercise, and community norms that do not support protective behaviors; *individual and behavioral factors*, including sedentary lifestyles, poor eating habits, not wearing seat belts, and participating in high-risk behaviors such as smoking; and *medical care factors*, including lack of access to health care, lack of quality health care, and lack of cultural competence among providers.

Among the variety of causes of racial and ethnic disparities in health, racism is the one factor that needs some explanation. Race is a social construct, not a biological reality (Jones, 2001). Both individuals labeled black and those labeled white represent a genetic admixture from many parts of the world. In general, in the United States, one is assigned to a race based on the color of one's skin, which does not begin to capture the genetic and cultural differences among, for example, those residing in the United States who are assigned to the racial category of black. Consider the cultural differences between black immigrants from Nigeria, Ethiopia, or Haiti and black people raised in the rural South or urban North.

While we often characterize our American society as a great melting pot and while the relationships between individuals assigned to different racial categories have improved dramatically, race still governs the distribution of risks and opportunities in our society to a great degree. Jones (2001) describes three types of racism that affect health outcomes: institutionalized racism, personally mediated racism, and internalized racism. *Institutionalized racism* is described as differential access to goods, services, resources, and opportunities by race. For example, 60 percent of minority children attend high-poverty, underresourced schools, while less than 20 percent of white children attend this type of school (Orfield & Lee, 2005). *Personally mediated racism* is discrimination in which the majority racial group treats members of a minority group as inferior and views the minorities' abilities, motives, and intents through a lens of prejudice based on race. This type of racism is what most individuals think of when they hear the term *racism*. It manifests as lack of respect, suspicion, devaluation, scapegoating, and dehumanizing. *Internalized racism* is acceptance of negative messages from others about one's own worth and abilities by members of the stigmatized race. It manifests as self-devaluation, helplessness, and hopelessness, potentially leading to risky behaviors that can endanger a person's health.

## PROGRAM STRATEGIES TO ELIMINATE HEALTH DISPARITIES AMONG MINORITIES

Health promotion programs that are designed with the goal of eliminating health disparities need to facilitate program participation. In order to do this, they first must promote rapport and cooperation and increase people's involvement in the program. Second, they must honor the program participants' autonomy, including people's right to retain their own cultural orientation in regard to their health (Gregory, 1995).

Designing health promotion programs that address health disparities is important and fundamental work in changing people's health status and health care. In each phase of program planning, implementation, and evaluation, eliminating health disparities needs to be a constant theme and consideration that permeates the process down to the smallest details and staff actions. To succeed, a health promotion program needs to be tailored to the people it serves. Successful customization of programs requires that program staff be aware of and sensitive to the culture of the program participants as well as incorporate and use culturally appropriate methods and interventions in the context of the culture.

To support the planning, implementation, and evaluation process discussed in this text, several strategies are available to health promotion program staff, stakeholders, and participants for reducing health disparities among racial and ethnic minorities. The four strategies discussed in this section are overarching strategies to support program planning, implementation, and evaluation. These strategies are engaging minority groups and communities directly in addressing health issues, improving cross-cultural staff training, recruiting and mentoring a diverse program staff, and addressing root causes of health disparities. As you move through the succeeding chapters of this text, think of these strategies as foundations on which to build and deliver health promotion programs.

The driving force for the strategies is the Office of Minority Health in the U.S. Department of Health and Human Services, which in 2008 released a strategic framework for eliminating health disparities (Exhibit 2.1). In 2009, the Office of Minority Health launched the National Partnership for Action to End Health Disparities, identifying twenty strategies that should be implemented in health promotion programs (Table 2.2). While there is general acknowledgment that there needs to be equity in access to culturally and linguistically appropriate health care, there is a growing recognition that equitable health care in and by itself will not reduce health disparities. Attention must be directed to the economic, educational, and environmental inequities at the individual and the community level.

## Engage Minority Groups and Communities Directly in Addressing Health Issues

Discussed throughout this text is the strategy of engaging stakeholders and program participants in all aspects of the program. Simply stated, talking with program participants and understanding their personal, cultural, social, and environmental realities provides the foundation for making sure that a program addresses the needs of the people it serves. Project REACH (Racial and Ethnic Approaches to Community Health) is one example of how the federal government has encouraged local communities to engage their vulnerable populations who are experiencing racial disparities as a resource for helping to reduce existing health disparities. The project has implications for health promotion programs across all types of sites (schools, workplaces, health care organizations, and communities). Its primary focus on eliminating health disparities is a model for health promotion programs working to affect the health status and health care of diverse populations.

Beginning in 2000, the Centers for Disease Control and Prevention, through Project REACH, funded the efforts of forty communities to eliminate health disparities by (1) empowering and mobilizing community members to seek better health, (2) bridging gaps between the health care system and community members, (3) changing the social and physical environments of communities to overcome barriers to good health, (4) implementing evidenced-based strategies and public health programs, and (5) studying community systems changes. Funding was provided to address a variety of priority health concerns in which disparities exist: cardiovascular disease, diabetes, breast and cervical cancer, immunizations, HIV/AIDS, and infant mortality. The Centers for Disease Control and Prevention provided training, technical assistance, and support to the forty communities. In turn, the funded communities have built and sustained effective long-term partnerships across community agencies, provided individuals with the tools to

# EXHIBIT 2.1

# A Strategic Framework for Improving Racial/Ethnic Minority Health and Eliminating Racial/Ethnic Health Disparities

*Long-Term Problems*

1. Racial/ethnic (R/E) minority health status issues (that is, preventable morbidity and premature mortality)
2. Racial/ethnic health disparities
3. Need for a systems approach

*Contributing Factors*

1. Individual level:
   - Knowledge
   - Attitudes
   - Skills
   - Behaviors
   - Biological/genetic risks
2. Environmental/setting (for example. community, school, workplace) level:
   - Physical environment
   - Social environment
     - Values
     - Assets
     - Involvement
   - Economic barriers
3. Systems level:
   - Components and resources
   - Coordination and collaboration
   - Leadership and commitment
   - User-centered design
   - Science and knowledge

*Strategies and Practices*

1. Individual level:
   - Efforts to increase knowledge
   - Efforts to promote attitudes conducive to good health
   - Efforts to build skills
   - Efforts to promote health behaviors
   - Efforts to address biological or genetic risks
2. Environmental/setting (for example, community, school, workplace) level:
   - Efforts to promote a healthy physical environment
   - Efforts aimed at the social environment
   - Efforts to address economic barriers

3. Systems level:
   - Efforts to strengthen components and resources
   - Efforts to promote coordination and collaboration
   - Efforts to foster leadership and commitment
   - Efforts to promote user-centered design to address racial/ethnic minority needs through
     - Racial/ethnic minority participation
     - Health care access/coverage
     - Culturally and linguistically appropriate service
     - Workforce diversity
     - Racial/ethnic data collection
   - Efforts to improve science and knowledge

## Outcomes and Impacts

1. Individual level; for example:
   - Increased awareness/knowledge about disease prevention or risk reduction
   - Increased health care provider skills in providing culturally and linguistically appropriate services
   - Increased patient adherence to prescribed treatment regimens
   - Reduced morbidity and mortality
2. Environmental/setting (for example, community, school, workplace) level; for example:
   - Decreased exposure to risks in the physical environment
   - Increased public awareness about racial/ethnic health disparities
   - Increased health care access and appropriate utilization
   - Increased plans and policies that promote health and well-being at the local, state, and national levels
   - Reduced morbidity and mortality
3. Systems level; for example:
   - Increased inputs and other resources for racial/ethnic minority health/health disparities-related priorities
   - Increased partnerships and collaborations for greater effectiveness and efficiency
   - Increased strategic planning, with goals and objectives, evaluation, and performance monitoring
   - Increased system design characteristics to minimize barriers for minority users
   - Increased knowledge development/science base about "what works"

## Long-Term Objectives and Goals

1. Increased quality and years of healthy life for racial/ethnic minorities
2. Reduced and, ultimately, eliminated racial/ethnic health disparities
3. Systems approach to racial/ethnic minority health improvement and health disparities reduction

---

*Source*: Adapted from U.S. Department of Health and Human Services, Office of Public Health and Science, Office of Minority Health, 2008.

TABLE 2.2    Regional and National Blueprint Strategies

| Objective | Strategies |
|---|---|
| **1. AWARENESS**<br>Increase awareness of the significance of health disparities, their impact on the nation, and the actions necessary to improve health outcomes for racial and ethnic minority populations. | **1. Health Care Agenda.** Ensure that ending health disparities is a priority on local, state, regional, tribal, and federal health care agendas.<br>**2. Partnerships.** Develop and support partnerships among public and private entities to provide a comprehensive infrastructure for awareness activities, drive action, and ensure accountability in efforts to end health disparities across the life span.<br>**3. Media.** Leverage local, regional, and national media outlets, using traditional and new media approaches (for example, social marketing, media advocacy) as well as information technology to reach a multi-tier audience—including racial and ethnic minority communities, rural populations, youth, persons with disabilities, older persons, and geographically isolated individuals—to compel action and accountability.<br>**4. Communication.** Create messages that are targeted toward and appropriate for specific audiences across their life spans, and present varied views of the consequences of health disparities that will compel individuals and organizations to take action and to reinvest in public health. |
| **2. LEADERSHIP**<br>Strengthen and broaden leadership for addressing health disparities at all levels. | **5. Capacity Building.** Support capacity building as a means of promoting community solutions for ending health disparities.<br>**6. Funding and Research Priorities.** Improve coordination, collaboration, and opportunities for soliciting community input on funding priorities and involvement in research.<br>**7. Youth.** Invest in young Americans, to prepare them to be future health leaders and practitioners, by actively engaging and including them in the planning and execution of health initiatives. |
| **3. HEALTH AND HEALTH SYSTEM EXPERIENCE**<br>Improve health and health care outcomes for racial and ethnic minorities and underserved populations and communities. | **8. Access to Care.** Ensure access to quality health care for all.<br>**9. Health Communication.** Enhance and improve health service experiences through improved health literacy, communications, and interactions.<br>**10. Education.** Substantially increase, with a goal of 100 percent, high school graduation rates by establishing a coalition of schools, community agencies, and public health organizations to promote |

TABLE 2.2   (Continued)

| Objective | Strategies |
|---|---|
| | the connection between educational attainment and long-term health benefits; and ensure health education and physical education for all children. **11. At-Risk Children.** Ensure the provision of needed services (for example, mental, oral and physical health, and nutrition) for at-risk children. |
| **4. CULTURAL AND LINGUISTIC COMPETENCY** Improve cultural and linguistic competency. | **12. Workforce Training.** Develop and support broad availability of cultural and linguistic competency training for physicians, other health professionals, and administrative workforces that are sensitive to the cultural and language variations of racially and ethnically diverse communities. **13. Diversity.** Increase diversity of the health care and administrative workforces through recruitment and education of racial/ethnic minorities and through leadership action by health care organizations and systems. **14. Standards.** Require interpreters and bilingual staff providing services in languages other than English to adhere to the National Center on Interpreting for Health Care Code of Ethics and Standards of Practice. **15. Interpretation Services.** Improve financing and reimbursement for medical interpretation services. |
| **5. RESEARCH AND EVALUATION** Improve coordination and utilization of research and evaluation outcomes. | **16. Data.** Ensure the availability of health data on all racial and ethnic minority populations. **17. Authentic Community-Based Research.** Invest in authentic community-based participatory research in order to enhance implementation and capacity development at the local level. **18. Community-Originated Intervention Strategies.** Fund the evaluation of community-originated intervention strategies for ending health disparities. **19. Coordination of Research.** Support and improve coordination of research that enhances understanding about and proposes methodology for reducing health and health care disparities. **20. Knowledge Transfer.** Expand and enhance knowledge transfer regarding successful programs that are addressing social determinants of health (for example, housing, education, poverty). |

*Source:* U.S. Department of Helath and Human Services, 2009.

seek and demand better health care, shared lessons learned and best practices with other communities, and improved health care and reduced disparities in numerous communities, proving that health care disparities are not inevitable and can be overcome (Centers for Disease Control and Prevention, 2007). Two examples from the REACH communities are featured in Exhibit 2.2.

---

### EXHIBIT 2.2
## Examples of REACH Community Projects

#### Vietnamese REACH for Health Initiative Coalition

A coalition in Santa Clara County, California, was organized to address the high incidence of cervical cancer among Vietnamese women, which is five times higher than that for non-Hispanic white women. Individuals with well-established ties and a good reputation in the Vietnamese community were trained as lay health workers. The lay health workers served as a bridge between the community and health services, providing information, advice, and solutions to address health problems affecting this population. After meeting with a community health worker and receiving information through a media information campaign, almost 48 percent of a group of women who had not previously had a Pap test had received a Pap test by the time of the follow-up. In contrast, among a group of women who had not previously received a Pap test and who learned about Pap testing through a media information campaign but did not meet with a community health worker, fewer than 25 percent had had a Pap test at follow-up.

#### REACH 2010 Charleston and Georgetown Diabetes Coalition

The coalition organized more than forty partner agencies in order to address diabetes in the African American community in two South Carolina counties. The partners in the coalition implemented a variety of strategies—for example, creating walk and talk groups, providing diabetic medicines and supplies, improving the quality of diabetes care, and creating learning environments in which health professionals and individuals with diabetes learned together. At the beginning of the intervention, there was a 21 percent gap between African Americans and whites in the community in hemoglobin A1c testing (the annual test that ascertains average blood sugar level, lipid profile, and kidney function). Two years after the start of the program, this gap was virtually eliminated. Furthermore, those with diabetes were physically more active and eating healthier foods at group activities. Amputations of lower extremities among African American men with diabetes declined 36 percent in Charleston County and by 44 percent in Georgetown County.

## Improve Cross-Cultural Staff Training

Studies have noted that minorities generally receive lower-quality health care than non-minorities (Hasnain-Wynia, Baker, & Nerenz, 2007); however, researchers have also found a major difference in where minorities seek health care. Arthur Keinman, a Harvard psychiatrist and anthropologist, has said that every encounter between a health care provider and a client is a cross-cultural experience (National Alliance for Hispanic Health, 2001). This cross-cultural situation is particularly salient when the interaction is between minority and non-minority individuals or when older adults, people who are poor, or people for whom English is a second language are involved. These categories of individuals often have low health literacy skills. Those with low health literacy skills have difficulty understanding health care directions, completing complex health forms that provide the basis for treatment, sharing their medical history with physicians, and even locating providers and services.

Culture can be thought of as a shared worldview. Culture is the ways in which a group of people organize their beliefs and make sense of life. Culture can be the glue that holds a community or group together. Cultural variations reflect what people hold to be worthwhile and help to determine what is believed about what is worth knowing and doing. There is wide variability between cultures, and there is diversity within cultures. Being a member of a culture means that you are in unity with your community, but you also have individual characteristics, tastes, experiences, and desires. Generalizing about persons within a culture is not useful. In any one culture, for instance, there are age differences, race differences, differences in sexual orientation, gender differences, religious differences, class differences, and educational differences. In addition, most persons inhabit several cultures simultaneously, existing within layers and collections of cultural identities. Sometimes those different cultural identities clash or conflict with each other. Mistakes to avoid in thinking about culture include having a deficit perspective (that is, thinking less of a person's abilities for no reason), stereotyping, victim blaming, and confusing culture with other concepts. The concept of culture is sometimes confused with concepts of race, color, or ethnicity. Culture is a much broader concept, encompassing all of the aspects that have been discussed earlier in this section, and skin color can vary greatly within cultural groups.

The Health Resources and Services Administration has defined cultural competence as a set of behaviors, attitudes, and policies that come together in an institution or agency or among a group of individuals and allow people to work effectively in cross-cultural situations. A culturally competent system of care acknowledges and incorporates the dynamics of culture, an analysis of potential cross-cultural misunderstanding, a focus on interactions that can result from cultural differences and ethnocentric approaches, and the adaptation of services to meet specific cultural needs (National Alliance for Hispanic Health, 2001). Cross, Bazron, Dennis, and Isaacs (1989) wrote about a variety of stages or phases toward becoming competent to work with persons of other cultures. They call this five-step journey a "continuum." Not only can individual helpers travel along this continuum but so can agencies and organizations. The first three stages relate to being unaware, and the final two involve being more appropriate and responsive.

1. Cultural destructiveness
2. Cultural incapacity
3. Cultural blindness
4. Cultural pre-competence
5. Cultural competence

Part of being culturally competent is understanding that some universal human experiences (such as joy and grief) transcend culture and that commonalities between cultural groups are just as important as differences. A culturally competent person or organization validates similarities as well as celebrates differences. Some of the signs of a culturally competent person and organization include

- Being aware of personal assumptions, values, and biases
- Changing personal perceptions and behaviors as needed in order to respect the beliefs and values of others
- Respecting others' definitions of *family*
- Feeling and communicating empathy
- Being aware of barriers that the organization presents to persons from various cultures and addressing those barriers
- Seeking information about other cultures by reading, observing consultants from other cultures, and respectfully asking questions
- Using language that is deemed to be respectful by members of' the group served
- Respectfully negotiating plans and approaches if there are differences of opinion
- Avoiding acting on stereotypes and unverified assumptions
- Striving to avoid offensive or hurtful language
- Approaching each person, family, culture, community, or group tentatively, seeking more information

Furthermore, organizations also have certain values and ways of doing things—their own culture. The assumptions of organizations and people sometimes negatively influence the helping relationship. Here are some examples of ideas from organizational culture that may get in the way of open dialogue or relationships:

- People who ask for help must be on time.
- Eye contact from the person seeking help is desirable.
- Technology is useful and not to be feared.
- Paperwork is essential.
- The individual is more important than his or her family, neighborhood, or community.
- Workers should be distant and uninvolved with service recipients or applicants.
- All services are suitable for all persons.
- Everyone should be treated exactly the same.
- Persons seeking help should follow our rules.
- The causes of illness are logical and rational.
- Experts know what is best for persons who ask for help.
- Drop-in care is impossible.
- Formal settings such as hospitals and clinics are the best places in which to provide medical care.
- Visiting hours in institutions should be limited.
- Medication is good.
- Mental health problems can be dealt with by strangers.
- People should be responsible for paying for their health care.
- People should go to the doctor even when they are not sick.

## Recruit and Mentor Diverse Staff

One of the strategies proposed for reducing health disparities is to boost the representation of minorities in the health care workforce (including health promotion programs). Having staff that look like the program participants is critical (staff selection is described later in this book, during the discussion of program implementation). Cohen, Gabriel, and Terrel (2002) argue that increasing the racial and ethnic diversity of the health care workforce is essential to the adequate provision of high-quality care to minority communities. The cultural competency gap of health care providers and any overt or latent racism is reduced when the health care providers are of the same racial or ethnic background as their clients. Here are a number of examples of initiatives to increase the pool and mentor minorities in a range of health professions.

The Institute of Medicine and the American Medical Association (AMA) are actively seeking approaches to attract more minorities to medical schools. The AMA's Doctors Back to School program aims to increase awareness of the need for more minority physicians and to encourage children from underrepresented minority groups to consider pursuing a medical career. Through the program, physicians and medical students visit schools and community organizations to talk with young minority children and help them realize that they also can become doctors (http://www.ama-assn.org/ama/pub/physician-resources/public-health/eliminating-health-disparities/doctors-back-school.shtml).

The Science Education Partnership Award (SEPA) program is a federal initiative to increase the interest of young students in health and biomedical careers. SEPA is sponsored by the National Center for Research Resources, which is part of the National Institutes of Health and funds partnerships among biomedical and clinical researchers; K–12 teachers, media experts and schools; museums and science centers; and other educational organizations (http://www.ncrrsepa.org).

Pathways to Health Professions, sponsored by the Bureau of Health Professions, which is part of the Health Resources and Services Administration, supports innovative, culturally competent approaches that encourage underrepresented minority and disadvantaged students to pursue a career in a health or allied health field. The ultimate goal of the program is to "strengthen the national capacity to produce a health care workforce that includes clinicians, researchers and faculty members whose diversity is representative of the U.S." population (http://bhpr.hrsa.gov/diversity).

## Address Root Causes of Health Disparities

There are those who encourage health promotion program staff as they plan, implement, and evaluate their advocacy efforts to consider moving upstream and addressing the social determinants of health disparities. A number of strategies are recommended. All health promotion programs will benefit from including these strategies because they contribute to the overall quality of life in any setting (community, school, workplace, health care organization, and so forth).

1. *Increase access to health care coverage and services.* Lack of access to quality care contributes to health disparities. However, health care coverage is only the first step to accessing quality care. Many of the root causes of health disparities act as barriers to utilizing health care services, even when insurance coverage becomes available. As part of all health promotion programs, people can work to help individuals to navigate and access health services (Center for Health Improvement, 2009).

2. *Increase access to prevention, screening, and treatment for chronic diseases.* Many health promotion programs are available to people with health care coverage; prevention, screening, and self-management services are readily available and affordable. However, for many minority populations who have limited health care coverage and financial resources or who may be new to this country opportunities to access such services are greatly limited. When working with minority populations, programs should consider the fact that chronic diseases are both highly costly and highly preventable and advocate for and develop chronic disease prevention resources in the community (as well as in schools, workplaces, and so forth) (Center for Health Improvement, 2009).

3. *Support healthy behaviors through increased opportunities to engage in physical activity and to access healthy foods.* Because physical activity is key to preventing disease and promoting health, policies are needed to encourage physical activity for students in school and facilitate after-hours use of school grounds and gyms to improve community access to physical activity facilities. Zoning laws and general plans should be developed to improve the safety of parks, walking paths, and other recreational facilities in high-crime and low-income communities. In addition, support should be provided to ensure access to healthy foods in all communities, through development of grocery stores in low-income communities, incentives for existing stores to offer more healthy food options, especially fresh produce, and also incentives for alternative venues, such as farmers' markets and community or school-based produce stands (Health Trust, 2009).

4. *Improve housing options.* High-quality, affordable, stable housing located close to resources leads to reduced exposure to toxins and stress, stronger relationships and willingness to act collectively among neighbors, greater economic security for families, and increased access to services (including health care) and resources (such as parks and supermarkets) that influence health. Policies should be implemented that support transit-oriented development, along with incentives for mixed-use and mixed-income development. Affordable housing should be protected (for example, via rent control laws), along with funding for emergency housing assistance (Health Trust, 2009).

5. *Improve transit options by providing incentives for use of mass transit and non-motorized vehicle transportation.* Designing streets that are safe and accessible for all users (that is, *complete streets*) will encourage walking and bicycling. Enhancing the safety, accessibility, and affordability of mass transit is also essential. Increased use of these types of transit will decrease air pollution and increase physical activity, which will lead to healthier individuals and communities (Health Trust, 2009).

6. *Improve air, water, and soil quality.* Environmental toxins adversely affect health. For example, a healthier environment can be achieved by reducing exposure to

diesel particulates by prohibiting diesel trucks in residential neighborhoods, enforcing the no-idling law near schools, requiring the use of clean technology in new ships and trucks, reducing emissions in existing fleets, and implementing existing state and federal emissions regulations. Monitoring the impacts of trucking and shipping activities should be expanded among low-income and vulnerable populations. Input from public health professionals on the impact of air pollution should also be incorporated in local land use and development decisions, using such tools as health impact assessments during planning phases (Health Trust, 2009).

7. *Increase high school graduation rates of poor and minority students.* In general these students do not receive equitable resources at the schools they attend. Sixty percent of minority students attend high-poverty, high-minority schools, while less than 20 percent of whites attend high-poverty, high-minority schools (Orfield & Lee, 2005). High-poverty schools often have inadequate, run-down facilities (Acevedo-Garcia, Osypuk, McArdle, & Williams, 2008) or receive lower per-pupil spending allocations from federal, state, and local districts. Furthermore, these schools often lack curriculum rigor; have fewer advanced placement courses (Nelson, 2006; Acevedo-Garcia, Osypuk, McArdle, & Williams, 2008); use fewer credentialed or qualified teachers (Halfron & Hochstein, 2002); have more inexperienced teachers; have teachers who are absent more often; experience higher teacher turnover; and have larger class sizes (Acevedo-Garcia, Osypuk, McArdle, & Williams, 2008). To address educational inequities, the local health department and the local education agency could establish a community-wide school health council to coordinate the health promotion activities of the school district and the various health, social service, juvenile justice, and youth development agencies in the community. In addition to ensuring that inequities in education are eliminated, the coordinating council could ensure that children and youth, particularly those from vulnerable communities, receive needed health interventions as well as other services that have been linked with some evidence of increasing academic success: (a) quality preschool education (Zaza, Briss, & Harris, 2005); (b) high-quality neighborhood schools (Blank & Shah, 2004); and (c) quality school health programs (Society of State Directors of Health, Physical Education, and Recreation, 2002).

## SUMMARY

Health disparities occur among various demographic groups in the United States, including groups delineated by gender, income and education, disability, geographic location, sexual orientation, and race or ethnicity. The federal government has led efforts to raise awareness of and identify potential solutions to alleviate these disparities. *Healthy People 2020* has identified reducing health disparities as one of the Healthy People initiative's four main goals.

Culturally sensitive health promotion programs acknowledge that cultural differences affect individuals' health status and health care. Effective health promotion programs address diversity with sensitive practice and awareness of program participants' cultural values and attitudes, resist stereotyping, and allow participants to communicate their views. Culturally sensitive programs designed to eliminate health disparities assess cultural practices that affect health status and health care. The stance of such programs is nonjudgmental about cultural differences, leading program staff to select interventions that respect cultural differences.

The four strategies for eliminating health disparities discussed in this chapter are overarching strategies that support program planning, implementation, and evaluation. These strategies are offered as foundations on which to build and deliver health promotion programs.

## FOR PRACTICE AND DISCUSSION

1. Following are some examples of staff actions used in a health promotion program focused on engaging and involving a culturally diverse group of individuals who are negatively affected by health disparities:
   - When asking a program participant his or her name, also ask how he or she wants to be addressed.
   - Be aware that people in the program may be more formal than typical Americans or those in other cultures.
   - Individuals may believe that foods can assist in healing disease, so inquire about a person's food choices and preferences.
   - Given that health decisions are often made by family members, include all family members in health discussions if the person desires.
   - Be aware of the importance of saving face and pride in a participant's culture.
   
   How do health promotion program staff learn what is correct and respectful in building relationships with program participants?
2. Investigate and discuss the consequences of being a member of two or more of the population groups who experience health disparities (for example, being a low-income African American with little education who is homosexual).
3. Discuss the relative merits of implementing a health promotion program that addresses the major cause of death of a specific population or of

implementing a health promotion program that addresses the root causes of that disease.

4.  Culturally competent health promotion programs are not designed with the notion that one size fits all; rather, such programs offer a variety of alternatives and options to fit a variety of people. Culturally competent health promotion programs have an underlying philosophy that each and every person deserves dignity and has value. What are some ways that a health promotion program can be culturally sensitive and respectful?

## KEY TERMS

Access

Cross-cultural staff training

Cultural competence

Cultural sensitivity

Culturally appropriate

Disability

Diversity

Education

Environmental factors

Equity

Ethnicity

Gender

Geographic location

Health disparities

Income

Individual and behavioral factors

Institutionalized racism

Internalized racism

Medical care factors

National Partnership for Action to End Health Disparities

Office of Minority Health

Personally mediated racism

Race

Racism

REACH communities

Root causes of health disparities

Sexual orientation

Societal factors

Staff diversity

## REFERENCES

Acevedo-Garcia, D., Osypuk, T. L., McArdle, N., & Williams, D. R. (2008). Toward a policy-relevant analysis of geographic and racial/ethnic disparities in child health. *Health Affairs, 27*(2), 321–333.

Agency for Healthcare Research and Quality. (2005). *National healthcare disparities report, 2005: Full report.* Retrieved November 3, 2009, from http://www.ahrq.gov/qual/nhdr05/fullreport.

Blank, M. J., & Shah, B. P. (2004, January). Community schools: Educators and community sharing responsibility for student learning. *Infobrief,* No. 36. Retrieved November 3, 2009, from http://www.ascd.org/publications/newsletters/infobrief/jan04/num36/toc.aspx.

Brault, M. (2008). *Americans with disabilities: 2005* (Current Population Report No. 70-117). Washington, DC: U.S. Census Bureau.

Center for Health Improvement. (2009). *Targeting root causes to address inequities and improve health: Implications for health reform.* Retrieved October 20, 2009, from http://www.chipolicy.org/pdf/6166.HealthInequities2009.pdf.

Centers for Disease Control and Prevention. (2006). *Women with disabilities.* Atlanta, GA: Centers for Disease Control and Prevention, National Center on Birth Defects and Developmental Disabilities. Retrieved November 3, 2009, from http://www.cdc.gov/ncbddd/women/default.htm.

Centers for Disease Control and Prevention. (2007). *REACHing across the divide: Finding solutions to heath disparities.* Atlanta, GA: U.S. Department of Health and Human Services, Centers for Disease Control and Prevention.

Cohen, J. J., Gabriel, B. A., & Terrel, C. (2002). The case for diversity in the health care workforce. *Health Affairs, 21*(5), 90–102.

Cristancho, S., Garces, D. M., Peters, K. E., & Mueller, B. C. (2008). Listening to rural Hispanic immigrants in the Midwest: A community-based participatory assessment of major barriers to health care access and use. *Qualitative Health Research, 18*(5), 633–646.

Cross, T., Bazron, B., Dennis, K., & Isaacs, M. (1989). *Towards a culturally competent system of care: Vol. 1.* Washington, DC: Georgetown University Child Development Center, Child and Adolescent Service System Program, Technical Assistance Center.

Eisenberg, M. E., & Resnick, M. D. (2006). Suicidality among gay, lesbian and bisexual youth: The role of protective factors. *Journal of Adolescent Health, 39*(5), 662–668.

Fyhri, A., & Klæboe, R. (2009). Road traffic noise, sensitivity, annoyance, and self-reported health—A structural equation model exercise. *Environmental International, 35*(1), 90–97.

Gay and Lesbian Medical Association. (2001). *Healthy People 2010: Companion document for lesbian, gay, bisexual, and transgender (LGBT) health.* San Francisco: Gay and Lesbian Medical Association. Retrieved November 3, 2009, from http://www.lgbthealth.net/downloads/hp2010doc.pdf.

Gregory, D. R. (1995). Modern medicine in a multicultural setting. *Bioethics Forum, 11*(2), 9–14.

Grindel, C. G., McGehee, L. A., Patsdaughter, C. A., & Roberts, S. J. (2006). Cancer prevention and screening behaviors in lesbians. *Women & Health, 44*(2), 15–39.

Halfron, N., & Hochstein, M. (2002). Life course health development: An integrated framework for developing health, policy, and research. *Milbank Quarterly, 80*(3).

Hasnain-Wynia, R., Baker, D. W., & Nerenz, D. (2007). Disparities in health care are driven by where minority patients seek care. *Archives of Internal Medicine, 167*(12), 1233–1239.

Health Trust. (2009). *Racial and ethnic health disparities.* Retrieved October 20, 2009, from http://www.healthtrust.org/initiatives/communities/facts.php#1.

Henderson, H. J. (2009). Why lesbians should be encouraged to have regular cervical screening. *Journal of Family Planning & Reproductive Health Care, 35*(1), 49–52.

Iceland, J. (2003). Why poverty remains high: The role of income growth, economic inequality, and changes in family structure, 1949–1999. *Demography, 40*(3), 499–519.

Jones, C. P. (2001). Race, racism, and the practice of epidemiology. *American Journal of Epidemiology, 154*(4), 299–304.

Jones, G. C., & Sinclair, L. B. (2008). Multiple health disparities among minority adults with mobility limitations: An application of the ICF framework and codes. *Disability and Rehabilitation, 30*(12–13), 901–915.

Kim, C. H., & Sakamoto, A. (2008). The rise of intra-occupational wage inequality in the United States, 1983 to 2002. *American Sociological Review, 73*(1), 129–157.

King, M., Semlyen, J., Tai, S. S., Killaspy, H., Osborn, D., Popelyuk, D., et al. (2008). A systematic review of mental disorder, suicide, and deliberate self harm in lesbian, gay and bisexual people. *BMC Psychiatry, 8*, 70–86.

Kroll, T., Jones, G. C., Kehn, M., & Neri, M. T. (2006). Barriers and strategies affecting the utilisation of primary preventive services for people with physical disabilities: A qualitative inquiry. *Health & Social Care in the Community, 14*(4), 284–293.

Marrazzo, J. M. (2004). Barriers to infectious disease care among lesbians. *Emerging Infectious Diseases, 10*(11). Retrieved June 12, 2009, from http://www.cdc.gov/ncidod/EID/vol10no11/pdfs/04-0467.pdf.

McBride, C., & Bagby, M. (2006). Rumination and interpersonal dependency: Explaining women's vulnerability to depression. *Canadian Psychology, 47*(3), 184–194.

Miniño, A. M., Heron, M. P., Murphy, S. L., & Kochanek, K. D. (2007, August). Deaths: Final data for 2004. *National Vital Statistics Reports, 55*(19).

Mirowsky, J., & Ross, C. E. (1995). Sex differences in distress: Real or artifact? *American Sociological Review, 60*(3), 449–468.

Mravcak, S. A. (2006). Primary care for lesbians and bisexual women. *American Family Physician, 74*(2), 227–229.

National Alliance for Hispanic Health. (2001). *Quality health services for Hispanics: The cultural competency component* (DHHS Publication No. 99-21). Washington, DC: U.S. Department of Health and Human Services.

Nelson, A. (2006, Fall). Closing the achievement gap: Overcoming the income gap. Alexandria, VA: *Infobrief*, No. 47. Retrieved November 3, 2009, from http://www.ascd.org/publications/newsletters/infobrief/fall06/num47/toc.aspx.

Orfield, G., & Lee, C. (2005). *Why segregation matters: Poverty and educational inequality*. Cambridge, MA: Harvard University, Civil Rights Project.

Prevention Institute. (2006). *The imperative of reducing health disparities through prevention: Challenges, implications and opportunities*. Retrieved June 12, 2009, from http://www.preventioninstitute.org/documents/DRA_ReducingHDthruPrx.pdf.

Robert Wood Johnson Foundation. (2009). *Beyond health care: New directions to a healthier America*. Retrieved November 3, 2009, from http://www.rwjf.org/files/research/commission2009executive summary.pdf.

Satcher, D., & Higginbotham, E. J. (2008). The public health approach to eliminating disparities in health. *American Journal of Public Health, 98*(3), 400–403.

Slifkin, R., Goldsmith, L., & Ricketts, T. (2000). *Race and place: Urban-rural differences in health for racial and ethnic minorities*. Retrieved November 3, 2009, from http://www.shepscenter.unc.edu/rural/pubs/finding_brief/fb61.pdf.

Society of State Directors of Health, Physical Education, and Recreation. (2002). *Making the connection: Health and student achievement*. Reston, VA: Society of State Directors of Health, Physical Education, and Recreation & Association of State and Territorial Health Officials.

Subramanian, S. V., & Kawachi, I. (2006). Whose health is affected by income inequality? A multilevel interaction analysis of contemporaneous and lagged effects of state income inequality on individual self-rated health in the United States. *Health & Place, 12*(2), 141–156.

U.S. Census Bureau. (2003). *Current population survey, 2003 annual social and economic (ASEC) supplement.* Retrieved June 15, 2009, from http://www.census.gov/apsd/techdoc/cps/cpsmar03.pdf.

U.S. Census Bureau. (2007). *Current population survey, 2007 annual social and economic (ASEC) supplement.* Retrieved June 15, 2009, from http://www.census.gov/apsd/techdoc/cps/cpsmar07.pdf.

U.S. Department of Agriculture. (2008). *Rural population and migration* (Briefing Room). Retrieved November 3, 2009, from http://www.ers.usda.gov/Briefing/Population.

U.S. Department of Health and Human Services. (2000). *Healthy People 2010: Understanding and improving health* (2nd ed.). Washington, DC: U.S. Government Printing Office.

U.S. Department of Health and Human Services. (2005). *Disability and health in 2005: Promoting the health and well-being of people with disabilities.* Retrieved November 3, 2009, from http://www.cdc.gov/ncbddd/factsheets/Disability_Health_AtAGlance.pdf.

U.S. Department of Health and Human Services. (2009). *Regional and national blueprints for action: Executive summary.* Retrieved from http://www.omhrc.gov/npa.

U.S. Department of Health and Human Services, Office of Public Health and Science, Office of Minority Health (2008). *A strategic framework for improving racial/ethnic minority health and eliminating racial/ethnic health disparities.* Retrieved October 14, 2009, from http://www.omhrc.gov/npa/templates/content.aspx?lvl=1&lvlid=13&id=78.

Waldrop, J., & Stern, S. M. (2003). *Disability status: 2000* (Census 2000 brief). Retrieved November 3, 2009, from http://www.census.gov/prod/2003pubs/c2kbr-17.pdf.

Wheeler, C. H. (2005). Evidence on wage inequality, worker education, and technology. *Federal Reserve Bank of St. Louis Review, 87*(3), 375–393.

Williams, D. R., & Jackson, P. B. (2006). Social sources of racial disparities in health. In R. Hofrichter (Ed.), *Tackling health inequities through public health practice.* Washington, DC: National Association of County Health Officials.

Wilson, A. M., Armstrong, C. D., Furrie, A., & Walcot, E. (2009). The mental health of Canadians with self-reported learning disabilities. *Journal of Learning Disabilities, 12*(1), 24–40.

Wong, S. T., & Regan, S. (2009). Patient perspectives on primary health care in rural communities: Effects of geography on access, continuity and efficiency. *Rural and Remote Health, 9*(1), 1142–1153.

World Health Organization. (2001, February). *Occupational and community noise* (Fact Sheet No. 258). Retrieved November 3, 2009, from http://www.who.int/mediacentre/factsheets/fs258/en/index.html.

World Health Organization. (2007, August). *Climate and health* (Fact Sheet No. 266). Retrieved November 3, 2009, from http://www.who.int/mediacentre/factsheets/fs266/en/index.html.

Zawaiza, T., Walker, S., Ball, S., & McQueen, M. F. (2003). Diversity matters: Infusing issues of people with disabilities from underserved communities into a trans-disciplinary research agenda in the behavioral sciences. In F. E. Menz & D. F. Thomas (Eds.), *Bridging the gaps: Refining the disability research agenda for rehabilitation and the social sciences—Conference proceedings* (pp. 279–312). Menomonie: University of Wisconsin–Stout, Stout Vocational Rehabilitation Institute, Research and Training Centers.

Zaza, S., Briss, P., & Harris, K. W. (Eds.) (2005). *The guide to community preventive services: What works to promote public health?* New York: Oxford University Press.

# CHAPTER THREE

# THEORY IN HEALTH PROMOTION PROGRAMS

LEONARD JACK JR.

MELISSA GRIM

TYRA GROSS

SARA LYNCH

CARLEN MCLIN

## LEARNING OBJECTIVES

- Define and explain the role of ideas, concepts, constructs, and variables in the development and support of a theory

- Discuss foundational health theories that reflect an ecological perspective (that emphasize interactions among factors)

- Summarize the essential constructs of intrapersonal, interpersonal, and population-level theories and models

- Describe the leading models of contemporary health promotion program planning, implementation, and evaluation and suggest how they might be used in practice

T**HE MOST EFFECTIVE** health promotion programs are based on health theories. Theories are used for two purposes. First, they provide the conceptual basis on which health promotion programs are built. Second, they guide the actual process of planning, implementing, and evaluating a program. The strongest programs will focus on both these purposes. The theories used in the field of health promotion have been derived from multiple disciplines, including education, sociology, psychology, anthropology, and public health. Health promotion program staff recognize that if programs do not use tested theories they may not produce the desired improvements in health. Specifically, in the absence of theories it is difficult to identify how health promotion programs affect factors that influence health at individual, family setting, or societal levels. Health promotion theories are used to guide interventions that are delivered in multiple settings, including schools, communities, work sites, health care organizations, homes, and the consumer marketplace (Glanz & Rimer, 2005). This chapter discusses some of the prominent health theories (Goodson, 2010). Understanding the history, purpose, constructs, and use of each theory provides the knowledge necessary to select the most appropriate theory to guide the development, implementation, and evaluation of health promotion programs.

## THEORY IN HEALTH PROMOTION PROGRAMS

Kerlinger (1986) defines a *theory* as "a set of interrelated concepts, definitions and propositions that present a systematic view of events or situations by specifying relationships among variables in order to explain and predict the events or situations" (p. 25). Theories help us articulate assumptions and hypotheses regarding the strategies and targets of interventions. In health promotion we are primarily interested in predicting or explaining changes in behaviors or environments. Glanz, Rimer, and Lewis (2002) have classified theories as explanatory theories (or the theories of the problem) and change theories (or theories of action). Explanatory theories help us describe and identify why a problem exists and search for modifiable constructs. Change theories guide the development of interventions and form the basis of evaluation. Sometimes health promotion practitioners and researchers combine two or more theories to address a specific problem, event, or situation; when this occurs, health models are formed (Glanz, Rimer, & Lewis, 2002).

Theories have their roots in concepts or ideas that are abstract entities. They are not measurable or observable. Concepts are adopted and formed in theories. They are the building blocks or primary elements of a theory (Glanz, Rimer, & Lewis, 2002). Concepts that have been developed and tested over time are referred to as *constructs*. For example, in the theory of reasoned action and theory of planned behavior, behavioral intention is a construct. And when a construct is assigned a specific property and can be measured, it becomes an indicator or *variable*. For example, the construct of behavioral intention is usually measured on a 7-point bipolar scale that includes the categories of extremely probable ($+3$), quite probable ($+2$), slightly probable ($+1$), neither probable nor improbable (0), slightly improbable ($-1$), quite improbable ($-2$), and extremely improbable ($-3$). Converting a theory construct into variables allows the construct to be refined through empirical testing. The constructs of theories must be able to explain phenomena, which for health promotion are behaviors and environmental conditions.

Theories in the early 1970s and 1980s focused primarily on the characteristics, risk factors, demographic characteristics, and life stages of individuals. Theories in the 1980s evolved to focus not only on characteristics of individuals but also on an increased recognition that behaviors take place in a social, physical, and environmental context. Prominent in the 1990s were models that identify steps in planning, implementing, and evaluating health promotion programs. The health theories and models presented in this chapter reflect this evolution of health promotion. The theories are dynamic. Health is not static but rather dynamic and so are health theories. Likewise, these theories represent different paradigms. They were formed to address a range of health concerns, needs, and situations, and therefore they are used in different ways. Theories are an important tool for health practitioners and researchers as they address health concerns, problems, and situations.

First, this chapter presents foundational health theories that reflect the ecological perspective of health promotion, which emphasizes the interaction between and interdependence of factors within and across all levels of a health problem. In other words, people are influenced at a number of levels and an individual's behavior both shapes and is shaped by the social environment. These theories are used to shape and plan interventions. They provide a program's theoretical foundation. These foundational theories focus on the three levels of influence to consider in developing health promotion programs: intrapersonal (individual), interpersonal, and population (McLeroy, Bibeau, Steckler, & Glanz, 1988; Glanz & Rimer, 2005). By considering the three levels of influence, practitioners are able to clarify the intent of their initiative and find appropriate theories to serve as a program's theoretical foundation.

Second, this chapter presents health models that focus on the process of developing a health promotion program. They are guides for how to plan, implement, and evaluate health promotion programs. The strongest health promotion programs will use both theories and models.

No theory or model is perfect. Each was designed to address a particular need or with a specific conceptualization of how best to address a health problem. Practitioners typically combine elements from different theories and models in their work. Furthermore, effective programs educate program stakeholders and participants on the health theories and models in order to help them be more fully engaged in the program. The theories and models are the first element of an effective health promotion program and provide the foundation for evidence-based programs based on science, research, and practice across settings.

# FOUNDATIONAL THEORIES: INTRAPERSONAL LEVEL

The most basic level of health theory is the intrapersonal level. When we are designing or working in a program, it is critical to understand how the theory underlying or directing the program would work at an individual level. Ideally, individual health theories provide the framework for the approach (that is, methodology) in the classroom, in the group setting, and in the development of health promotion materials. In addition to structuring the interventions, the theories help us address intrapersonal factors such as knowledge, attitudes, beliefs, motivation, self-concept, and skills. Four of the major intrapersonal health theories are highlighted in this section: the health belief model, the theory of planned behavior, the theory of reasoned action, and the transtheoretical model and stages of change.

## Health Belief Model

The health belief model, one of the more widely researched models, originated in the 1950s as a way to understand health-seeking behaviors (Rosenstock, 1974). In particular, it grew from work that sought to understand why very few people were participating in preventive and disease detection programs. The Public Health Service was sending out chest X-ray units to local neighborhoods to conduct free screenings for tuberculosis, yet very few people were taking advantage of these services. According to this model, a person's action to change his or her behavior (or lack of action) results from the person's evaluation of several constructs. First, a person decides if he or she is susceptible (*perceived susceptibility*) to a disease or condition, and weighs this against the severity of the disease or condition (*perceived severity*). For example, if a person believes that he or she is susceptible and the disease is severe enough to motivate him or her to change, he or she is more likely to take action to change. Alternatively, if a person does not believe he or she is susceptible, even though the disease might be severe, he or she will likely not act. A person also weighs the benefits of action to change (*perceived benefits*) versus the barriers to change (*perceived barriers*), and this analysis is the strongest predictive factor for behavior change (Janz, Champion, & Strecher, 2002). If a person believes that the benefits outweigh the barriers, then he or she is more likely to take action to change. *Cues to action*, such as instructions or reminders, can also be used to facilitate change. The health belief model also takes other factors, such as age, gender, and personality, into account, with the assumption that these factors can influence a person's motivation to change behavior. *Self-efficacy*, a person's belief that he or she can engage in a behavior (Bandura, 1986), was added later as a factor in behavior maintenance (Rosenstock, Strecher, & Becker, 1988); the original health belief model was tested on short-term health-seeking behaviors.

## Theory of Planned Behavior and Theory of Reasoned Action

The theory of planned behavior, a derivative of the theory of reasoned action, postulates that people are motivated to change based on their perceptions of norms, attitudes, and control over behaviors. Each of these factors can either increase or decrease a person's intent to change his or her behavior. Intention to change behavior, then, is thought to be directly related to behavior change. Table 3.1 shows several important constructs that are involved in these value-expectancy theories: *attitude, subjective norm, perceived behavioral control, intention,* and *behavior* (Montano & Kasprzyk, 2008). Figure 3.1 shows the theory of planned behavior explanation of how behavioral intention determines behavior, and how attitude toward behavior, subjective norm, and perceived behavioral control influence behavioral intention. According to the theory, attitudes toward behavior are shaped by beliefs about what is entailed in performing the behavior and outcomes of the behavior. Beliefs about social standards and motivation to comply with those norms affect subjective norms. The presence or lack of things that will make it easier or harder to perform the behaviors affects perceived behavioral control. Thus a chain of beliefs, attitudes, and intentions drives behavior.

The strength of the relationship between the first three constructs in Table 3.1 and intention and behavior varies, depending on the population and the specific topic being studied. Research is currently being conducted on the magnitude of the relationship between intention and behavior; so far, only a modest connection has been shown (Hardeman, Kinmonth, Michie, Sutton, & the ProActive Project Team, 2009). Recent research points to the impact that distal variables such as culture, personality, and stereotypes have on the more proximal constructs (attitude, subjective norm, and perceived behavioral control) (Yzer et al., 2004). Distal variables are those that are further removed from the person, behavior, or

TABLE 3.1    Constructs in the Theory of Planned Behavior
and Theory of Reasoned Action

| Attitude | Comprises a person's beliefs that the behavior will lead to certain outcomes as well as the value the individual places on those outcomes |
| --- | --- |
| Subjective norm | Comprises a person's perception of a social norm and his or her motivation to comply with that perceived norm |
| Perceived behavioral control | Comprises beliefs about facilitators or barriers and how easy or difficult it would be to change behavior in the face of those facilitators or barriers |
| Intention | The probability that a person will perform a behavior |
| Behavior | Single, observable action performed by an individual, or a category of actions with a specification of target, action, context, and time (TACT) |

FIGURE 3.1    Theory of Planned Behavior
and Theory of Reasoned Action

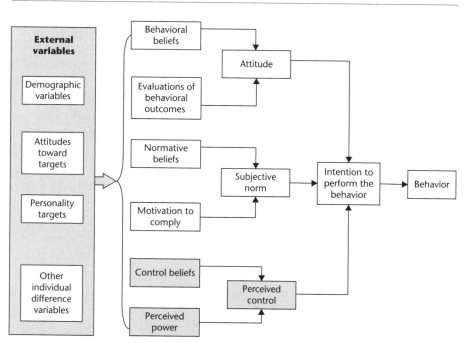

*Source*: "Theory of Reasoned Action, Theory of Planned Behavior, and the Integrated Behavioral Model," by Daniel E. Montano and Danuta Kasprzyk. In *Health Behavior and Health Education: Theory, Research, and Practice* (4th ed.), edited by K. Glanz, B. K. Rimer, & K. Viswanath, San Francisco: Jossey-Bass, 2008. Reprinted with permission of John Wiley & Sons, Inc.

health status. These variables can have a direct influence on health behaviors and health status or can have an indirect influence on health behaviors and health status (for example, culture might affect attitudes or subjective norms, which influence a person's behavior). Proximal constructs are those that directly influence either intention or behavior.

## Transtheoretical Model and Stages of Change

The transtheoretical model was developed in the early 1980s as a way to understand behavior change—in particular, change associated with addictive behavior (Prochaska, DiClemente, & Norcross, 1992). The transtheoretical model proposes that behavior change is a process that occurs in stages; a person moving through these stages in a very specific sequence constitutes the change. Thus the transtheoretical model is also known as *stages of change*. However the stages are one of the theory constructs. The stages are pre-contemplation, contemplation, preparation, action, and maintenance (Table 3.2). People move forward or backward (relapse) through the stages. The dimension of time—that is, each of the stages being associated with a specific time frame—is unique to the transtheoretical model.

Throughout the entire process of changing behavior, people weigh the benefits and drawbacks of behavior change. This construct, called *decisional balance*, is fluid throughout the process. For example, in the pre-contemplation stage, a person might associate more negatives than positives with a behavior change. A person moving through this stage to subsequent stages and to the action stage might find there are more positives than negatives associated with behavior change. When the perceived benefits outweigh the perceived barriers, action occurs.

### TABLE 3.2 Transtheoretical Model Construct: Stages of Change

| | |
|---|---|
| Pre-contemplation | Person is not planning a behavior change within the next six months. |
| Contemplation | Person begins to consider behavior change and is intending to change within six months. |
| Preparation | Person is planning a behavior change within the next month. |
| Action | Person has initiated a behavior change but has done so for six months or less. |
| Maintenance | Person has maintained the behavior change for at least six months but less than five years. |

This model postulates that *processes of change* (construct) can be used to facilitate behavior change during different stages of change (Prochaska, Redding, & Evers, 2002). For example, consciousness raising (increasing awareness of health factors), dramatic relief of symptoms (no longer experiencing negative emotions), or environmental reevaluation (realizing the impact of a behavior on one's environment) might help people move from pre-contemplation to contemplation. Self-reevaluation (understanding the personal impact of the behavior change) is useful in moving people from contemplation to preparation. Self-liberation (making a commitment to change) is used to move people from preparation through action to maintenance. During the maintenance phase, counter-conditioning (behavioral substitution), helping relationships (social support), reinforcement management, and stimulus control (manipulating cues for behavior change) can be used to help people maintain the changed behavior.

Other transtheoretical model constructs include *self-efficacy* (Bandura, 1986) and *temptation*. Temptation refers to the urge to engage in unhealthy behavior when confronted with a difficult situation (Prochaska, Redding, & Evers, 2002). Temptation is represented by three factors that denote the most common types of tempting situations: negative affect or emotional distress, positive social situations, and craving.

## FOUNDATIONAL THEORIES: INTERPERSONAL LEVEL

The second level of health theories focuses on individuals within their social environment. Our social environment includes the people with whom we interact and live our daily life (for example, family members, co-workers, friends, peers, teachers, clergy, health professionals). The theories recognize that we are influenced and influence others through personal opinions, beliefs, behavior, advice, and support, which in turn influence our health and that of others. This section discusses two theories that explore these reciprocal effects of relationships on our health behavior: social cognitive theory and social network and social support theory.

### Social Cognitive Theory

Social cognitive theory evolved from social learning theory, which was created by Albert Bandura in the early 1960s (Bandura & Walters, 1963). In 1986, Bandura officially launched social cognitive theory with his book *Social Foundations of Thought and Action: A Social Cognitive Theory*. Social cognitive theory defines human behavior as an interaction of personal factors, behavior, and the environment. Social cognitive theory is the most frequently used paradigm in health promotion. This theory is based on the reciprocal determinism between behavior, environment, and person; their constant interactions constitute the basis for human action. Bandura posits that individuals learn from their interactions and observations (Bandura, 1986). According to this theory, an individual's behavior is uniquely determined by each of these three factors (Bandura, 1986):

- **Personal factors**:  A person's expectations, beliefs, self-perceptions, goals, and intentions shape and direct behavior.
- **Environmental factors**:  Human expectations, beliefs, and cognitive competencies are developed and modified by social influences and physical structures within the environment.
- **Behavioral factors**:  A person's behavior will determine the aspects of the person's environment to which the person is exposed, and behavior is, in turn, modified by that environment.

Bandura has identified several important constructs of social cognitive theory, including the *environment, situations, behavioral capacity, outcome expectations, outcome expectancies, self-control, observational learning, self-efficacy,* and *emotional coping.* Each of these constructs is defined in Table 3.3.

#### TABLE 3.3    Constructs of Social Cognitive Theory

| Construct | Definition |
| --- | --- |
| Environment | Social or physical circumstances or conditions that surround a person |
| Situations | A person's perception of his or her environment |
| Behavioral capability | The knowledge and skill needed to perform a given behavior |
| Outcome expectations | Anticipation of the probable outcomes that would ensue as a result of engaging in the behavior under discussion |
| Outcome expectancies | The values that a person places on the probable outcome that results from performing a behavior |
| Self-control | Personal regulation of goal-directed behavior or performance |
| Observational learning | Behavioral acquisition that occurs through watching the actions of others and the outcomes of their behaviors |
| Self-efficacy | A person's confidence in performing a particular behavior |
| Emotional coping | Personal techniques employed to control the emotional and physiological states associated with acquisition of a new behavior |

According to Bandura (1986), these constructs are important in understanding health behaviors and planning interventions to change them. The construct of self-efficacy is among the most analyzed psychosocial constructs in research. Bandura (1995) defines self-efficacy as the confidence a person has in his or her ability to pursue a behavior. Self-efficacy is behavior specific and is in the present. It is not past or future. Self-efficacy plays a central role in behavior change. It serves as a guide for and motivator of health behaviors and is rooted in the core belief that one has the power to produce desired effects through one's actions. Unless people believe that they can produce the desired changes by their own effort, there will be very little incentive to put in that effort (Bandura & Locke, 2003).

## Social Network and Social Support Theory

It is widely recognized that social networks and the social relationships that are derived from them have powerful effects on important aspects of both physical and mental health. *Social network* refers to the existence of social ties. Research into how aspects of social networks influence health (positively or negatively) offers insight into the pathways through which social ties influence health. There are at least five primary pathways through which social ties influence health: (1) provision of social support; (2) social influence; (3) social engagement; (4) person-to-person contact; and (5) access to resources and material goods (Ayres, 2008; Twoy, Connolly, & Novak, 2007; Csorba et al., 2007).

Most obviously, the structure of network ties influences health via the provision of social support. *Social support* has been defined as the physical and emotional comfort given to us by our family, friends, co-workers, and others (House, 1981). Social support is typically divided into five subtypes (constructs): emotional, instrumental, appraisal, sharing points of view, and informational support. Each of these subtypes is defined in Table 3.4. Equally important are the ways in which social relationships provide a basis for intimacy and attachment. Intimacy and attachment have meaning not only in relationships that are traditionally thought of as intimate (for example, between couples or between parents and children) but also in more extended ties to the community. For instance, scholars have recently focused on the role of social capital in overall health (Stephens, 2008). *Social capital* refers to the degree to which a community or society collaborates and cooperates (through such mechanisms as networks, shared trust, norms, and values) in order to achieve mutual benefits (Baum & Ziersch, 2003). When relationships are solid at the community level, individuals feel strong bonds and attachment to places (for example, a neighborhood) and organizations (for example, voluntary or religious organizations)—bonds that may lead to improvements in psychological and physical health.

TABLE 3.4    Subtypes of Social Support

| Subtypes | Definition |
|---|---|
| Emotional support | Conveying that a person is being thought about, appreciated, or valued enough to be cared for in ways that are health-promoting |
| Instrumental support | Provision of tangible aid and services such as gifts of money, moving furniture, food, assistance with cooking, or child care |
| Appraisal | Provision of information that is useful for self-evaluation purposes: constructive feedback, affirmation, and social comparison |
| Sharing points of view | Offering opinions about how one views a particular situation or how one would handle a situation, in order to suggest ways that a person can address a particular situation |
| Informational support | Provision of advice, suggestions, or information that a person can use to address a particular situation |

# FOUNDATIONAL THEORIES: POPULATION LEVEL

Health promotion programs for diverse settings and populations, not just a specific group of individuals, are at the heart of the health promotion field. Theories at the population level explore how social systems function and change and how to mobilize individuals at the different settings. They offer strategies that work across settings such as schools, work sites, health care organizations, and communities. Embodying an ecological perspective, theories at the population level address individual, group, and setting issues.

The conceptual frameworks in this section offer strategies for intervening at the population level. This section discusses how communication theory, diffusion of innovations, and community mobilization can be used to affect health behavior.

## Communication Theory

Communication theory focuses on two main areas: (1) message production, which involves both the creation of a message and the way the message is delivered, and (2) media effects, in which the impact that a message has on one or more levels (individual, group, or society) is investigated (Finnegan & Viswanath, 2002). Effective message production requires that messages be tailored to the target audience (Rimer & Kreuter, 2006). Tailoring messages has four components: content, context, design and production, and amount and type of channels (shown in Table 3.5).

TABLE 3.5   Tailoring Messages

| Components | Definition |
|---|---|
| Content | Message content aligns with an individual's wants and needs |
| Context | Message is framed to be applicable to an individual |
| Design and production | Message is interesting to an individual |
| Amount and type of channels | Appropriate channels of delivery are used, and the amount of exposure is acceptable to an individual |

Topics of research on health communication theory range from interpersonal communication (for example, communication between program participants and health promotion program staff) to media campaigns and messages on behavior. The research falls into four categories: knowledge gap, agenda setting, cultivation studies, and risk communication (Finnegan & Viswanath, 2002). Knowledge gap research looks to decrease disparities in health knowledge by targeting individuals or groups and by carefully selecting the message channel in order to reach those most in need of the message. Research on agenda setting aims to influence the audience's thoughts in regard to health policy. Cultivation studies analyze the impact of the media or message on individuals' perceptions of reality. Finally, risk communication research involves investigating the delicate balance between communicating risk and promoting behavior change. Much of the research on health communication theory is limited to investigations of message type and level of interest in specific populations; how people internalize and react to messages is still not well understood (Fishbein & Cappella, 2006).

## Diffusion of Innovations Model

The diffusion of innovations model focuses both on the adopter and on innovative characteristics of the intervention. This theory uses marketing strategies to target specific segments of the population. People are grouped into adopter categories (Rogers, 1995) based on when they buy in to an innovation (such as a new product, program, or service): innovators, early adopters, early majority, late majority, and laggards. Marketing strategies are then tailored toward each group in order to maximize adoption of an innovation. The innovators are the first group to adopt an innovation; they are the first to adopt because they want to be on the cutting edge. Early adopters, the next group, typically adopt an innovation after seeing how it works for the innovators. The early majority and late majority are the next two groups to adopt; they usually wait to see the longer-term benefits and drawbacks of an innovation before adopting it. The last group to adopt an innovation, if they do adopt it, is the laggards. Table 3.6 shows key concepts in the diffusion of innovations model, along with questions that illustrate their application (Oldenburg & Parcel, 2002).

The concepts of the diffusion of innovations model help to define and structure the communications related to an intervention. The concepts guide program staff in how to pitch a program to a potential group of participants. For example, using the concept of complexity, the staff for a walking program to encourage employees at a particular work site to engage in physical activity might frame the idea of fitting walking into a busy schedule as something that is relatively simple to do. A staff member might advocate for employees to hold meetings while walking, or she might promote quick ten-minute walking breaks during the day. The message would change depending on the characteristics of the adopter group (for example, innovators, early adopters) that is being targeted.

TABLE 3.6    Concepts in the Diffusion of Innovations Model and Illustrations of Their Application

| Concept | Questions Used to Make Decisions About Adoption |
|---|---|
| Relative advantage | Is the innovation easier or more cost-effective to use than other options? |
| Compatibility | Is the innovation compatible with the adopter's lifestyle? |
| Complexity | Is the innovation relatively simple to adopt and use? |
| Trialability | Can adopters try the innovation out before adopting? |
| Observability | Can the innovation's benefits be easily observed? |
| Impact on social relations | Will the innovation have a positive impact on the adopter's social structure? |
| Reversibility | Can an adopter discontinue the innovation easily? |
| Communicability | Is the innovation understandable? |
| Time | How much time must be committed in order to adopt the innovation? |
| Risk and uncertainty level | How much risk is associated with adoption of the innovation? |
| Commitment | How much commitment is needed for adoption of the innovation? |
| Modifiability | Will there be opportunities for modifications after adoption has occurred? |

## Community Mobilization

Community mobilization is broadly defined as individuals taking action that is organized around specific community issues. Community mobilization focuses on community-based strategies to improve health outcomes. Grounded and guided by the seminal works of Cloward and Ohlin (1961), Alinsky (1971), Arnstein (1969), and Freire (1972), early community mobilization efforts attempted to view the individual in relationship to the community (for example, the individual's family or neighborhood) in order to better understand the interplay of individual characteristics, health conditions, and environmental factors. Concepts associated with community mobilization include community empowerment, community participation, capacity building, community coalitions, and community organization and development.

As originally developed, community mobilization focused on communities as defined in Chapter One—that is, both as physical locations (for example, neighborhoods, towns, or villages) and as groups of people with common interests (for example, cultural, racial, faith, or hunger action groups). The community mobilization phases discussed in this section are now widely used in all types of settings (for example workplaces, schools, health care organizations, and communities).

Community mobilization attempts to engage all sectors of a community or setting in a community-wide (or setting-wide) effort to address a health, social, or environmental issue. Desired results of mobilizing stakeholders may include promoting collaboration between individuals and organizations; creating a public awareness; promoting shared ownership between individuals and organizations; expanding the base of support for an issue; promoting networking, training, and education; increasing opportunities for training and education; and increasing access to funding opportunities to support community (or setting) programming (Centers for Disease Control and Prevention, 2002).

The literature discusses four phases in mobilizing a community or a setting: (1) planning for mobilization, (2) raising awareness, (3) building a coalition, and (4) taking action (Centers for Disease Control and Prevention, 2002).

In the first phase, *planning for mobilization*, organizers initiate a planning process to determine the many factors that may affect the overall mobilization process. The second phase, *raising awareness*, focuses on the key individuals and organizations to contact in order to stimulate interest, participation, and collaboration. The third phase, *building a coalition*, emphasizes the need to build a coalition that includes key organizations and individuals like health care providers, clergy members, community-based organization leaders, housing authorities, members of the local media, school and university administrators, local police forces, local businesses, and, most important, citizens of the community.

Once an active, participatory coalition, along with formal goals and objectives, is put in place, the final phase, *taking action*, is critical to actualizing results. This phase involves the development and implementation of an action plan. The action plan is based on the results of a needs assessment of the community or setting (see Chapter Four) and the effective use of coalition members' strengths and talents. The action plan would address, for example, efforts to educate members of the community or people in the setting about important health issues that affect the community or setting and ways to reduce or eliminate health problems.

## HEALTH PROMOTION PROGRAM PLANNING MODELS

The health promotion planning models discussed in this section have common elements, although the elements may have different labels. In fact, all the approaches involve three basic steps:

1. Planning the program, including conducting a needs assessment of a health problem and its related factors and influences, prioritizing actions, selecting interventions, and making decisions to create and develop the program
2. Implementation of the program interventions and activities that are based on health theory, eliminate disparities, and are rooted in a needs assessment
3. Evaluation of the program to determine whether it has been implemented as planned and whether it has actually affected the health problem or related factors (identified in assessment) that it was intended to affect

This general three-part process makes sense; the three parts work together to give continual feedback and opportunities to adjust the program. The remainder of this section presents several prominent models that are used by health promotion professionals across the four settings that are the focus of this text: schools, workplaces, health care organizations, and communities. In this chapter, we will discuss the PRECEDE-PROCEED model, the MATCH model, intervention mapping, the community readiness model, and social marketing. These represent a wide range of models that share the three basic elements of planning, implementation, and evaluation.

## PRECEDE-PROCEED Model

One of the most well-known approaches to planning, implementing, and evaluating health promotion programs is the PRECEDE-PROCEED model (Green & Kreuter, 1999). The PRECEDE portion of the model (Phases 1–4) focuses on program planning, and the PROCEED portion (Phases 5–8) focuses on implementation and evaluation. The eight phases of the model guide planners in creating health promotion programs, beginning with more general outcomes and moving to more specific outcomes. Gradually, the process leads to creation of a program, delivery of the program, and evaluation of the program. (Figure 3.2 presents the PRECEDE-PROCEED model for health program planning and evaluation; the direction of the arrows shows the main lines of progression from program inputs and determinants of health to outcomes.)

### Phase 1: Social Assessment

In the first phase, the program staff are looking for quality of life outcomes—specifically, the main social indicators of health in a specific population (for example,

## FIGURE 3.2　PRECEDE-PROCEED Model

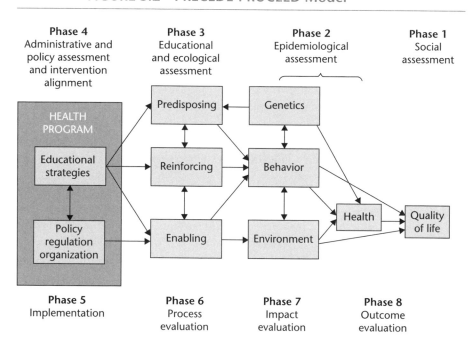

*Source*: Green & Kreuter, 2005, p. 10. Reproduced with permission.

poverty level, crime rates, absenteeism, or low education levels) that affect health outcomes and quality of life. For example, in a dirty and dangerous industrial work site with high rates of accidents, few medical services, and limited food services beyond vending machines, employees may feel unsafe and be unhealthy due to the working conditions.

## Phase 2: Epidemiological Assessment

In this second phase, after specifying the social problems related to poor quality of life in the first phase, the program staff identify which health problems or other factors play a role in impaired quality of life. The health problems would be analyzed according to two factors: importance in terms of how related the health problems are to the social indicator identified in the social assessment and how amenable to change the health problems are. After a first-priority health problem is established, identification of the determinants that can lead to that health problem occurs. Specifically, which environmental factors, behavioral factors, and genetic indicators lead to a specific health problem? The same importance and changeability analysis would be performed to identify which factors to target in a health promotion program. Continuing with the work site example, the program staff would gather data on health problems in the population that might lead to absenteeism, such as obesity, heart disease, cancer, and communicable disease. After ranking the diseases according to importance and amenability to change, the planner might select one health problem. The next step in this assessment would be to investigate the underlying causes of these diseases, such as environmental factors (for example, toxins, stressful working conditions, or no control over working conditions), behavioral factors (for example, lack of physical activity, poor diet, smoking, or alcohol use), and genetic factors (for example, family history). Data on importance and changeability would be analyzed, and then one or several of these risk factors might be selected to focus on. To complete this phase, a health status goal, behavioral objective (or objectives), and environmental objective (or objectives) would be constructed.

## Phase 3: Educational and Ecological Assessment

The focus of phase 3 shifts to mediating factors that help or hinder a positive environment or positive behaviors. These factors are grouped into three categories: predisposing factors, enabling factors, and reinforcing factors (Green & Kreuter, 2005). Predisposing factors are those that can either promote or detract from *motivation* to change, such as attitude or knowledge. Enabling factors are those that can promote or detract from change, such as resources or skills. Reinforcing factors are those that help continue motivation and change by providing feedback or rewards.

These factors are analyzed according to importance, changeability, and feasibility (that is, how many factors is it feasible to include in a program). Factors are then selected to serve as a basis for program development, and educational objectives are composed.

## Phase 4: Administrative and Policy Assessment and Intervention Alignment

The main focus of the administrative and policy assessment and the intervention alignment in the fourth phase is a reality check, to be sure that at the setting (the school, workplace, health care organization, or community) all of the necessary support, funding, personnel, facilities, policies, and other resources are present to develop and implement the program. In the previous workplace example, site policies and procedures would be reviewed, revised, created, and implemented. Likewise at this point, there is an assessment at the site to clarify exactly what staff are needed to implement the program as well as to determine funding levels, space requirements (maybe a classroom, a gym, changing rooms, or showers are needed, for example), and materials and also to examine the details of associated program logistics, such as how to recruit and retain program participants.

## Phase 5: Implementation

Delivery of the program occurs during phase 5. Also, the process evaluation (phase 6), which is the first evaluation phase, occurs simultaneously with implementation of the program.

## Phase 6: Process Evaluation

The process evaluation is a formative evaluation, one that occurs during implementation of the program. The goals of this type of evaluation are to collect both quantitative and qualitative data to assess feasibility of the program as well as to ensure quality delivery of the program. For example, participant attendance and attitudes toward the program might be recorded, as well as an assessment of how well the written lesson plans (describing what content is to be delivered, how it will be delivered, and how much time is allotted) align with actual delivery of the lesson (what content actually was delivered, how it was delivered, and how much time it took to deliver it). Achievement of educational objectives is also measured in this phase.

## Phase 7: Impact Evaluation

The focus of phase 7's summative evaluation, which occurs after the program ends, is to determine the intervention's impact on behaviors or environment.

Timing may vary from immediately after the completion of all the intervention activities to several years later.

## Phase 8: Outcome Evaluation

The focus of the last evaluative phase is the same as the focus when the entire process began—evaluation of indicators of quality of life and health status.

## Multilevel Approach to Community Health (MATCH) Model

The MATCH model, developed in the 1980s, was created in response to a perceived lack of focus in the PRECEDE-PROCEED model on implementation of health programs (Simons-Morton, Simons-Morton, Parcel, & Bunker, 1988). Though it is not widely used, it can guide health professionals in developing, implementing, and evaluating health programs. The MATCH model delineates five main phases, which are subdivided into steps. Table 3.7 provides a general summary of the model.

## Intervention Mapping

Intervention mapping is another approach to planning health promotion programs. According to Bartholomew, Parcel, Kok, and Gottlieb (2006), the purpose of intervention mapping is to provide health promotion program planners with a framework for effective decision making at each stage of intervention planning, implementation, and evaluation. Interventions using this model have addressed health issues such as nutrition and physical activity, sexually transmitted infections, and mental health (Brug, Oenema, & Ferreira, 2005; van Oostrom et al., 2007; Wolfers, van den Hoek, Brug, & de Zwart, 2007). The intervention mapping process consists of six steps: (1) needs assessment, (2) matrices, (3) theory-based methods and practical strategies, (4) program, (5) adoption and implementation plan, and (6) evaluation plan. Although the model is presented in steps, program planners often go back and forth between steps as needed (Bartholomew, Parcel, Kok, & Gottlieb, 2006).

Before planning the intervention, a needs assessment of the target population is conducted (step 1 of the intervention mapping process). Based on the assessment of the health issues, quality of life, and behavioral and environmental concerns of a given population, the desired program outcomes are established. Step 2 involves stating who and what will change at each ecological level as a result of the intervention. This step also involves crossing performance objectives for each ecological level with personal and external determinants in matrices in

TABLE 3.7    Description of the MATCH Model

| Phase | Step |
|---|---|
| 1. Goal selection | 1. Health status indicators are selected and prioritized according to importance (that is, prevalence of health problem, severity of health problem), changeability, and resource availability, and health status goals are written.<br>2. Populations most at risk are identified.<br>3. Behaviors relevant to modifying the health status goals are selected, and behavioral goals are written.<br>4. Environmental factors related to the health status goals and behavioral goals are identified, and environmental goals are written. |
| 2. Intervention planning | 1. Main intervention targets are identified (that is, individuals who have some level of control over behaviors or environmental factors related to the health status goals).<br>2. Intervention objectives are written.<br>3. An intervention framework, including theoretical variables and other mediating variables, is created.<br>4. Intervention approaches—for example, media advocacy, health communication, or educational sessions—are identified. |
| 3. Program development | 1. Main programmatic components are identified.<br>2. Curricula are obtained or created.<br>3. Lesson plans are developed.<br>4. Materials, supplies, and other resources are gathered. |
| 4. Implementation preparation | 1. A support structure—including advocacy in the community, support from key stakeholders, and promoting the program to population—is developed.<br>2. Personnel who will implement the program are trained. |
| 5. Evaluation | 1. A process evaluation—including feasibility, acceptability, impact on learning outcomes—is conducted.<br>2. An impact evaluation—including change in environment, behaviors, theoretical variables, and cognitive variables such as knowledge and attitudes—is conducted.<br>3. In an outcome evaluation, changes in health status are assessed. |

order to help write the change objectives (Bartholomew, Parcel, Kok, & Gottlieb, 2006).

In step 3, theory-based methods for bringing about changes at each ecological level are identified. In addition, practical strategies for realizing the change objectives are selected or designed. Step 4 involves consulting the intended program participants and implementers for their input, delineating the program's scope and sequence, compiling a list of needed materials, and developing and pretesting program materials with the target population (Bartholomew, Parcel, Kok, & Gottlieb, 2006).

Step 5 focuses on developing a program implementation plan. Matrices are created, similar to those in step 2, by crossing adoption and implementation performance objectives with personal and external determinants. Last, step 6 is to finalize the evaluation plan for the program. This step involves describing the program and its intended outcomes, writing questions for the process evaluation based on the matrices from step 2, developing indicators and measures, and specifying the evaluation design (Bartholomew, Parcel, Kok, & Gottlieb, 2006).

## Community Readiness Model

The community readiness model is a theory-based model that is designed both to assess and to build a community's capacity to take action on social issues (Donnermeyer, Plested, Edwards, Oetting, & Littlethunder, 1997). It can and is applied in any setting (for example, school, workplace, healthcare organization, or community). It provides a framework for assessing the social contexts in which individual behavior takes place by measuring changes in readiness related to community-wide efforts. The model integrates a community's culture, resources, and level of readiness to more effectively address an issue. The model consists of nine stages that can be used as a guide to assess readiness and to determine the best intervention (or interventions) that align with a particular stage (see Table 3.8). Using the community readiness model will help increase community (as well as other settings), partnership, participation, and investment in the delivery of interventions at a site.

## Social Marketing

*Social marketing* is not a theory but an approach to promoting health behavior. Social marketing uses commercial marketing techniques to influence the voluntary behavior of target audience members for a health benefit. Social marketing promotes a behavior change to a targeted group of individuals in several ways. It encourages persons to accept a new behavior, reject a potential behavior, modify a current behavior, or abandon an old behavior. Advising women of childbearing age to take a folic acid supplement (accept a new behavior) would help reduce the incidence of birth defects. Discouraging the use of toxic fertilizers (rejection of a potential behavior) would enhance water supply and quality. Promoting the consumption of eight or more glasses of water daily (modification of a current behavior) would prevent dehydration. Encouraging smokers to quit smoking (abandon an old behavior) would reduce the incidence of lung illnesses (Green & Kreuter, 2005).

TABLE 3.8   Community Readiness Model

| Stage | Description |
|---|---|
| 1. Community tolerance | Issue is not generally recognized by the individuals at the site or leaders as a problem (or it may truly not be an issue). |
| 2. Denial, resistance | There is recognition by individuals at the site that there is a local problem, but little concern is occurring locally. |
| 3. Vague awareness | There is recognition by individuals at the site that there is a local problem but little or no specific knowledge of its extent. Leadership to do something about the problem is minimal. |
| 4. Pre-planning | There is clear recognition that there is a local problem; however, efforts to address it are not focused and detailed. |
| 5. Preparation | Individuals at the site are actively engaged in developing a plan of action to address an issue. |
| 6. Initiation | Enough information is available to justify efforts to address an issue. |
| 7. Institutionalization | A program to address a social issue is up and running. Staff either are trained or have recently been trained to lead the effort. |
| 8. Confirmation, expansion | Program continues to receive support and is perceived by individuals and leaders as useful. Data on the extent of the problem locally are collected regularly. |
| 9. Professionalism | Data on prevalence rates and risk factors are collected periodically and used by staff to adjust program goals and target high-risk groups. |

It is important to differentiate social marketing from commercial marketing. Marketing, in general, focuses on the process in which goods or services are exchanged for a profit, which may be financial or for other goods and services. Social marketing is similar to commercial marketing in that both have a customer-centered approach (Oldenburg & Parcel, 2002), which includes the following:

- **Audience segmentation**: the process of dividing larger markets of dissimilar individuals into a smaller market of more similar individuals for which an appropriate intervention can be designed (Rogers, 1995)
- **Market research**: research to understand the behaviors of the target audience—for example, to understand how they perceive their needs, benefits to change, barriers, and opportunities (Green & Kreuter, 2005)

- **Exchange theory**: the idea that people will accept, reject, maintain, or modify a new behavior if the benefits exceed the cost of the behavior (Oldenburg & Parcel, 2002)

In addition, both commercial marketing and social marketing involve competition and are designed by using the *marketing mix*: product, price, place, and promotion (Oldenburg & Parcel, 2002). Commercial marketing seeks to make money by selling certain goods and services, while social marketing seeks to resolve certain social problems by targeting behaviors. Social marketing competes with the "preferred behavior of the target market and [its] perceived benefits" (Oldenburg & Parcel, 2002). Commercial marketing competes with other groups or organizations that sell similar goods and services. Social marketing often has limited funding available from taxes and donations, while commercial marketing is funded through investments. Social marketing is accountable to the public, and its performance is difficult to assess. Commercial marketing, on the other hand, measures performance through financial profits and is accountable to parties in the private sector. Table 3.9 outlines the differences that have been discussed in this section (Finnegan & Viswanath, 2002).

As in commercial marketing, an appropriately designed social marketing program has four basic elements: product, price, place, and promotion. These elements are known as the *four P's of marketing*.

- **Product**: the good, service, or idea being marketed in order to change behavior (for example, hand washing, safe sex, wearing a seat belt)
- **Price**: the costs of and barriers to behavior change (for example, money, time, discomfort)
- **Place**: the physical location and time in which the behavior change will take place (for example, at home, at school, in the car)
- **Promotion**: the tactics used to communicate the message of behavior change (for example, media, brochures, billboards)

## USING HEALTH THEORIES AND PLANNING MODELS

Health theories provide guidance and support for planning, implementing, and evaluating a health promotion program. Programs drawn from health theories use a body of knowledge and experience that allows health promotion staff, stakeholders, and participants to be confident that a program is not just made up but rather is based on current research and best practices.

TABLE 3.9    Differentiating Social Marketing from Commercial Marketing

|  | Social Marketing | Commercial Marketing |
|---|---|---|
| Goal | Resolve certain social problems | Financial profit |
| Focus | Behaviors | Selling goods and services |
| Product | Often intangible (ideas) | Tangible (physical goods) |
| Funding | Taxes, donations (often limited) | Investments |
| Accountability | Public | Private |
| Performance | Hard to measure | Measured by financial profits |

The theories are the foundation for evidence-based health promotion programs. All the theories have the potential to contribute to the process of planning, implementing, and evaluating a health promotion program. To aid in the process, Table 3.10 summarizes the foundational health promotion theories that are identified

TABLE 3.10    Foundational Health Promotion Theories:
Focus and Key Concepts

| Level | Theory | Focus | Constructs and Key Concepts |
|---|---|---|---|
| Individual (intrapersonal) level | Health belief model | Individuals' perceptions of the threat posed by a health problem, the benefits of avoiding the threat, and factors influencing the decision to act | Perceived susceptibility<br>Perceived severity<br>Perceived benefits<br>Perceived barriers<br>Cues to action<br>Self-efficacy |
|  | Theory of planned behavior<br><br>Theory of reasoned action | Individuals' attitudes toward a behavior, perceptions of norms, and beliefs about the ease or difficulty of changing | Behavior<br>Intention<br>Attitude<br>Subjective norm<br>Perceived behavioral control |
|  | Transtheoretical model | Individuals' motivation and readiness to change a problem behavior across time | Stages of change<br>Process of change<br>Decisional balance<br>Self-efficacy<br>Temptation |

TABLE 3.10   (Continued)

| Level | Theory | Focus | Constructs and Key Concepts |
|---|---|---|---|
| Interpersonal level | Social cognitive theory | Personal factors, environmental factors, and human behavior, which each exert influence on the other | Reciprocal determinism<br>Environment<br>Situations<br>Behavioral capability<br>Outcome expectations<br>Outcome expectancies<br>Self-control<br>Observational learning<br>Self-efficacy<br>Emotional coping |
| | Social network and social support theory | Social influences on health and behavior | Emotional support<br>Instrumental support<br>Appraisal<br>Sharing points of view<br>Informational support |
| Population level | Communication theory | How different types of communication affect health behavior | Content<br>Context<br>Design and production<br>Amount and type of channels |
| | Diffusion of innovations model | How new ideas, products, and practices spread within a society or from one society to another | Relative advantage<br>Compatibility<br>Complexity<br>Trialability<br>Observability<br>Impact of social relations<br>Reversibility<br>Communicability<br>Time<br>Risk and uncertainty level<br>Commitment<br>Modifiability |
| | Community mobilization | Community-driven (or setting-driven) approaches to assessing and solving health and social problems | Planning for mobilization<br>Raising awareness<br>Building a coalition<br>Taking action |

*Source*: Adapted from Glanz & Rimer, 2005.

in this chapter. Likewise, Table 3.11 lists examples of theory-based strategies that can be used at all levels of influence.

Developing health promotion programs can be an overwhelming task. The theories have been developed and tested to guide professionals in the development of health promotion programs. Not all theories and their concepts are appropriate for all settings and behaviors. Program staff members, stakeholders, and participants need to consider the setting, population, behavior, their desired level of influence, and practical issues such as resources when planning health promotion programs.

The planning models for developing health programs focus on the big picture. Health promotion programs develop and grow over time. In the most effective

**TABLE 3.11   Using Theory to Plan Multilevel Interventions**

| Change Strategies | Examples of Strategies | Ecological Level | Useful Theories |
|---|---|---|---|
| Change people's behavior | • Educational sessions<br>• Interactive kiosks<br>• Print brochures<br>• Social marketing campaigns | Individual (intrapersonal) | • Health belief model<br>• Theory of planned behavior<br>• Theory of reasoned action<br>• Transtheoretical model |
| | • Mentoring programs<br>• Lay health advising<br>• Goal setting<br>• Enhancing social networks or improving social support<br>• Creating new organizational policy and procedures | Interpersonal | • Social cognitive theory<br>• Social network and social support theory |
| Change the environment | • Media advocacy campaigns<br>• Advocating changes to public policy | Population | • Communication theory<br>• Diffusion of innovations model<br>• Community mobilization |

*Source*: Adapted from Glanz & Rimer, 2005.

health promotion programs, staff members have a sense of the program's growth and development. These models of the program development cycle provide this type of program perspective. They provide a guide to where a program is in its development and what might be next as it grows. Without such a guide, staff as well as program participants and stakeholders may lose sight of the particular health concerns and problems that the program is attempting to address. Table 3.12 provides a summary of the program planning models and their key concepts.

### TABLE 3.12 Models and Key Concepts for Developing Health Promotion Programs

| Model | Key Concepts |
|---|---|
| PRECEDE-PROCEED model | Phase 1: Social assessment<br>Phase 2: Epidemiological assessment<br>Phase 3: Education and ecological assessment<br>Phase 4: Administrative and policy assessment<br>Phase 5: Implementation<br>Phase 6: Process evaluation<br>Phase 7: Impact evaluation<br>Phase 8: Outcome evaluation |
| Multilevel approach to community health (MATCH) model | Goal selection<br>Intervention planning<br>Program development<br>Implementation preparation<br>Evaluation |
| Intervention mapping | Needs assessment<br>Matrices<br>Theory-based methods and practical strategies<br>Program<br>Adoption and implementation plan<br>Evaluation plan |
| Community readiness model | Community tolerance<br>Denial, resistance<br>Vague awareness<br>Pre-planning<br>Preparation<br>Initiation<br>Institutionalization<br>Confirmation, expansion<br>Professionalism |
| Social marketing | Product<br>Price<br>Place<br>Promotion |

By becoming familiar with the theories and models, program staff, stakeholders, and participants gain access to tools that will allow them to generate creative solutions to unique situations. They are able to go beyond acting on instinct or repeating earlier ineffective interventions to adopt a systematic, scientific approach to their work. Theories and models help staff, stakeholders, and participants to ask the right questions and zero in on factors that contribute to a problem. The theories help everyone to understand the dynamics that underlie real situations and to think about solutions in new ways.

## SUMMARY

Prominent health theories and planning models were discussed in this chapter to encourage their use throughout the planning, implementing, and evaluating of health promotion programs. No theory or model is perfect. Each was designed to address a particular need or conceptualization of how best to manage a health problem. Practitioners typically combine elements from different theories and models in their work. The process of selecting and combining the elements is creative and dynamic, changing over time as health promotion staff, stakeholders, and participants plan, implement, and evaluate health promotion programs.

Health theories and models are dynamic, and the range of theories and models available for application in health promotion programs is rapidly expanding. Health theories describe, explain, and predict behavior at the intrapersonal, interpersonal, and population levels. Health theories reflect the ecological perspective of health promotion, which emphasizes the interaction between and interdependence of factors within and across all levels of a health problem. Health planning models can and should guide the building and delivering of health promotion programs through planning, implementing, and evaluating. The strongest health promotion programs will use both health theories and planning models.

## FOR PRACTICE AND DISCUSSION

1. A senior center serving healthy Hispanic male and female seniors, ages sixty-five to seventy-five, wants to use social cognitive theory to encourage these seniors to change their habits in order to meet cancer risk reduction guidelines (behavior). Use the social cognitive theory concept of reciprocal

determinism and the constructs of environment, situation perceptions, outcome expectations and expectancies, self-control, observational learning, self-efficacy, and emotional coping to discuss potential intervention points for the program activities.

2. Risky drinking among college students is a problem. The health belief model can be useful in developing strategies to deal with college students who drink too much. College programs to prevent risky drinking among students often identify students who are at high risk for substance abuse but say they have not experienced any symptoms or problems. Use the health belief model to detail and discuss the challenges of addressing risky drinking among college students.

3. You are hired by the local Target store to plan, implement, and evaluate a program to promote nutritional health among its 250 employees. The plan is to offer nutrition education activities (for example, cooking classes, home gardening workshops), personal nutrition counseling, a group weight management program, and improved employee food services (for example, low-calorie vending machine options) to employees at varied times. Several months pass, and only 50 employees have participated. The store manager is concerned. She wants you to explain why 200 employees are not participating. She also wants you to change or revise the nutrition education program to make sure it is helping employees maintain and improve their nutritional health. Using the stages of change model, propose questions to assess employees' stages of change in regard to nutritional health in order to answer the store manager's questions.

4. A group of stakeholders want to plan an innovative diabetes prevention program that targets elementary school students and uses a range of activities and strategies. Using the PRECEDE-PROCEED model, discuss what would be involved with each phase of planning the program. In addition discuss key concepts from the other planning models (Table 3.12) and how they might clarify for the stakeholders what to expect as they plan, implement, and evaluate their program.

5. Using the same innovative diabetes prevention program discussed in Question 4, apply the concepts from the diffusion of innovations model to discuss strategies the program developers can use to ensure that the program will be adopted and will change elementary school practices.

6. A hospital that serves a large farming population wants to increase childhood vaccinations among the families it serves. Using the four P's of marketing (product, price, place, promotion), design a social marketing mix for the hospital to use in order to increase childhood vaccinations among children living in rural farming communities.

## KEY TERMS

Behavior

Communication theory

Community mobilization

Community readiness
 model

Concept

Construct

Diffusion of innovations
 model

Health belief model

Ideas

Intervention mapping

Model

Multilevel approach
 to community health
 (MATCH) model

PRECEDE-PROCEED
 model

Social cognitive theory

Social marketing

Social network and social
 support theory

Stages of change model

Theory

Theory of planned
 behavior

Theory of reasoned
 action

Transtheoretical model

Variable

## REFERENCES

Alinsky, S. (1971). *Rules for radicals*. New York: Random House.

Arnstein, S. (1969). A ladder of citizen participation. *Journal of Institutional Planning, 35*, 216–224.

Ayres, C. G. (2008). Mediators of the relationship between social support and positive health practice
　　in middle adolescents. *Journal of Pediatric Health Care, 22*(2), 94–102.

Bandura, A. (1986). *Social foundations of thought and action: A social cognitive theory*. Englewood Cliffs, NJ:
　　Prentice Hall.

Bandura, A. (1995). Exercise of personal and collective efficacy in changing societies. In A. Bandura
　　(Ed.), *Self-efficacy in changing societies* (pp. 1–45). New York: Cambridge University Press.

Bandura, A., & Locke, E. A. (2003). Negative self-efficacy and goal effects revisited. *Journal of Applied
　　Psychology, 88*(1), 87–99.

Bandura, A., & Walters, R. H. (1963). *Social learning and personality development*. New York: Holt, Rinehart
　　& Winston.

Bartholomew, L. K., Parcel, G. S., Kok, G., & Gottlieb, N. H. (2006). *Planning health promotion programs:
　　An intervention mapping approach*. San Francisco: Jossey-Bass.

Baum, F. E., & Ziersch, A. M. (2003). Social capital. *Journal of Epidemiology and Community Health, 57*,
　　320–323.

Brug, J., Oenema, A., & Ferreira, I. (2005). Theory, evidence and intervention mapping to improve
　　behavior nutrition and physical activity interventions. *International Journal of Behavioral Nutrition
　　and Physical Activity, 2*(1), 2.

Centers for Disease Control and Prevention. (2002). *Community mobilization guide: A community-based effort
　　to eliminate syphilis in the United States*. Retrieved April 14, 2008, from www.cdc.gov/std/see/
　　Community/CommunityGuide.pdf.

Cloward R., & Ohlin, L. (1961). *Delinquency and opportunity: A theory of delinquent gangs*. New York: Free
　　Press, 1961.

Csorba, J., Sörfozo, Z., Steiner, P., Ficsor, B., Harká Any, E., Babrik, Z., et al. (2007). Maladaptive strategies, dysfunctional attitudes and negative life events among adolescents treated for the diagnosis of "suicidal behaviour." *Psychiatria Hungarica, 22*(3), 200–211.

Donnermeyer, J. F., Plested, B. A., Edwards, R. W., Oetting, E. R., & Littlethunder, L. (1997). Community readiness and prevention programs. *Journal of the Community Development Society, 28*(1), 65–83.

Freire, P. (1972). *Pedagogy of the oppressed.* London: Sheed & Ward.

Finnegan, J. R., & Viswanath, K. (2002). Communication theory and health behavior change. (2002). In K. Glanz, B. K. Rimer, & F. M. Lewis (Eds.), *Health behavior and health education: Theory, research, and practice* (3rd ed., pp. 361–388). San Francisco: Jossey-Bass.

Fishbein, M., & Cappella, J. N. (2006). The role of theory in developing effective health communications. *Journal of Communication, 56*(1), S1–S17.

Glanz, K., & Rimer, B. K. (2005). *Theory at a glance: A guide for health promotion practice.* Retrieved April 16, 2008, from http://www.cancer.gov/PDF/481f5d53-63df-41bc-bfaf-5aa48ee1da4d/TAAG3.pdf.

Glanz, K., Rimer, B. K., & Lewis, F. M. (2002). *Health behavior and health education: Theory, research, and practice* (3rd ed.). San Francisco: Jossey-Bass.

Goodson, P. (2010). *Theory in health promotion research and practice.* Sudbury, MA: Jones & Bartlett.

Green, L. W., & Kreuter, M. W. (1999). *Health promotion planning: An educational and ecological approach* (3rd ed.). New York: McGraw-Hill.

Green, L. W., & Kreuter, M. W. (2005). *Health program planning: An educational and ecological approach* (4th ed.). New York: McGraw-Hill.

Hardeman, W., Kinmonth, A. L., Michie, S., Sutton, S., & the ProActive Project Team. (2009). Impact of a physical activity intervention program on cognitive predictors of behaviour among adults at risk of type 2 diabetes (ProActive randomized controlled trial). *International Journal of Behavioral Nutrition and Physical Activity, 6*(11), 6–16.

House, J. S. (1981). *Work stress and social support.* Reading, MA: Addison-Wesley.

Janz, N., Champion V., & Strecher, V. (2002). The health belief model. In K. Glanz, B. K. Rimer, & F. M. Lewis (Eds.), *Health behavior and health education: Theory, research, and practice* (3rd ed., pp. 45–66). San Francisco: Jossey-Bass.

Kerlinger, F. N. (1986). *Foundations of behavioral research* (3rd ed.). New York: Holt, Rinehart & Winston.

McLeroy, K. R., Bibeau, D., Steckler, A., & Glanz, K. (1988). An ecological perspective on health promotion programs. *Health Education & Behavior, 15*(4), 351–377.

Montano, D., & Kasprzyk, D. (2008). Theory of reasoned action, theory of planned behavior, and the integrated behavioral model. In K. Glanz, B. K. Rimer, & K. Viswanath (Eds.), *Health behavior and health education: Theory, research, and practice* (4th ed., pp. 67–96). San Francisco: Jossey-Bass.

Oldenburg, B., & Parcel, G. (2002). Diffusion of innovations. In K. Glanz, B. K. Rimer, & F. M. Lewis, (Eds.), *Health behavior and health education: Theory, research, and practice* (3rd ed., pp. 312–334). San Francisco: Jossey-Bass.

Prochaska, J. O., DiClemente, C. C., & Norcross, J. C. (1992). In search of how people change: Applications to addictive behaviors. *American Psychologist, 47*(9), 1102–1114.

Prochaska, J. O., Redding, C. A., & Evers, K. E. (2002). The transtheoretical model and stages of change. In K. Glanz, B. K. Rimer, & F. M. Lewis (Eds.), *Health behavior and health education: Theory, research, and practice* (3rd ed., pp. 99–120). San Francisco: Jossey-Bass.

Rimer, B. K., & Kreuter, M. W. (2006). Advancing tailored health communication: A persuasion and message effects perspective. *Journal of Communication, 56*(1), S184–S201.

Rogers, E. (1995). *Diffusion of innovations* (4th ed.). New York: Free Press.

Rosenstock, I. (1974). Historical origins of the health belief model. *Health Education Monographs, 2,* 328–335.

Rosenstock, I., Strecher, V., & Becker, M. (1988). Social learning theory and the health belief model. *Health Education Quarterly, 15*(2), 175–183.

Simons-Morton, D. G., Simons-Morton, B. G., Parcel, G. S., & Bunker, J. F. (1988). Influencing personal and environmental conditions for community health: A multilevel intervention model. *Family and Community Health, 11*(2), 25–35.

Stephens, C. (2008). Social capital in its place: Using social theory to understand social capital and inequalities in health. *Social Science Medicine, 66*(5), 1174–1184.

Twoy, R., Connolly, P. M., & Novak, J. M. (2007). Coping strategies used by parents of children with autism. *Journal of American Academic Nurse Practitioners, 19*(5), 251–260.

van Oostrom, S. H., Anema, J. R., Terluin, B., Venema, A., de Vet, H. C., & van Mechelen, W. (2007). Development of a workplace intervention for sick-listed employees with stress-related mental disorders: Intervention mapping as a useful tool. *BMC Health Services Research, 7,* 127.

Wolfers, M. E., van den Hoek, C., Brug, J., & de Zwart, O. (2007). Using Intervention Mapping to develop a programme to prevent sexually transmittable infections, including HIV, among heterosexual migrant men. *BMC Public Health Services Research, 7,* 141.

Yzer, M. C., Cappella, J. N., Fishbein, M., Hornik, R., Sayeed, S., & Ahern, R. K. (2004). The role of distal variables in behavior change: Effects of adolescents' risk for marijuana use on intention to use marijuana. *Journal of Applied Social Psychology, 34*(6), 1229–1250.

# PART TWO

# PLANNING HEALTH PROMOTION PROGRAMS

# CHAPTER FOUR

# ASSESSING THE NEEDS OF PROGRAM PARTICIPANTS

JAMES H. PRICE

JOSEPH A. DAKE

BRITNEY WARD

## LEARNING OBJECTIVES

- Define *needs assessment*, and explain its relevance to health promotion programming

- Evaluate sources of needs assessment data and information in terms of scope, timeliness, cost, and relevance to program recipients

- Describe the four-step needs assessment process and the role of program stakeholders at each step

- Describe how to report needs assessment findings in a way that meets stakeholders' requirements and uses for the data

CCORDING TO the health theories and models for developing health promotion programs in Chapter Three (Table 3.12), the first phase in the process of creating, operating, and sustaining a health promotion program is program planning. In all of the models, one of the first steps in planning a health promotion program is conducting a needs assessment. A needs assessment gathers information about individuals' health needs and a site's support and resources to inform the process of planning, implementing, and evaluating a program. Critical to a successful health promotion program is making sure the program addresses the needs of the people at the program site, whether it is a school, workplace, health care organization, or community. Although there are many methods of conducting a needs assessment, following some basic principles is essential in order to secure quality information upon which a health promotion program that will increase the well-being of the individuals at a particular site can be developed. This chapter explains what a needs assessment is and identifies what might be measured when a needs assessment is conducted. Also covered are the processes for conducting a needs assessment and the types of primary and secondary data that can be useful in establishing priorities. Finally, we discuss the importance of reporting the results of a needs assessment in a manner that the staff, stakeholders, and target audience of the health promotion program will understand and find useful.

## DEFINING A NEEDS ASSESSMENT

Understanding how the health of a group of individuals at a site might be improved requires information on both their current health status and their ideal health status. Collection of that information is called a *needs assessment*. Traditionally, needs assessments have been associated with individuals living in a specific geographic area such as a city, county, state, or nation (commonly known as a community needs assessment, a reflection of health promotion's roots in health education). However, needs assessments are completed for all groups of individuals who participate in a health promotion program at a site. Needs assessments describe the program participants (for example, they identify the demographic characteristics of a group of individuals in terms of race, gender, age, and sexual orientation and identify individuals with health problems such as diabetes and obesity) (Centers for Disease Control and Prevention, 1995). Needs assessments can reflect the three levels of influence in the ecological health perspective: intrapersonal, interpersonal, and population (McLeroy, Bibeau, Steckler, & Glanz, 1988; Glanz & Rimer, 2005). Consistent with the goal of eliminating health disparities (see Chapter Two), the assessment needs to be culturally appropriate. Finally, the health theories and models discussed in Chapter Three will influence the questions asked and the information sought during the needs assessment.

The results of a needs assessment provide a foundation for the work of planning a health promotion program that addresses identified health problems and concerns. Furthermore, the results can be used to help allocate health resources and to establish a baseline against which to gauge the effectiveness of the program (through evaluation of interventions).

Finally, to fully answer the question, what is a needs assessment? we need to answer the question, what is a need? A *need* is usually conceptualized as the difference between "what is" at the present time and "what should be" under more ideal circumstances (Witkin & Altschuld, 1995). A *needs assessment* is a formalized approach to collecting data in order to identify the needs of a group of individuals.

## What Is Measured in Assessing Health? Focus on the Individuals

The first dimension of health that almost everyone would agree is part of health is physical health. Most individuals would define *physical health* as being free from pain, physical disability, chronic and infectious diseases, and bodily discomforts that require the attention of a physician, and perhaps also as having increased longevity. A population's physical health problems are likely to be assessed in terms of the number and variety of diseases (morbidity), number and variety of deaths (mortality), office visits to clinicians, hospitalizations, and many other indicators (see Exhibit 4.1). As you examine the partial list of potential indicators of physical health in Exhibit 4.1, consider what other indicators should be listed. Are these indicators measures of physical health, or are they measures of the level of disease within the population?

*Mental health* is characterized by an ability to deal constructively with reality, adapt to change, and cope with adversity. In contrast, *mental illness* is characterized by alterations in thinking, mood, or behaviors that impair a person's relationships with others in their environment. Mental health and mental illness are not polar opposites but exist along a continuum of impairment. Mental illness typically affects about 20 percent of the population at any point in time (U.S. Department of Health and Human Services, 1999). Assessing the mental health status of a population requires that associations be made between the numbers of individuals with various mental disorders and, for example, the number who obtain care from mental health professionals, receive psychotropic medications, or are institutionalized for some period of time for their disorders (see Exhibit 4.1). However, because mental health insurance coverage is far less comprehensive than traditional health insurance coverage (Carter & Landau, 2009), assessments based on

# EXHIBIT 4.1
## Dimensions of Health

### Indicators of Physical Health

- Morbidity rates
- Life span
- Number of prescriptions
- Nutritional status
- Health care expenditures
- Environmental quality
- Level of physical disability
- Self-assessed health status
- Prevalence of health risk factors
- Number and types of health procedures
- Rate of premature births
- Prevalence of health insurance
- Health promotion or disease prevention programs
- Number and types of health professionals
- Number and types of health institutions

### Indicators of Mental Health

- Mortality rates
- Morbidity rates
- Life span
- Number of psychotropic prescriptions
- Mental health care expenditures
- Number and types of mental health services
- Prevalence of insurance coverage for mental illness
- Self-assessed mental health status

- Hospitalization rates for mental illness
- Number and types of mental health professionals
- Number and types of mental health institutions

### Indicators of Social Health

- Poverty levels
- Educational status
- Crime rates
- Divorce rates
- Out-of-wedlock pregnancies
- Social supports
- Social roles
- Drug abuse
- Unemployment rates
- Number and type of social service agencies

### Indicators of Environmental Health

- Built environment
- Environmental toxins
- Pollutants (air, water, noise)
- Population density
- Transportation options
- Recreational facilities
- Housing facilities

### Indicators of Spiritual Health

- Level of sense of purpose in life
- Number and types of religious institutions
- Level of life satisfaction
- Level of prejudice

the volume of mental health care use are likely to underestimate the actual need for such services in a community.

A third dimension of health has been termed *social health*. This area has been variously conceptualized by using variables such as educational status of a population, level of poverty and near poverty, crime rates, and a wide variety of other indicators (see Exhibit 4.1). A fourth dimension of health that can be measured is *environmental health*, which includes external conditions and influences that affect healthy growth and development.

The final dimension of health that some feel needs to be examined is *spiritual health* (see Exhibit 4.1). The spiritual dimension of health has not been explored or assessed in populations with the same intensity or depth as the other dimensions of health that we have discussed. People who conduct needs assessments have historically ignored this dimension of health because of the difficulty of assessing this concept.

## What Is Measured in Assessing Health? Focus on the School, Workplace, Health Care Organization, Community

Needs assessments also focus on the health promotion program site: a school, workplace, health care organization, or community. This part of a needs assessment is known as a capacity assessment (Gilmore & Campbell, 2005). A *capacity assessment* is a thorough and accurate assessment of the site to determine what resources are available in the setting to address the identified health concerns and problems—for example, health promotion materials, technology (computers, software packages, Internet access, DSL, Web sites, and so on), staff, programs, funding, and services, as well as the gaps and needs in these areas. A key element of a capacity assessment is the empowerment of potential program participants, staff, and stakeholders to mobilize forces to address and solve the health problems or concerns identified in the needs assessment.

Tools for assessing capacity at each type of site are available. For example, for school sites, the *School Health Index: A Self-Assessment and Planning Guide* has been developed by the National Center for Chronic Disease Prevention and Health Promotion (2008) at the Centers for Disease Control and Prevention, in partnership with school administrators and staff, school health experts, parents, and national nongovernmental health and education agencies for the purpose of

- Enabling schools to identify strengths and weaknesses of health and safety policies and programs
- Enabling schools to develop an action plan for improving student health, which can be incorporated into the school improvement plan

- Engaging teachers, parents, students, and the community in promoting health-enhancing behaviors and better health

The *School Health Index* has two activities that are completed by teams from a school: the eight self-assessment modules and a planning for improvement process. The self-assessment process involves members of the school community coming together to discuss what the school is already doing to promote good health and to identify strengths and weaknesses. The *School Health Index* assesses the extent to which a school implements the types of policies and practices recommended by the Centers for Disease Control and Prevention's research-based guidelines for school health and safety policies and programs.

In Part Five of this book, tools and resources for assessing capacity in schools, workplaces, health care organizations, and communities that are specific to each type of site are discussed. The areas covered by the assessments can be quite broad. For example, they might include policies, procedures, health services and health promotion resources (for example, staff, space, materials, technology, and funding), service gaps and linkages, networks, health insurance and benefits, legal requirements and compliance, and accreditations. Furthermore, assessments might cover an organization's experience and lessons learned from its own growth and development and incorporating change and trying new initiatives, such as a health promotion program (Senge, 1990).

Assessing the capacity of a site to operate and support a health promotion program provides early insight into the culture and climate of a setting. According to Moos (1979), climate is the social atmosphere of a setting or the learning environment, in which individuals have different experiences, depending on the protocols set up by the staff and administrators. In addition to the items already discussed, examples of areas that could be explored as part of a capacity assessment include relationships that support health, opportunities to promote personal health for everyone at the site, and support systems for and barriers to implementation of the program.

## Data Collection for Needs Assessments

Data collection plays a pivotal role in assessing the quality of life of the population of interest and in establishing priorities for health promotion programs. There are two major categories of data: primary data and secondary data.

- **Primary data** are new, original data that did not exist before, obtained directly from individuals at the site, usually by means of surveys, interviews, focus groups, or direct observation. Primary data constitute new information that will be used to answer specific questions.

- **Secondary data** already exist because they were collected by someone for another purpose. The data may or may not be directly from the individual or population that is being assessed. Secondary data sources include *Healthy People* information, vital records, census data, and peer-reviewed journals.

Primary data are more expensive and time consuming to collect than secondary data. Collection of quality primary data requires technical expertise in order to identify representative samples, design instruments, and complete data analysis. The problems with secondary data are that some information may not exist for some settings, the data may be old, or the data may not have been correctly collected.

Information to be collected can be divided into two broad categories: quantitative and qualitative. *Quantitative data* are statistical information (for example, percentages, means, or correlations) such as one would typically find in professional journals. However, numbers alone do not provide sufficient insights to allow program staff to completely understand health problems or decide how to intervene in order to reduce a health problem. *Qualitative data* are more narrative, with fewer numbers. They include the perceptions and misperceptions of community members in regard to quality of life issues in the community. Qualitative methods include one-on-one interviews with key informants, focus groups, public hearings, and observational methods. The two forms of data (quantitative and qualitative) complement one another, each type informing the other as staff derive conclusions and establish goals for community interventions.

Specific data-gathering techniques to be used depend on what one wants to know, the resources available, and the constraints of the target population (for example, lack of reading ability, absence of telephones, or mobility problems). For initial phases of primary data collection, interactive group processes are recommended (for example, focus groups) because they allow those conducting the needs assessment to clarify both their own questions and respondents' answers. Interactive methods also provide the opportunity to collect specific words that members of the population group use to describe health issues, which can later be used to form questions for a final questionnaire that can be used to survey even more individuals. Later, these written questionnaires can be used to collect large amounts of data from many people over a wide geographic area. Such a large quantity of data will need to be aggregated and analyzed by computer.

## CONDUCTING A HEALTH NEEDS ASSESSMENT

Needs assessments consist of four basic steps: (1) determining the scope of the assessment, (2) gathering data, (3) analyzing the data, and (4) reporting the findings.

Before you do anything, it is best to think about each of the steps and map out to the best of your ability what will happen in each step. This planning is important so that you can explain to stakeholders what they can expect from the process as well as how long it will take to complete the needs assessment.

1. *Determine the scope.* Work with the key informants and stakeholders (that is, an advisory committee) to determine the scope of the work and the purpose of the needs assessment. Ask who will be involved and what decisions will be based on the needs assessment. Think carefully and critically about what information is needed in order to make the decisions. Who ultimately will use the results to make decisions about the intervention or prevention programs? Whenever possible, take an ecological approach to the needs assessment. Assess both the stakeholders and their environment. In the environmental assessment, include an analysis of organizational and community assets and capacity.

2. *Gather the data.* Gather only the needed data. Consider culturally appropriate data-gathering approaches tailored to the target population and setting (see Chapter Two). Gather multiple types of data—both qualitative and quantitative. Exhibit 4.1 provides an overview of types of data that could be secured in order to address the various dimensions of health.

3. *Analyze the data.* Use clear methods that people can understand.

4. *Report and share the findings.* Identify your options for sharing the findings of the needs assessment. Think about how best to communicate the findings. In sharing the information, identify any factors that are linked to the health problem. Validate the need for the program before continuing with the planning process. Tailor all communications to the program participants, stakeholders, and staff.

Many approaches can be used to conduct a needs assessment. Often, the methods that can be used will be limited by a lack of time, personnel, or money or by political constraints.

## PROMOTING A NEEDS ASSESSMENT

Conducting a needs assessment is an exciting event in the development of a health promotion program. It is often the first public acknowledgment that a school, workplace, health care organization, or community is working to address health problems at a site. Publicity to promote the needs assessment creates awareness of the needs assessment, enhances the chances that individuals and groups who have been asked to participate will respond, and increases the visibility of the organizations that form the advisory committee. Have a media kickoff for the needs assessment, and distribute press releases and information packets. Use e-mail and telephone messages to let people know about the needs assessment. For a needs assessment that is focused on a community, attempt to reach as many forms of mass media as possible (for example, local radio or TV programs, local newspapers, and newsletters of various community organizations). Numerous service clubs (for example, Rotary, Kiwanis, or Chamber of Commerce) may provide a forum in which to communicate the importance of the health needs assessment. Finally, be sure to obtain copies of newsletter articles and newspaper clippings to share with the advisory committee. This form of sharing can bolster support from the advisory committee.

## USING PRIMARY DATA METHODS AND TOOLS

The sections that follow briefly describe a series of methods and tools that can be used to collect primary data for the needs assessment. Each method or tool has specific strengths and weaknesses.

### Key Informant (One-on-One) Interviews

The idea underlying the qualitative technique of key informant interviews is that certain individuals possess unique and important information that can provide insights into the health issues at a site. These *key informants* may be selected on the basis of their position at the site (Centers for Disease Control and Prevention, 1995). For example, at schools, key informants might include teachers, principals, parents, school nurses, and students. Examples of key informants at work sites are human resource directors, company owners, supervisors, and union leaders. In communities, key informants might be local government officials, ministers, medical personnel, or agency directors. Another type of key informant is people who are chosen because of their reputation. Such individuals usually include opinion leaders, activists, or other socially prominent individuals. A needs assessment should include interviews with both types of individuals.

It is important that a specific set of questions be created ahead of time in order to create a uniform interview format. (See Exhibit 4.2 for some questions that key informants in a community might be asked.) Pilot-testing the interview questionnaire is essential. Again, remember that each person will share opinions (and biases) with the interviewer as if they were facts. Usually, not all key informants are interviewed, so the opinions collected will represent limited insights into the issues being assessed.

**EXHIBIT 4.2**
**Interview or Focus Group Questions for a**
**Community Assessment**

1. What do you think the main health problems are in the community?
2. What do you think are the causes of these health problems?
3. How can these problems be reduced or eliminated in the community?
4. Are there any special health problems or issues affecting children and adolescents in the community?
5. Are there any special health problems or issues affecting the elderly in the community?
6. Is there a particular group of community residents that you would consider more unhealthy than the rest of the residents? If so, why are they less healthy?
7. Which one of the previously mentioned problems do you consider to be the most important one in the community?
8. If you were given $1 million to correct the health problems of the community, what would you spend it on?

In-depth interviews with key informants typically take the form of conversation between the interviewer and the respondent. This type of interaction gathers the views of the respondents in their own terms. Through probing questions, a well-trained interviewer can clarify statements made by an informant.

## Focus Groups

A focus group is a qualitative data collection technique in which a small group of individuals meet to share their views and experiences on some topic. The ideal size of the group depends, in part, on the skills of the facilitator (Krueger & Casey, 2000). Usually the ideal group size is six to twelve participants who are similar in some way. The subjects should not know one another personally because that might affect the willingness of some members to share different opinions and values. The groups should be of the same race or ethnicity, gender, educational status, and socioeconomic status. This technique capitalizes on the interaction of the group members. The greater the diversity of the demographic characteristics of the group, the greater is the chance that dialogue may be inhibited (Krueger & Casey, 2000). For example, males have often been found to dominate the discussions in mixed-gender focus groups. If you have great disparity in education levels among members, those who are not as educated may feel intimidated about expressing their opinions.

Usually, the number of focus groups sufficient to study the perceptions of individuals at a site is determined by the diversity of the population at the site. People of different ages (youths, middle-aged people, elderly people), sexes, and racial or ethnic groups (African Americans, Asians, Hispanics, Caucasians) all need their own focus groups. Focus groups bring together preselected individuals; usually a greater number than is needed is invited because often there are no-shows. Focus groups typically take sixty to ninety minutes (Krueger & Casey, 2000).

Besides the group moderator, it is usually helpful to have an observer who serves as a recorder in order to capture the specific comments and unique words of the participants. The focus group leader should not try to take extensive notes because that might cause him or her to miss important elements of nonverbal communication (for example, facial expressions, gestures, or other body language). Respondents are usually provided with drinks and, sometimes, a snack and are paid for the time they spend to participate in a focus group. The themes found in their comments and, in some cases, the specific wording can give important insights into their perceptions of the site and provide the specific wording that can be used to form survey questions, if a survey is going to be used afterward to assess more individuals within the target population (Henderson, 1995).

## Delphi Technique

The Delphi technique has been used to solicit information from individuals who cannot easily be brought together for, say, a focus group. This technique might be used with a group of health experts (for example, physicians or dentists) who cannot conveniently meet in person. First, a group of professionals are asked to respond to a few open-ended questions. Their responses are returned and are compiled into one list. Second, the experts are asked to respond to the combined list and add more items, eliminate items they do not support, and reword items that they think need to be clarified. The experts send their responses back, and again, the responses are compiled into one master list. The process can be stopped at this point, or the list of responses can be sent to the experts again in order for them to rate or rank the items. This process can be cumbersome if postal mail is used, or it can be simplified by using electronic or Web-based communication.

## Survey Questionnaires

Surveys, especially written questionnaires, are the most common form of gathering data for a needs assessment (public perceptions and behaviors in regard to issues). Questionnaires can be administered in four ways—as mail surveys, as telephone surveys, face to face (as discussed earlier), or as electronic surveys (Fowler, 2002; Dillman, 2007). If an anonymous and confidential mail survey is used, one is more likely to obtain truthful responses, even to sensitive questions. Mail surveys allow a large quantity of data to be collected in a relatively short period of time. The main disadvantages are that special expertise is required to create valid and reliable mail surveys and to sample the population correctly. Techniques to increase the likelihood that one will obtain a satisfactory return rate can be employed (King, Pealer, & Bernard, 2001); too low a return rate increases the likelihood of biased data (nonresponse error).

In contrast to mail surveys, telephone surveys are more time consuming, more expensive to conduct, and often result in a lower response rate (due to screening by telephone answering machines and the difficulty of interviewing people on cell phones). Recent research indicates that 92.8 percent of households have a land-line telephone and 5.6 percent have only cellular phone service. Fewer than 2 percent have no phone service at all (Blumberg, Luke, & Cynamon, 2006).

Some subjects may feel intimidated in a telephone interview and give socially desirable responses rather than authentic answers to some questions. However, the response rate for telephone surveys may be higher than that for mail surveys for groups of individuals who do not read well (for example, some elderly people, people of low socioeconomic status, and non-native English language speakers). The longer the survey, the less likely it is that respondents will complete the questionnaire by phone.

Electronic surveys can be conducted by e-mail or through a Web site. When e-mail is used (which is less common), the questionnaire is provided as an attachment. However, because many computer viruses are transmitted by attachments, many potential respondents may not open the e-mail or the attachment. In contrast, Web surveys contact community members through an e-mail message and embed a URL in the message. Clicking on the URL takes the respondent directly to the Web site so that the questionnaire can be completed online. Unfortunately, the digital divide means that many of the economically disadvantaged and the elderly do not use computers as a method of communication. Another concern is that it seems to be easier for people to decline an Internet survey, even with a promise of a mailed incentive, in contrast to mail surveys, which can and should contain a modest financial incentive. This incentive can be as simple as a one- or two-dollar bill (King, Pealer, & Bernard, 2001). Regardless of the survey method, it is essential to have a good survey instrument. Questionnaires should have overall visual appeal; for example, they should use large enough print and adequate white space, have directions at the beginning of the questionnaire, and present the most important questions first and the demographic questions at the end.

Two very important attributes of a questionnaire are validity and reliability. A valid questionnaire is one that correctly measures what you want it to measure. The higher the validity, the more complex the assessment is. Face validity, in which the questions are based on previous questions or a review of the literature, is the weakest form of validity to use. Content validity is based on how well the questionnaire items reflect all of the content areas that one is attempting to measure (DeVon et al., 2007). To establish content validity, the questionnaire is sent to a panel of six to eight experts on the topic of the survey and on survey research. The experts are asked to add any other items needed, delete unneeded items, and reword any items that are unclear. More complex forms of establishing questionnaire validity, such as the procedures used to establish criterion-based validity or construct validity, are usually the most appropriate for health needs assessments.

Test-retest reliability (stability) of an instrument means that the same results will be obtained each time the instrument is given to the same sample of subjects (DeVon et al., 2007). To determine this form of reliability score, the instrument is given to a group of subjects ($n$ = 30 to 50) and then the same instrument is given to the same subjects a second time, one to two weeks later. The results of the respondents' first and second surveys must be matched and are generally entered into a computer software program that can calculate the reliability score. In the case of parametric data, the score generated is a Pearson product-moment correlation coefficient. The reliability score can vary from $-1.0$ to $+1.0$; the preferred score is 0.7 or higher. If the needs assessment items are nonparametric in nature, then other more appropriate analyses such as kappa coefficients or percent agreements should be calculated in order to determine the test-retest reliability.

Two other attributes of questionnaires to consider are readability and acceptability. A number of readability formulas—for example, the SMOG or the Dale-Chall formulas—can be applied to a written questionnaire to assess reading level. Another one is the Flesch-Kincaid formula, which is included in some popular word processing software, making it easy to obtain a reading level. Needs assessment instruments should be created with text at a reading level of seventh grade or lower. Acceptability relates to questionnaire wording and formatting (for example, the print is easy to read, the questionnaire is not too long, the instructions appear at appropriate places); the creators should also ensure that there are no offensive statements or material that unnecessarily touches on sensitive issues. To assess acceptability, one should pilot-test the questionnaire with ten to twenty people.

## Selecting a Sample

Three techniques of survey research are key to obtaining results that represent the health-related perceptions, behaviors, and needs of the group being assessed at a site. First is correctly selecting the people who will receive the questionnaire. Second is selecting a large enough sample that the results will be representative of the entire population. Third is making sure the return rate is high enough (better than 50 percent) to reach this adequate sample size.

Because limited resources usually prohibit surveying the entire population, obtaining a representative sample is an acceptable alternative. A representative sample can be accomplished through random selection of individuals, which involves selecting members of the population in such a way that each member has an equal chance of being selected to receive the questionnaire. In practice, true random selection for a needs assessment is unlikely to occur, but choosing methods that are as close as possible to random is ideal. Getting as close to randomization as possible helps to ensure that the responses are characteristic of the responses that would be obtained from the entire population of people (internal validity of the findings).

The second factor to be considered is power analysis (Price, Dake, Murnan, Dimmig, & Akpanudo, 2005). Power analysis deals with having an adequate number of individuals to be able to generalize the findings from the sample to the population. To determine the necessary size of the random sample, one needs to know the following: how much sampling error (variation in how accurately the sample represents the entire population) one is willing to accept, the size ($n$) of the population, and how much variation there is in the population with respect to the outcome variables (for example, health beliefs or behaviors) being surveyed. Table 4.1 shows various population sizes and the number of sample responses needed in order to be able to generalize findings to that population. For example, if one wanted to survey a community of 50,000 people in regard to perceptions and practices of smoking behaviors and secondary data indicated homogeneous perceptions or practices within that population, then one would use the categories that best represent that level of variation (a 90/10 split is the most homogeneous scenario available, representing a population in which 90 percent engage in the behavior and 10 percent do not, or vice versa). If, however, the community survey was more general and asked a wide variety of questions on various health behaviors and perceptions (as a general needs assessment typically would), then one might assume maximum heterogeneity in the responses and thus use the column labeled "50/50 Split." If the 50/50 split category is used and an error level of ±3 percent is determined to be acceptable, then one would need a sample of 1,045 completed surveys. If the survey team is willing to accept a larger sampling error, say, ±5 percent, then one would need only 381 completed surveys. Note that in Table 4.1, even when surveying very large populations (for example, 1 million or more), the samples needed are close to each other in size.

TABLE 4.1    Sample Sizes for Two Levels of Sampling Error at the
95 Percent Confidence Interval

| | Sample Error ± 3% | | Sample Error ± 5% | |
| | Variation in Responses | | Variation in Responses | |
| Population Size | 50/50 Split | 80/20 Split | 50/50 Split | 80/20 Split |
| --- | --- | --- | --- | --- |
| 100 | 92 | 87 | 80 | 71 |
| 250 | 203 | 183 | 152 | 124 |
| 500 | 341 | 289 | 217 | 165 |
| 750 | 441 | 358 | 254 | 185 |
| 1,000 | 516 | 406 | 278 | 198 |
| 2,500 | 748 | 537 | 333 | 224 |
| 5,000 | 880 | 601 | 357 | 264 |
| 10,000 | 964 | 639 | 370 | 240 |
| 25,000 | 1,023 | 665 | 378 | 243 |
| 50,000 | 1,045 | 674 | 381 | 245 |
| 100,000 | 1,056 | 678 | 383 | 245 |
| 1,000,000 | 1,066 | 682 | 384 | 246 |
| 10,000,000 | 1,067 | 683 | 384 | 246 |

*Note*: Numbers in table refer to completed questionnaires returned.

*Source*: Price, Dake, Murnan, Dimmig, & Akpanudo, 2005.

The third factor is survey return rates. In the aforementioned example on smoking behaviors in which 381 surveys were needed, if the survey were sent to a random sample of 3,000 and 381 surveys were returned, the response rate would be 13 percent (381/3000). However, if the questionnaire were sent to a random sample of 700 and there were 381 returned, the response rate would be 54 percent (381/700). Does it make a difference what the return rate is as long as the number of questionnaires returned meet the number needed for power? The answer depends on two issues: potential for sampling bias and potential for response bias.

Sampling bias occurs when the sample is selected in a manner (for example, a convenience sample) that results in people being left out who have unique characteristics (for example, race or ethnicity, health beliefs or behaviors, or socioeconomic status), which results in the final survey responses being uncharacteristic of the population. In contrast, response bias occurs when people who respond to the survey are different in their health beliefs or behaviors from those who do not respond to the survey. The more beliefs and behaviors reflected in the responses differ from the beliefs and behaviors of the nonrespondents, the greater the magnitude of the response bias. Another way of stating this is that a low return rate is a potential threat to external validity (being able to generalize the findings to the population from which the sample was drawn).

## USING SECONDARY DATA METHODS AND TOOLS

Secondary data already exist because they were collected by someone for another purpose. No health promotion program should be undertaken without a prior search of secondary sources. From secondary sources, you can get the big picture as well as an overview of how to proceed to address a health problem. Working with secondary data, you can view a variety of approaches to defining and analyzing a problem. There are many other reasons for using secondary data:

- It is far cheaper to collect secondary data than to obtain primary data. In other words, you can get a lot of information for your money and time—usually, more than you would get using the same amount of money to collect primary data.
- National, state, and local health data are publicly available and accessible electronically. The time involved in searching these sources is much less than that needed to collect primary data.
- Secondary sources of information usually yield more accurate data than those obtained through primary research. A government agency that has undertaken a large-scale survey or a census is likely to produce far more accurate results than custom-designed surveys that are based on relatively small sample sizes. However, not all secondary sources are more accurate.
- Secondary sources help define the population. Secondary data can be extremely useful both in defining the population and in structuring the sample to be taken. For instance, government statistics on a county's demographics will help decide how to stratify a sample and, once sample estimates have been calculated, these can be used to project those estimates to the population.
- Sometimes sufficient secondary data may be available that are entirely adequate for drawing conclusions and answering the questions, making primary data collection unnecessary.

## Internal Sources of Secondary Data

Working in a particular setting may have the advantage of allowing the use of internal sources of secondary information. All organizations collect information in the course of their everyday operations. Attendance rates, performance scores (grades, annual tests), number of sick days taken, production statistics, sales figures, and expenses are some of the data that might be available. Health data that are collected as a by-product of health services—for example, clinic records, data from immunization programs, data from water pollution control programs, clinical indicators, or data from health office visits and insurance claims—are possible internal sources of secondary data. Much of this information is of potential use in planning a health promotion program. Even being aware of people's work schedules or amounts of vacation and sick days might be important in order to know when people work and when they would be available to participate in a program.

## External Sources of Secondary Data

Large numbers of organizations provide health data, including national and local government agencies, trade associations, universities, research institutes, financial institutions, specialist suppliers of secondary marketing data, and professional health policy research centers. The main external sources of secondary information are government (federal, state, and local), voluntary health associations, private foundations, national and international institutions, professional associations, and universities. Some of the many sources of publicly available data can be found in Exhibit 4.3.

## Problems with Secondary Information

The benefits of using secondary information are considerable; however, the quality of both the source of the data and the data themselves should be evaluated. When deciding whether to use a particular source of secondary data, it may be helpful to ask the following questions: How easy will it be to access and use the data source? Do the data help address the desired specific program area? Do the data apply to the target population? Are the data relatively current? Are the data collection methods acceptable? Finally, are the data biased? Are the data trustworthy? If the answer to these questions is yes, the data source is good to use.

Whenever possible, use multiple sources of secondary data. In this way, different sources can be cross-checked and used to confirm one another. When differences occur, an explanation for the differences must be found or the data should be set aside.

## EXHIBIT 4.3
## Publicly Available Health Data Sources

| | |
|---|---|
| Behavioral Risk Factor Surveillance System | http://www.cdc.gov/brfss/technical_infodata/surveydata.htm |
| General Social Survey | http://www.norc.org/GSS+Website/Download |
| Healthcare Cost and Utilization Data | http://www.ahrq.gov/data/hcup/ |
| Henry A. Murray Research Archive | http://dvn.iq.harvard.edu/dvn/dv/mra/faces/HomePage.jsp |
| Joint Canada/United States Survey of Health | http://www.cdc.gov/nchs/about/major/nhis/jcush_mainpage.htm |
| Longitudinal Studies of Aging | http://www.cdc.gov/nchs/lsoa.htm |
| Medical Expenditures Panel Survey | http://www.meps.ahrq.gov/mepsweb/data_stats/download_data_files.jsp |
| Monitoring the Future | http://www.icpsr.umich.edu/cocoon/SAMHDA/SERIES/00035.xml |
| National Ambulatory Medical Care Survey and the National Hospital Ambulatory Medical Care Survey | http://www.cdc.gov/nchs/about/major/ahcd/ahcd1.htm#Micro-data |
| National Health and Nutrition Examination Survey | http://www.cdc.gov/nchs/about/major/nhanes/datalink.htm |
| National Health Interview Survey | http://www.cdc.gov/nchs/about/major/nhis/quest_data_related_doc.htm |

## REPORTING AND SHARING THE FINDINGS

The last step in the process of needs assessment is to report and share the findings. What are your options for sharing the findings of a needs assessment? Think about how best to communicate. In sharing the information, identify any factors that are linked to the health problem. Identify the focus for the program, and validate the need for the program before continuing with the planning process. Tailor all communications to the program participants, staff, and stakeholders.

### Analyzing Results

How the results of a needs assessment are analyzed will largely depend on the purpose of the needs assessment. The data may be largely descriptive in order

| | |
|---|---|
| National Hospital Discharge Survey | http://www.cdc.gov/nchs/about/major/hdasd/nhds.htm |
| National Immunization Survey | http://www.cdc.gov/nis/datafiles.htm |
| National Mortality Followback Survey | http://www.cdc.gov/nchs/about/major/nmfs/nmfs.htm |
| National Survey of Children's Health | http://www.cdc.gov/nchs/about/major/slaits/imputed_data.htm |
| National Survey of Family Growth | http://www.cdc.gov/nchs/NSFG.htm |
| National Survey on Drug Use and Health | http://www.icpsr.umich.edu/cocoon/SAMHDA/STUDY/21240.xml |
| Pregnancy Risk Assessment Monitoring System | http://www.cdc.gov/PRAMS/index.htm |
| Surveillance Epidemiology and End Results Program | http://seer.cancer.gov/data/access.html |
| Treatment Episode Data Set | http://www.icpsr.umich.edu/cocoon/SAMHDA/STUDY/21540.xml |
| U.S. Census | http://factfinder.census.gov/servlet/DatasetMainPageServlet |
| Youth Risk Behavior Surveillance System | http://www.cdc.gov/HealthyYouth/yrbs/data/index.htm |

to provide a baseline assessment from which to do comparisons, write grants, plan programs, and so on. It is often useful when reporting descriptive statistics (percentages, means, standard deviations, and so on) to make comparisons with other appropriate data sources. For example, if the assessment of a site includes a question on the percentage of adults who are current smokers, it would be useful to report the findings not only for that site but also for the state or nation, if the secondary data exist. This comparison could be presented in tabular format or graphical format (Figure 4.1). The data could also be separated by important characteristics such as gender, race, or socioeconomic indicators (Figure 4.2).

If data beyond descriptive statistics are desired, it would be important to hire a statistician to determine what types of analyses are possible and appropriate based on the sample obtained for the needs assessment. If more in-depth analyses that

FIGURE 4.1   Comparisons to State and Federal Data

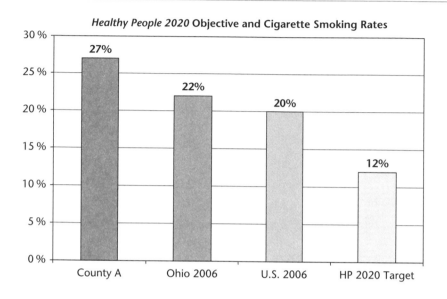

FIGURE 4.2   Data Comparisons to Subgroups

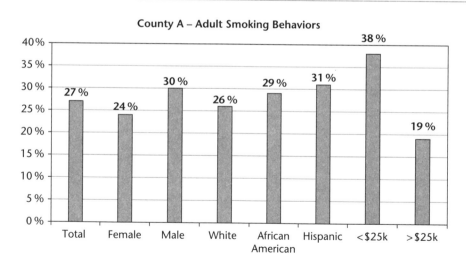

compare subgroups are desired, increased sample sizes may be needed. It is sometimes inappropriate to calculate statistical comparisons on every subgroup that can
be derived from needs assessment data. If an advisory committee wants to investigate a specific subgroup, it is important that this be decided prior to beginning

the assessment so that oversampling of that subgroup is built into the assessment, ensuring adequate power in the subsample to calculate needed statistics.

One new technique that can be used in reporting the results of needs assessments is a geographic information system (GIS) (Metzler et al., 2008). GIS technology is becoming popular in a wide variety of fields for numerous reasons. In the field of public health, a GIS can be used to visualize health data that are gathered and processed in a software program that presents the data in a spatial format, allowing interpretation and analysis that may be different from what is possible through tabular or other graphical methods. Uses of GIS technology in health include determining the geographic distribution of various diseases (both infectious and chronic), analyzing spatial trends in health, analyzing needs assessment data to help plan the most effective interventions, and analyzing health outcomes based on distances between individual homes and health care institutions.

## Establishing Priorities

The advisory board (Chapter One) plays an important role during the needs assessment to establish program priorities Most board members will come together (sometimes with program staff and other program stakeholders) to look at the needs assessment data (for example, numbers, summaries of interviews, and secondary data reports) and to discuss and decide on program priorities based on the data. Frequently the needs assessment produces a lot of information (such as numbers, tables, and charts). So the first task is to reduce the information to a manageable number of health concerns and topics. One way to group the data to facilitate ratings is to divide them into three areas: types of death or disability, behavioral risk factors, and nonbehavioral risk factors. (Social, physical, and environmental factors that affect health are considered nonbehavioral risk factors.) Once the data are grouped, then the advisory board can prioritize what to address within each group and among groups. Identifying which problems to address will require that criteria (for example, importance, feasibility of change, magnitude of problem, and cost) be established by the advisory board. These priorities provide justification for starting new programs and continuing or terminating existing programs. The following issues might be factors to consider in establishing program priorities at a site.

- How large is the discrepancy between the incidence of the health problem locally and the incidence at state or national levels?
- How many individuals are affected by the health problem?
- Which problem has the greatest impact on disability or mortality?
- What are the leading perceived health problems of the stakeholders?

- What will be the consequences if the health problem is not corrected?
- Would not correcting the problem cause other health-related problems?
- Would other health-related problems be reduced if this health problem were reduced?
- What is the potential impact on others at the site if the health problem is reduced?
- How difficult would it be to correct the health problem?
- Which problems are already being addressed by other groups and organizations?
- How many resources would be required to solve the health-related problem?
- How effective are available interventions in preventing or reducing the health-related problem?
- Do you have the expertise to resolve the health-related problem?
- What are the barriers (obstacles) to correcting the health-related problem?
- Will the stakeholders want and accept the proposed solution to the health-related problem?
- Do current laws permit the proposed health-related program activities to be conducted?

These questions can guide the board's thinking when it is establishing priorities. Eventually, however, the criteria will probably need to be weighed numerically. One simple method of establishing priorities is to use only two categories to assess each health-related problem: importance and feasibility (Table 4.2). Importance factors include the number of people affected, mortality rate, and potential impact on the population. Feasibility factors include how difficult it will be to correct the problem, availability of resources, effectiveness of available interventions, and potential acceptance of solutions at the site. Each member of the advisory board rates the health-related problems that have been identified in the target population. The aggregated ratings of all board members are then used to determine the final priorities.

### TABLE 4.2    Process for Determining Health Priorities

|  |  | Feasibility | | |
|---|---|---|---|---|
|  |  | High (3) | Moderate (2) | Low (1) |
|  | High (3) | 6 points | 5 points | 4 points |
| Importance | Moderate (2) | 5 points | 4 points | 3 points |
|  | Low (1) | 4 points | 3 points | 2 points |

On the basis of the priorities it has set, the advisory board then establishes program goals. In other words, program goals are directed toward reducing a particular health problem. Which programs will actually be implemented is not based just on the results of an analysis but depends on a variety of issues. Figure 4.3 shows four factors that most often affect which actions are taken. Initially, it would seem that the most serious health problems (based on data from the needs assessment) should be the ones to be addressed first. In reality, other factors—for example, insufficient resources, a lack of available effective interventions, or the political and social values of the school, workplace, health care organization, or community—may play significant roles in determining which needs are addressed.

A second approach to making decisions on which interventions to pursue is to use the PEARL model (Vilnius & Dandoy, 1990). PEARL is an acronym that represents five feasibility factors that have a high degree of influence in determining how a particular problem can be addressed. Board members (and maybe staff and other stakeholders too) answer the following questions in order to determine a score for a particular option:

**Propriety**: Does the problem fall within the organization's overall mission?
**Economic feasibility**: Does it make economic sense to address the problem? Will there be economic consequences if the problem is not addressed?

FIGURE 4.3   Factors in Decisions on Actions to Take After a Needs Assessment

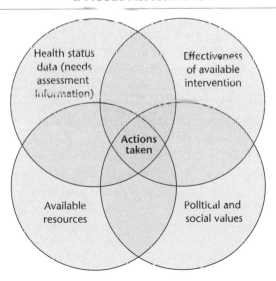

**Acceptability**: Will the community or target population accept an intervention to address the problem?

**Resources**: Are resources available to address the problem?

**Legality**: Do current laws allow the problem to be addressed?

Each of these five PEARL factors is scored. The score is 1 if the answer is yes and 0 if the answer is no. When scoring is complete, the five scores for that option are multiplied to obtain a final score. Because the scores are multiplied, not added, if the answer on any of the five factors is no, then the product will equal 0 and the health problem will not be addressed in the overall priority rating, regardless of the rank of the problem on each individual factor.

A third approach to making program priority decisions, often used in combination with the two just mentioned, is consensus building. Essentially, *consensus building* (also called collaborative problem solving or collaboration) is bringing together advisory board members, program staff, program participants, and stakeholders to use the needs assessment results and data to express their ideas, clarify areas of agreement and disagreement, and develop shared program direction. Consensus can be difficult to reach. However, developing program priorities through consensus maximizes the opportunities to gain input and support from a wide range of individuals, groups, and organizations for the subsequent program planning decisions (discussed in Chapter Five) as well as program implementation and evaluation.

## Writing the Final Report and Disseminating Findings

Once analysis of the data is complete and the ranking of priorities has been agreed on, then it is time to write the final report on the needs assessment. The final report contains an executive summary, acknowledgments, a table of contents, demographics of the community, methods of data collection, main findings, established priorities, references, and appendixes. The final report will be the face of the needs assessment for the next several years. The executive summary is an abbreviated (typically four to six pages), stand-alone summary of the essential findings of the report. The demographics section is usually from secondary sources and describes the characteristics of the general population. The methods section of the report explains how the study was conducted. The findings section is the largest segment of the report; it is the section that is usually full of tables, graphs, and diagrams. Be careful to minimize the use of jargon and technical terminology that fails to communicate to a general audience. The section on priorities is the part of the final report that provides direction for the development of a health promotion program. Prioritizing the health needs at the site helps to focus the direction of the health promotion program. Be sure to have a person who is not directly related to writing the report proofread it for grammar problems and minor mistakes. Also make sure it is easy to read and use. (Chapter Eight has more information about the importance of making reports easy to read—often called writing in plain language—to make sure health promotion program materials, including reports, are easy to understand.) Expect the report to need revisions and perhaps to need some sections rewritten before it is printed and bound. Finally the choices for how the report is disseminated will influence how the report is used. Dissemination options include printing the entire report; preparing special reports or brochures for particular groups of individuals and stakeholders (such as funders or program participants); posting the report on the Web; and informing people about the report through e-mail, public meetings, board and staff meetings, newspaper reports, radio and television interviews by advisory board members and staff, press releases, and news conferences.

Here are three tips for writing the final report:

- **Start with a plan**. Think about the information that the audience needs and the format that is most appropriate. Both written and oral reports can be developed. Tailor presentations to program staff, participants, and stakeholders. Remember to plan ahead; don't wait until there are results to think about how to share them.

- **Keep it simple**. Needs assessment reports do not need to be elaborate. It is most important that the information shared be clear, simple, and timely. Use brief sections and subsections, and make titles clear and informative. Whenever possible, depict findings pictorially in charts, graphs, or figures, and combine these with explanations in the text. Mix didactic and data-rich information with supporting evidence and anecdotal descriptions. Varying the material in this way will make the report more interesting and readable and the findings more believable.

- **Respect adult learning styles**. Three principles of adult learning are important to keep in mind when communicating the findings of a needs assessment. First, adults are most interested in information that is directly relevant to the projects and problems they are dealing with in their own lives. Second, they are most likely to use information that relates to their own personal experiences. Third, different people learn in different ways; some are visually oriented, others prefer narrative text, and some learn best when they hear something instead of reading it. Therefore, it may be beneficial to combine a few different methods of information dissemination.

## SUMMARY

Conducting a needs assessment provides an unbiased look at a target population within a particular setting and provides a foundation for the work of putting together a program that is culturally appropriate and based on health theory in order to address identified health problems and concerns. When conducting a needs assessment, it is essential to use a variety of methods to collect and analyze data from both primary and secondary sources and to conduct a capacity assessment of the site: school, workplace, health care organization, or community. Then, working with the advisory board, program participants, staff, and stakeholders, establish program priorities using approaches such as PEARL and consensus building to maximize program support in the later program planning decisions as well during the program implementation and evaluation.

Tailor the needs assessment report to the program participants, staff and stakeholders, and the setting. In the report, in plain language, identify the diverse factors that influence health behaviors as well as the behaviors and environmental conditions that promote or compromise health. Likewise, identify factors that influence learning and behavior, foster or hinder the health promotion process, and determine the extent of existing and available health promotion programs and services.

## FOR PRACTICE AND DISCUSSION

1. Review the health theories in Chapter Three (Table 3.10). Select a theory and discuss how it might influence a needs assessment. Compare and contrast the theories. How do they help you to understand needs assessment for health promotion programs?

2. How would a needs assessment for a rural community of 5,000 people (including adults, children, and senior citizens) differ from a needs assessment for a large urban hospital with 1,500 employees working seven days a week, twenty-four hours a day, or for a school district with 4,000 students in kindergarten through twelfth grade? How might the use of the primary data methods discussed in this chapter differ at the sites? What would be the pros and cons of the methods at the sites?

3. A manufacturing company is planning a program to promote physical activity among 1,000 employees at one of its sites. The company's directors have expressed interest in a particular physical activity program that is based on the stages of change model. How might this fact influence the needs assessment?

4. The first step toward eliminating health disparities is a culturally appropriate needs assessment. If you were assigned the task of preparing a needs assessment of incoming college freshmen at the University of Texas at El Paso, what steps would you take to implement and ensure a culturally appropriate needs assessment?

5. What important information is added to a needs assessment by conducting a capacity assessment at a work site? Can you identify any resources that might help in completing the work site capacity assessment?

6. You are working on a student health needs assessment for a school district. Your job is to conduct a survey by administering a health needs questionnaire to 1,500 students in grades 9–12. The school directors and the superintendent want you to identify how much it will cost. What are the costs?

7. Dissemination options for a needs assessment report include printing the entire report, preparing special reports or brochures for particular groups of individuals and stakeholders (such as funders or program participants), posting the report on the Web, and informing people about the report through e-mail, public meetings, board and staff meetings, newspaper reports, radio and television interviews by advisory board members and staff, press releases, and news conferences. Which options do you think would work best, and why, at the different sites: schools, workplaces, health care organizations, and communities?

## KEY TERMS

| | | |
|---|---|---|
| Bias | Key informant interviews | Random selection |
| Capacity assessment | Need | Reliability |
| Climate | Needs assessment | Response bias |
| Content validity | Needs assessment report | Sample |
| Consensus building | PEARL model | Sampling bias |
| Delphi technique | Power analysis | School Health Index |
| Face validity | Primary data | Secondary data |
| Focus group | Priorities | Survey questionnaires |
| Geographic information system (GIS) | Qualitative data | Validity |
| | Quantitative data | |

# REFERENCES

Blumberg, S. J., Luke, J. V., & Cynamon, M. A. (2006). Telephone coverage and health survey estimates: Evaluating the need for concern about wireless substitution. *American Journal of Public Health, 96,* 926–931.

Carter, M., & Landau, R. (2009). Employers face challenges with new mental health parity act. *Compensation Benefits Review, 41,* 39–51.

Centers for Disease Control and Prevention. (1995). *Planned approach to community health: Guide for the local coordinator.* Atlanta, GA: U.S. Department of Health and Human Services, Centers for Disease Control and Prevention, National Center for Chronic Disease Prevention and Health Promotion.

DeVon, H. A., Block, M. E., Moyle-Wright, P., Ernst, D. M., Hayden, S. J., Lazzara, D. J., et al. (2007). A psychometric toolbox for testing validity and reliability. *Journal of Nursing Scholarship, 39,* 155–164.

Dillman, D. A. (2007). *Mail and internet surveys: The tailored design method.* Hoboken, NJ: Wiley.

Fowler, F. J. (2002). *Survey research methods.* Thousand Oaks, CA: Sage.

Gilmore, G., & Campbell, M. (2005). *Needs and capacity assessment strategies for health education and health promotion.* Sudbury, MA: Jones & Bartlett.

Glanz, K., & Rimer, B. K. (2005). *Theory at a glance: A guide for health promotion practice.* Retrieved April 16, 2008, from http://www.cancer.gov/PDF/481f5d53-63df-41bc-bfaf-5aa48ee1da4d/TAAG3 .pdf.

Henderson, N. R. (1995). A practical approach to analyzing and reporting focus group studies: Lessons from qualitative market research. *Qualitative Health Research, 5,* 436–477.

King, K. A., Pealer, L. N., & Bernard, A. L. (2001). Increasing response rates to mail questionnaires: A review of inducement strategies. *American Journal of Health Education, 32,* 4–15.

Krueger, R., & Casey, M. (2000). *Focus groups: A practical guide for applied research* (3rd ed.). Thousand Oaks, CA: Sage.

McLeroy, K. R., Bibeau, D., Steckler, A., & Glanz, K. (1988). An ecological perspective on health promotion programs. *Health Education & Behavior, 15*(4), 351–377.

Metzler, M., Kanarek, N., Highsmith, K., Bialek, R., Straw, R., Auston, I., et al. (2008). *Community health status indicators project: The development of a national approach to community health.* Retrieved September 8, 2008, from http://.cdc.gov/pcd/issues/2008/jul/07_0225.htm.

Moos, R. H. (1979). *Evaluating educational environments: Procedures, measures, findings, and policy implications.* San Francisco: Jossey-Bass.

National Center for Chronic Disease Prevention and Health Promotion. (2008). *School Health Index.* Atlanta, GA: Author. Retrieved October 20, 2009, from http://www.cdc.gov/HealthyYouth/ SHI/introduction.htm.

Price, J. H., Dake, J. A., Murnan, J., Dimmig, J., & Akpanudo, S. (2005). Power analysis in survey research: Importance and use for health educators. *American Journal of Health Education, 36,* 202–207.

Senge, P. (1990). *The fifth discipline: The art and practice of the learning organization.* New York: Doubleday/Currency.

U.S. Department of Health and Human Services. (1999). *Mental health: A report of the surgeon general*. Rockville, MD: U.S. Department of Health and Human Services, Substance Abuse and Mental Health Services Administration, Center for Mental Health Services & National Institutes of Health, National Institute of Mental Health.

Vilnius, D., & Dandoy, S. (1990). A priority rating system for public health programs. *Public Health Reports, 105*(5), 463–470.

Witkin, B. R., & Altschuld, J. W. (1995). *Planning and conducting needs assessments: A practical guide*. Thousand Oaks, CA: Sage.

# CHAPTER FIVE

# MAKING DECISIONS TO CREATE AND SUPPORT A PROGRAM

W. WILLIAM CHEN

JIUNN-JYE SHEU

HUEY-SHYS CHEN

## LEARNING OBJECTIVES

- Define *mission, goals,* and *objectives;* explain how they interact during program design and development

- Write measurable process, action, and outcome objectives

- Explain the link between measurable objectives and evidence-based practice approaches

- Identify health promotion interventions designed to change knowledge, attitudes, and behavior

- Create, write, and revise policies to support program implementation

- Be able to make the transition to program implementation

ONCE THE NEEDS ASSESSMENT for a health promotion program is complete, the focus shifts to developing a clear vision of what the program will try to accomplish—that is, a mission for the program. Decisions will be made about what strategies and interventions to use in order to achieve the identified goals, as well as about ways to address health disparities and which health theories or models to use as the program's foundation. Work will focus on developing criteria for selection of the health promotion interventions, searching for interventions that have already been conceived or tried (including evidence-based ones), and making decisions about whether to create, purchase, or adopt interventions. Furthermore, decisions will need to be made about the scope of the interventions and the support needed to execute those interventions. Some of the decisions about the support that is needed to create and implement a program will involve tending to policies and procedures at the site where the program is to be implemented. Effective policies provide infrastructure for the program; good policy decisions result in effective programs. With all of these decisions in place, the program's staff, stakeholders, and participants will be able to describe the program's mission as well as the program's goals, objectives, and interventions. The program supports (policies and procedures) will be in place and will be known. All stakeholders will have a shared understanding of the interventions and expected outcomes.

## IDENTIFYING A MISSION STATEMENT, GOALS, AND OBJECTIVES

A *mission statement* is usually a short statement that describes the general focus or purpose of a program (McKenzie, Neiger, & Thackeray, 2009). The mission statement answers the question of why a health promotion program is being developed and established. As such, a mission statement reflects the program's overall purpose and values. A mission statement is sometimes referred to as the *philosophy* of a health promotion program.

The following are samples of mission statements:

- The Employee Wellness Program was developed to increase productivity by encouraging employees to practice a healthy lifestyle.
- The mission of the American Lung Association is to prevent lung disease and promote lung health.
- The mission of the Brookfield Unified School District's Coordinated School Health Program is to prepare students to become healthy and productive individuals.

- Communities in Action for Peace's mission is to promote healthy communities by modeling peace and justice in action, as we strive to end violence and its causes in a nontraditional and culturally sensitive manner.

A *goal* sets a program's direction and intent (Gilbert & Sawyer, 2000). Goals clarify what is important in the health promotion program and state the end results of the program. A goal includes the program's target population and, in general, uses action words such as *reduce, eliminate,* or *increase.* Some examples of program goals are listed here:

- A goal of the Employee Walking Program is to increase regular exercise among staff and their family members.
- A goal of the American Lung Association's Freedom From Smoking program is to decrease the number of smokers by helping people who already smoke to stop smoking.
- A goal of Brookfield Unified School District's Coordinated School Health Program is to increase the numbers of students K to 12 who adopt healthy nutrition behaviors.

Program *objectives* are the specific steps (or subgoals) that need to be achieved in order to attain the goal. They are specific and measurable targets with a timeline that identifies by when the objective will be attained. An objective statement specifies who, what, when, and where and clarifies by how much, how many, or how often (U.S. Department of Health and Human Services, 1997). Each objective makes clear what is expected and is stated in such a way that the achievement can be measured. While achievement of objectives may not always be measured, the objectives must be measurable. If measurement is not possible, the objective is probably not clearly stated. Measurability is the major difference between goals and objectives. Goals provide an overview of the desired outcomes at the end of the program, while objectives provide specific and clear steps (tasks) that need to be achieved in order to attain the goal (or goals) of the program. Each goal may have several tasks (objectives) that need to be completed in order to achieve it. Different types of objective statements are used, depending on the needs of the program.

*Process* (or *administrative*) *objectives* are used to identify the needed changes or tasks in the administration of the program itself (for example, hiring staff, providing professional development for staff, seeking additional funding). These types of objectives are used to evaluate progress in the implementation of the program (process or formative evaluation). Here are some examples of process (administrative) objectives:

- By month 3 of the initiative, two qualified instructors will have been hired and received orientation in effectively delivering the curriculum of the initiative.
- By the end of the year, smoking cessation programs for college students will have been initiated in fifteen of the thirty-three institutions of higher education in the state.

*Action* (or *behavioral*) *objectives* are used to identify needed changes in the actions or behaviors of the target population. This type of objective is appropriate for impact evaluation or summative evaluation. Action (behavioral) objectives are similar to these examples:

- The percentage of binge drinkers among college students will decrease from 60 percent to less than 50 percent after completion of the health promotion program at the end of the year.
- By the end of the program, 50 percent of the participants will increase their exercise activities to at least thirty minutes a day, three times a week.

*Outcome objectives* are used to identify the long-term accomplishments of a health promotion program. Following are some examples of outcome objectives:

- The number of alcohol-related driving deaths and injuries will decrease by 25 percent within the city during the next two years.
- New cases of HIV among Hispanic women ages 18 to 25 will be reduced by 25 percent by the year 2015.

## WRITING PROGRAM OBJECTIVES

Writing a good objective takes skill and judgment. As we have discussed, objectives are the steps or tasks needed to achieve a goal. The objectives connect goals to the interventions that will facilitate achievement of the goals. When you begin to draft objectives, you ask questions like these:

- What does the target population need to know or do in order to achieve this goal?
- What changes in knowledge, attitudes, or skills need to occur?
- What social support is needed to facilitate behavioral changes?
- What policy or environmental changes are needed to achieve the goal?
- Specifically, who is expected to change, by how much, and by when?

Reviewing data from the needs assessment will help in establishing target numbers. Being very clear by specifying numbers and percentages facilitates monitoring progress.

When writing objectives, make sure that the objectives (1) are measurable, relevant, and achievable; (2) drive action and suggest a set of steps that will help to achieve the goals within a specific time frame; (3) include a range of measures directed toward achieving program goals; (4) are established at the outset of the program in order to make evaluation possible; (5) support short-term as well as long-term plans; and (6) are based on sound scientific evidence (U.S. Department of Health and Human Services, 1997).

One approach to writing program objectives uses the mnemonic SMART, which indicates objectives that are specific, measurable, achievable, realistic, and time-bound. SMART objectives allow you to proceed with your program, knowing that you have a strong foundation on which implementation and evaluation plans can be developed. The SMART mnemonic is described in more detail in the following sections.

## Specific

When you write an objective, clearly state exactly what you plan to achieve by providing the appropriate type and amount of detail. The details can be summarized with the following "four W's" rule:

- Who or what is expected to change or happen?
- What or how much change is expected? (amount or degree of change)
- Where will the change occur?
- When will the change occur? (often indicated by a date)

For example, an objective of a program to prevent obesity among youth might say, "By May 30, 2015, 80 percent of the students in grades 6–8 in the Riverside County Schools will engage in sixty minutes of moderate to vigorous physical activity each day as determined by an annual youth behavior risk survey (Baseline: 30 percent of students in 2010)."

- Who or what is expected to change or happen? Students will increase daily physical activity to sixty minutes.
- What or how much change is expected? Change from 30 percent to 80 percent of students.
- Where will the change occur? Riverside County Schools.
- When will the change occur? By May 30, 2015. (The change will occur over time, beginning in 2010.)

Some objectives do not have a quantifiable outcome and will not involve many numbers. However, this type of objective is still required to be specific, and the four W's rule still applies. Here is an example of this type of objective: "By June 30, 2015, Allegheny County commissioners will adopt and disseminate a policy to prohibit smoking in all restaurants and public eating establishments."

- What is expected to change or happen? Policy to prohibit smoking.
- What or how much change is expected? Policy to prohibit smoking in all restaurants and public eating establishments.
- Where will the change occur? Allegheny County.
- When will the change occur? By June 30, 2015.

## Measurable (or Observable)

In the first example in the preceding section, the measurable outcome is whether the students have increased their physical activity to sixty minutes per day. To measure the change that has occurred, you would compare the percentage of students engaging in sixty minutes of daily physical activity as shown in the youth risk behavior survey that the school administers in 2015 to the percentage that were exercising in 2010 (30 percent).

In the second example, the achievement of the objective is a one-time event—the adoption of the policy—that does not involve measuring a quantity. However, one can observe whether the policy has been adopted or not and whether the policy has been disseminated or not. The observable outcome is whether the policy has been adopted. To verify that the policy has indeed been adopted, you could obtain official documents. Verification of dissemination could occur after the policy has been enacted and publicized as part of the public health department's periodic sanitary inspection of all restaurants.

## Achievable (Reachable)

For objectives that have a quantifiable outcome, a baseline measure will assist in estimating the level of success that one might expect to achieve. Decide whether your objective is reachable by considering baseline measurements as well as by using your knowledge and experience in this area. For example, if at the start of the program, 30 percent of students engage in sixty minutes of physical activity per day, it may be too ambitious to aim to increase the number of students who exercise an hour daily to 80 percent by 2015. An increase to 45 percent might be more achievable. In practice, your estimation would depend on the strategies that you were planning to implement as part of the health promotion program. In the first example in the preceding section, if the intervention strategies focused only on instruction about the value of exercise, one would choose a smaller number. But if the intervention included a program in which all K–6 teachers provided exercise breaks for students at their desk for five to ten minutes several times a day, the number of students who achieved the goal would increase more than if the intervention were just instruction.

In the second example the objective is a step toward a smoke-free environment. However, achieving a smoke-free environment represents a large goal that will take time. The objective to adopt and disseminate a policy to prohibit smoking in all restaurants and public eating establishments is one of the items that need to be accomplished. Objectives related to public education about the new policy and enforcement might be subsequent steps (objectives) once this objective is achieved.

### Realistic, Meaningful, and Important

Objectives need to address concerns that are absolute priorities. Programs are expensive in terms of money and people's time and energy. Often, there is a limited window of opportunity in which to address a concern. A limited budget may force you to trim the scope of a program's activities. A program's objectives will determine its interventions and its advocacy agenda. For these reasons, from the beginning, you need to ask whether an objective is realistic and whether it is the most important and meaningful way to address a health concern.

### Time-Bound

Effective objectives are time-bound. By what date do you want the outcome to be achieved? A time frame is important to establish because the type and intensity of your interventions, activities, and evaluation will depend on how much time you think it will take to achieve your goal.

## DECIDING ON PROGRAM INTERVENTIONS

Once the goals and objectives of a program have been written, the health promotion program staff, stakeholders, and participants need to identify the interventions or strategies that will facilitate attainment of each objective and all goals. The most effective interventions are culturally appropriate and based on health theories and models. An intervention is any set of methods, techniques, or processes designed to effect changes in behaviors or the environment. Identifying the interventions explains how you intend to achieve the objectives.

In planning program interventions, first consider the range of interventions available to be used in health promotion programs—for example,

- Instruction: teacher-based lessons (for example, lecture, discussion, group work) and individual-based instruction (for example, computer-assisted learning or written or audiovisual materials)
- Counseling: individual or group sessions, behavioral modification, behavioral contracting
- Regulatory strategies: policy mandates, legislation, ordinances, rules, regulations
- Environmental change: changes in the physical, social, or economic environment that provide incentives or disincentives for behavior change
- Social support: support buddy, support group, social networks
- Direct interventions: screening, referral, treatment, and follow-up to stimulate needed changes
- Communication or media outreach: mass media, including radio, TV, newspapers; personal media, including text messages; printed media, including pamphlets, billboards, posters, direct mail, church bulletins
- Advocacy: organizing at the site, coalition building, community development, social action

In planning which interventions a health promotion program will use, it is important to match the intervention to the specific needs of the target population as well as choose interventions that represent a broad range of approaches in order to affect the target population in different ways, depending on whether individuals need knowledge, practice in specific skills, change of attitudes, change in behaviors, support by significant others, or broad environmental change. For example, drug abuse prevention programs for school-age adolescents can achieve significant reductions in the rates of social, behavioral, and academic problems when interventions are designed for youths who are at risk for beginning to experiment with drug use. However, this instructional program designed to prevent alcohol and drug use in adolescents would not be effective for adolescents who already have an addiction problem; the interventions that they would need would be quite different.

The Institute of Medicine (1994) identified preventive interventions for different target populations and different health problems and concerns. The model uses the range of identifiable risk to categorize preventive interventions. The three levels are:

- **Universal preventive interventions**: The target population is the general public or a population that has not been identified on the basis of individual risk. In other words, these interventions are designed for everyone. Universal preventive interventions are found to have mild to strong influences on different health concerns among different populations. Examples of this type of intervention include mass media campaigns via public service announcements on TV and social skills instruction provided to all K–12 students.

- **Selective preventive interventions**: The target population is individuals or a subgroup of the population whose risk of developing illness or disorders is significantly higher than average. Examples include an education program to encourage construction workers to wear earplugs or protective devices when operating noisy machinery and grief counseling sessions provided to students who are experiencing a traumatic loss.

- **Indicated preventive interventions**: The target population is high-risk individuals who have detectable signs or symptoms but have not reached the diagnostic criteria of a particular health problem. Indicated preventive interventions are found to have medium effects on health issues. An example would be a smoking cessation program for heavy smokers.

Weisz, Sandler, Durlak, & Anton (2005) expanded the Institute of Medicine's model of preventive intervention to five levels of strategies; health promotion and positive development strategies and treatment strategies are added to the components of the Institute of Medicine's model.

- **Health promotion and positive development strategies** target an entire population with the goal of enhancing strengths in order to reduce the risk of later problem outcomes or to increase prospects for positive development. Examples include programs that focus on building personal and social skills through teacher, parent, and youth training and development of individualized action plans to improve fitness levels after receiving the results of a fitness screening test.

- **Universal preventive strategies** are approaches designed to address risk factors in an entire population without attempting to distinguish who is at elevated risk. Examples include programs that address risk factors in broadly defined population groups (for instance, a program in which all children in a particular grade or age range receive anti-bullying instruction and improved recess supervision in which teachers intervene with guided discovery when there is bullying on the playground).

- **Selective preventive strategies** are approaches in which specific groups are targeted because they share a significant risk factor and interventions are designed to reduce that risk. An example of a selective preventive strategy is providing visits by a public health nurse to a young, unmarried, and economically disadvantaged pregnant woman to promote behaviors during and after pregnancy that will be healthy for both the woman and her child.

- **Indicated preventive strategies** are approaches aimed at individuals who have significant symptoms of a disorder but do not meet diagnostic criteria. An example of an indicated preventive strategy is a home-based and school-based intervention that focuses on disruptive boys in kindergarten.
- **Treatment interventions** are approaches that target those who have high symptom levels or a diagnosable illness or disorder. These interventions apply to those individuals' diagnosed illnesses and disorders. The interventions (treatment) usually take place in clinical settings.

Table 5.1 presents different types of interventions along with corresponding methods, techniques, or processes designed to effect changes in behaviors

**TABLE 5.1   Typology of Health Promotion Interventions**

| Level | Strategies |
|---|---|
| Health promotion interventions for individuals | Focus on information, modeling, education, and training in order to promote change in knowledge, attitudes, beliefs, and behavior in regard to health risks such as smoking, eating, and physical activity |
| Policy and practices of organizations | Focus on organizational change and consultancy in order to change organizational policies (rules, roles, sanctions, and incentives) and practices in order to produce changes in individuals' risky behavior and greater access to social, educational, and health resources that promote health |
| Environmental actions and social change at sites | Focus on social action and social planning at existing sites and on creating new sites (for example, organizations, networks, or partnerships) in order to produce change in organizations and redistribute resources that affect health |
| Public advocacy | Focus on social advocacy in order to change legislative, budgetary, and institutional settings that affect community, organizational, and individual levels |

*Source:* Adapted from Swerissen & Crisp, 2004.

or the environment. The four types of interventions focus on health promotion interventions for individuals, policy of organizations, environmental actions and social change at sites and beyond, and public advocacy. While the types are nested within one another, they involve different processes (Swerissen & Crisp, 2004).

Health promotion interventions are often created (designed) for a target population. Interventions that have already been developed can also be selected (or sometimes purchased) and used. Program staff can now select from an increasing number of evidence-based health promotion interventions that have been researched and reviewed for their effectiveness; we will discuss evidence-based interventions later in this chapter.

Regardless of whether an intervention is created, purchased, or selected from existing interventions, connecting the intervention to one or more of the health theories or models in Chapter Three (Table 3.10) provides the groundwork for the intervention and the program. Interventions based on health theories provide assurance to program participants that program staff were thoughtful and professional in their decisions about a particular intervention. When program staff are questioned about an intervention, knowing the health theories helps staff members communicate how and why activities are designed as well as communicate the expected outcomes. The theories provide guidance in translating insights gained from the needs assessment into actions that improve health. To make appropriate use of theory in a given situation, practitioners must consider both the social and health problems at hand and the context in which the health promotion intervention will take place.

## SELECTING HEALTH PROMOTION MATERIALS

Many health promotion intervention materials have been developed by government or commercial developers. Existing materials can be obtained from the catalogues published by government agencies or companies, but they should be reviewed before use. Even if the materials are considered acceptable, they still need to be pilot-tested by a sample group of the target population. The following questions in regard to the program objectives, theoretical foundation, interventions, and strategies should be examined:

- Do the program materials enable the objectives to be met?
- Do they deliver the intended theoretical methods and practical strategies?
- Do the materials fit with the target population?
- Are the materials attractive, appealing, and culturally appropriate?

- Are the messages delivered by the materials consistent with the program objectives?
- Will the materials be properly used in the planned intervention?

After the materials are determined to be appropriate, the following criteria should be considered:

- **Availability**. The availability of the material, in terms of quantity and time frame, should be considered in the planning stage. Reproduction may be possible if permission is granted. Companies that produce intervention materials may charge for them on the basis of quantity or frequency of use. Many materials are placed on the Web in formats such as Web pages, PDF documents, PowerPoint presentations, Word documents, videos, audio files, or graphics files. If modification is needed, permission should be obtained from the developer in advance and proper acknowledgment should be included in the materials.
- **Reading level**. The reading level of a piece of writing indicates how easy it is to read by assigning it a school grade level. The reading level often determines whether the intervention material is acceptable for the intended participants. Low reading literacy in the American general population has become a challenge in developing health promotion materials. Using graphics and short sentences helps to make materials accessible to populations with low levels of literacy.
- **Production quality and suitability**. To address the overall suitability of materials (including reading level), Doak, Doak, and Root (1996) developed the Suitability Assessment of Materials (SAM). Although the SAM was developed for use with print materials, it has also been used to assess videotaped and audio instructions. The SAM scores materials in six categories: content, literacy demand, graphics, layout and typography, learning stimulation, and cultural appropriateness. The SAM yields a final percentage score, which falls into one of three categories: superior, adequate, or not suitable. The SAM can be used to identify specific shortcomings that reduce the suitability of materials either in the developmental stage or in final form. (A full description of the SAM and a scoring sheet are available in Doak, Doak, & Root, 1996.)

## USING EVIDENCE-BASED INTERVENTIONS

Evidence-based health promotion interventions can be conceptualized as the delivery of optimal care through integration of current best scientific evidence, clinical expertise and experience, and preferences of individuals, families, organizations, and communities. They provide to practitioners interventions that are critically appraised and that incorporate scientific evidence into clinical practice. Evidence-based health promotion interventions identify the target populations that would benefit from the intervention and the conditions under which the intervention works and may indicate the change mechanisms that account for intervention effects. The interventions include various tested strategies that target different diseases or behaviors. A defining characteristic of evidence-based interventions is their use of health theory (Table 3.10) in both developing the intervention content (activities, curriculum, tasks) and evaluation (measures, outcomes).

Numerous health promotion interventions have been initiated and evaluated and found to be effective. Examples can be found in the published literature by using the free PubMed database (http://www.pubmed.gov) created by the National Library of Medicine and the National Institutes of Health. Use key words related to the health behavior that is of interest to you.

Two key sources of evidence-based health promotion interventions have been developed by the federal government. The first is the National Registry of Evidence-Based Programs and Practices (NREPP), which was developed and is maintained by the Substance Abuse and Mental Health Services Administration (SAMHSA) in the U.S. Department of Health and Human Services. NREPP (http://www.nrepp.samhsa.gov) is a searchable database of interventions for the prevention and treatment of mental and substance use disorders (Figure 5.1). NREPP uses a voluntary, self-nominating system in which intervention developers elect to participate. There will always be some interventions that are not submitted to NREPP, and not all that are submitted are reviewed. Nevertheless, new intervention summaries are continually being added to the site. The registry is expected to grow to a large number of interventions over time.

The second federal source of evidence-based health promotion interventions, Research-Tested Intervention Programs (RTIPs), was developed and is maintained by the National Cancer Institute. RTIPs (http://rtips.cancer.gov/rtips/index.do) is linked to the Guide to Community Preventive Services (http://www.thecom munityguide.org/index.html), a resource from the Centers for Disease Control and Prevention that evaluates the effectiveness of broad intervention categories through systematic research reviews. RTIPs is a database of actual programs and products that individuals, groups, and organizations can access and use (Figure 5.2).

## Identifying Appropriate Evidence-Based Interventions

Using sites like NREPP or RTIPs, you may have choices about interventions that you can use in your program. To identify evidence-based interventions that are appropriate for your health promotion program, consider the following:

- **Contexts for intervention**. The array of settings in which the intervention might be based should be considered when deciding which evidence-based interventions would be most appropriate to address specific goals. Settings to

FIGURE 5.1   Search Page on the Web Site of the National
Registry of Evidence-Based Programs and Practices

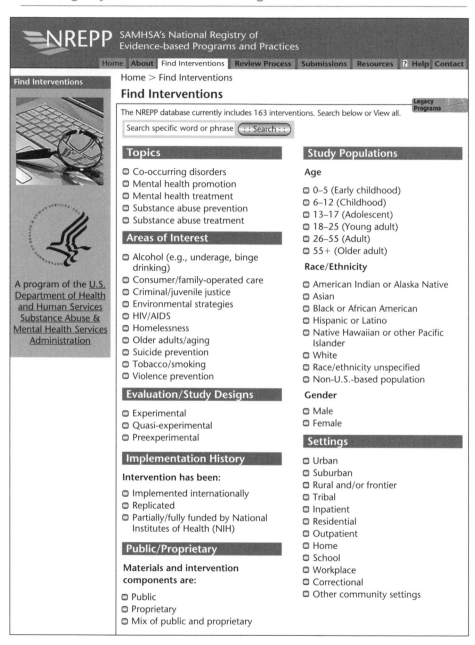

**FIGURE 5.2  Home Page of the Research-Tested Intervention Programs (RTIPs) Web Site**

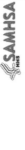

**Research-tested Intervention Programs** (RTIPs)

**SAMHSA** HHS

RTIPs: Moving Science into Programs for People

■ RTIPs Home  ■ Frequently Asked Questions  ■ RTIPs Home  ■ Frequently Asked Questions  ■ Fact Sheet  ■ Contact Us

🌎 Cancer Control PLA-N.E.T. Home

**Use this Web site to:**

- Find research-tested intervention programs and products.
- Review summary information and usefulness/integrity scores for each program.
- Order or download materials to adapt for use in your own program.
- Obtain readability scores for products distributed to the public.

**Program topics now available:**

- Breast cancer screening promotion
  - Community-based interventions
  - Physician-based curriculums
- Cervical cancer screening promotion
  - Community outreach programs
  - Direct mail interventions
- Colorectal cancer screening promotion
  - Physician-based intervention programs
- Diet/Nutrition
  - Community-based social support interventions
  - Small group education interventions
  - Fruit and vegetable behavior change programs
- Informed Decision Making
  - Patient decision-making programs
- Physical activity
  - Physical health enhancement programs
- Sun safety
  - Sun protection awareness programs
- Survivorship
- Tobacco control
  - Smoking prevention programs
  - Smoking cessation programs
  - Smoke-free environmental campaigns

**RTIPs and Research Reviews**

The Guide to Community Preventive Services evaluates the effectiveness of types of interventions (as opposed to individual programs) by conducting systematic reviews of all available research in collaboration with partners. The Task Force on Community Preventive Services then uses the systematic review findings as the basis for their recommendations for practice, policy and future research. The symbol below links to applicable Community Guide findings:

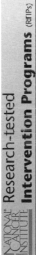

**New programs featured:**

- Sun Safety
  - ★ - Sun Safety Among US Postal Service Carriers ("Project SUNWISE") (Post date: October 2009)
    - Go Sun Smart (CSS) Post date: August 2009)
- Tobacco
  - Family Matters (Post date: September 2009)

★ New programs are released periodically. Please check for updates.

**New Adaptation Tool Available:**

- Using What Works: a train-the-trainer course that teaches users how to adapt a research-tested intervention program to the local community context

Register your program now and be part of the RTIPs Community.

We welcome your feedback on the Research-tested Intervention Programs Web site. To submit feedback or a program for review, please contact us. Thank you for helping to improve this site for the cancer control community.

Using What Works

consider include homes, schools, churches, primary care clinics, residential facilities, community centers, boys and girls clubs, after-school programs, teen social centers, sports team facilities, volunteer centers, and summer job settings. Preventive interventions can be sited in the places where the target population lives or at the sites of other activities.

- **Coverage across the range of populations or settings involved in a health concern**. Many of the most prevalent and significant risks and issues pertaining to specific health problems can now be identified through published empirical data, but significant gaps in coverage still remain, both in terms of information and appropriate interventions. For example, although anorexia interventions may have demonstrated effectiveness among the fifteen-to-twenty-four-year-old females who have the highest prevalence, the settings and program designs may not apply well to pre-adolescents. You should search extensively and find the most appropriate design for your target audience.

- **Knowledge of what populations interventions will be effective for—and under what conditions**. For each intervention that works, you need to know as much as possible about the population within which benefits accrue. You need to know in what settings an intervention works. Even the best-supported interventions are apt to be beneficial for some groups (defined by age, gender, socioeconomic status, or other demographic characteristics) but not for others and in some settings but not in others. Understanding factors (in terms of population groups and conditions) that moderate intervention effects is essential to understanding how and to whom to apply various health promotion interventions.

- **Role of race, ethnicity, and culture**. Factors of race, ethnicity, and culture—for example, norms, beliefs, and values derived from their respective cultures—influence the target population and program site. An effective intervention must be compatible with relevant norms, beliefs, and values or must incorporate the ability to understand, respect, and work with differences. Responses to health promotion interventions may differ on the basis of participants' ethnicity or culture.

- **Staff creativity, experience, and clinical expertise**. Evidence-based interventions have explicit protocols described in intervention manuals that may provide essential principles and guidelines but still allow considerable flexibility and use of staff's creativity, experience, and clinical expertise in the effort to achieve desired intervention outcomes. Specific elements of these interventions, combined in ways that fit the distinctive characteristics of the individuals targeted for intervention, may produce genuine benefits. For example, an element such as a role-playing activity to strengthen self-efficacy in refusing a cigarette could be modified and used in another intervention program to model how to ask friends to wear seat belts when one is driving.

## Balancing Fidelity and Adaptation

Evidence-based interventions usually have prescribed protocols to direct the implementation or use of the intervention, including a detailed set of instructions, materials, and staffing requirements. Furthermore, there is a prescribed implementation process as well as staff training and development. Developers of evidence-based health promotion interventions try to facilitate maximum fidelity to the essentials of intervention while still allowing maximal adaptation for the specific needs of a setting. Fidelity defines the extent to which the delivery of a health intervention conforms to the curriculum, protocol, or guidelines for implementing that intervention. Intervention fidelity is rated from high to low. A high-fidelity intervention would be delivered exactly as intended by the people who created it. A low-fidelity program would be delivered quite differently than intended by the people who created it. Adaptation defines the degree to which an intervention undergoes change in its implementation to fit the needs of a particular delivery situation. The apparent antithesis of fidelity, adaptation could alter program integrity if an intervention is adapted so drastically that it is not delivered as originally intended. However, it is possible for an intervention to be rendered more responsive to a particular target population through the adaptation process. For example, adaptation could increase an intervention's cultural sensitivity and its fit within a new setting.

Researchers have suggested that modifying an intervention is acceptable up to a *zone of drastic mutation*; after that point, further modification will compromise the program's integrity and effectiveness (Hall & Loucks, 1978). In working with evidence-based interventions, it is necessary to have a balance between fidelity and adaptation in order to fine-tune the complex, dynamic interaction between a health promotion intervention and its target population and environment. Schinke, Brounstein, and Gardner (2002) recommend guidelines to help balance fidelity and adaptation:

1. Identify and understand the theory behind an intervention. What are the intervention's theoretical underpinnings? Reading the published literature on the intervention and talking with the individuals who developed the intervention are two strategies for answering this question. Understanding the mission, goals, and objectives of a particular intervention can help program staff to persuade stakeholders of the current health promotion program of an intervention's utility to them in the given environment.

2. Assess fidelity and adaptation concerns for a particular site or setting. Determine what adaptation might be required to meet the needs of the target population and the environment where the intervention is to be implemented.

3. Involve the individuals who developed the intervention. Talk with them about their thinking as they shaped the intervention. Consultations with other groups that have implemented the intervention in similar environments may also be helpful.

4. Talk with the stakeholders at the site where the intervention will be implemented. Discuss your thoughts on the balance of fidelity and adaptation in order to understand concerns, build support, and generate input on how to achieve successful implementation.

5. Employ an analysis of core components. A core component analysis is a listing of an intervention's core ingredients followed by discussion with program staff, participants, and stakeholders about which are essential for success and which are more amenable to modification in order to meet local conditions and needs. Table 5.2 shows a list of core components for an intervention to prevent substance abuse in elementary school and areas to consider for

**TABLE 5.2   Core Component Analysis for an Intervention to Prevent Substance Abuse in an Elementary School**

| Core Component | Description of Areas to Consider for Adaptation |
|---|---|
| Content focus | Intervention focuses on generic life skills and specific skills for avoiding the use of alcohol and tobacco. Consider adding marijuana as a content area. |
| Modeling and behavioral rehearsal | Instructor demonstrates new skills using set scripts; participant then performs the skill within the session. Consider student-produced scripts and use of upper elementary and middle school students as peer leaders in sessions. |
| Homework assignments | Assignments (for example, journaling, practicing a skill at home with a parent or others) reinforce concepts. |
| Cueing | Instructor cues students to use new behavior in a specific situation. Consider having the upper elementary and middle school student peer leaders cue students during school activities (for example, during lunch or before and after school programs). |
| Self-monitoring | Participants log behavior in order to enhance awareness and enactment of desired behavior. Consider using Web postings and discussion boards. |

adaptation. A core component analysis can be a bridge between intervention developers and practitioners.

6. Develop an overall implementation plan based on these inputs. Include a strategy for achieving and measuring the balance between fidelity and adaptation as the intervention is implemented

These guidelines can inform and facilitate an implementation process that maintains fidelity to the concept of the intervention and makes necessary adaptations to facilitate effective delivery.

## DEVELOPING EFFECTIVE POLICIES AND PROCEDURES

Health promotion programs do not operate in a vacuum. They operate within the structure of their setting. Each setting (school, workplace, hospital, community) has its policies— operating rules that specify people's rights and responsibilities as well as spelling out the rights and responsibilities of the organization in regard to its stakeholders (for example, students, employees, clients, or members). Policies are the backbone of health promotion programs. Effective policies clearly state the health values and priorities of the organization and are tailored to the unique requirements and needs of the setting and stakeholders. Drawn from the policies are procedures, which typically address program logistics and day-to-day operating details such as recruitment, retention, and recognition of program participants.

The model smoke-free workplace policy in Exhibit 5.1 was promulgated and promoted by the New York City Health Department for use by businesses and organizations at their sites in order to clearly state that smoke-free workplaces are required by law and, furthermore, that each organization, by personalizing the policy through such action as adding its name and placing the policy on the organization's stationery, agrees with the policy and supports smoke-free workplaces. What makes this a good policy is its clarity, nonjudgmental approach, grievance alternatives, and resources for support and for having questions answered about the policy.

There are many reasons to put health policies in writing:

- It creates a supportive health-promoting environment.
- A written policy may be required by a law or by the organization's insurance carriers.
- It makes legal review possible.
- It provides a record of the organization's efforts and a reference if the policy is challenged. It may protect the employer from certain kinds of claims by stakeholders such as employees, families, or students.

## EXHIBIT 5.1
## Sample Smoke-Free Workplace Policy for New York City

**Purpose**. A smoke-free policy has been developed to comply with the New York City Smoke-Free Air Act (Title 17, Chapter 5 of the Administrative Code of the City of New York) and New York State Clean Indoor Air Act (Article 13-E of the New York State Public Health Law) and to protect all employees and visitors from secondhand smoke, an established cause of cancer and respiratory disease. The policy set forth below is effective March 30, 2003, for all [company name] locations.

**Smoke-Free Areas**. All areas of the workplace are now smoke-free without exception. Smoking is not permitted anywhere in the workplace, including all indoor facilities and company vehicles with more than one person present. Smoking is not permitted in private enclosed offices, conference and meeting rooms, cafeterias, lunchrooms, or employee lounges.

**Sign Requirements**. "No Smoking" signs must be clearly posted at all entrances and on bulletin boards, bathrooms, stairwells, and other prominent places. No ashtrays are permitted in any indoor area.

**Compliance**. Compliance with the smoke-free workplace policy is mandatory for all employees and persons visiting the company, with no exceptions. Employees who violate this policy are subject to disciplinary action. Any disputes involving smoking should be handled through the company's procedure for resolving other work-related problems. If the problem persists, an employee can speak to [company department and phone number for complaints] or lodge an anonymous complaint by calling the New York City Department of Health and Mental Hygiene's complaint line, 1-877-NYC-DOH7 (1-877-692-3647) or on the Web at nyc.gov/health. DOHMH's enforcement staff will take appropriate action to resolve the problem.

The law prohibits employers from retaliating against employees who invoke the law or who request management's assistance in implementing it in the workplace.

**Smoking Cessation Opportunities**. [Company name] encourages all smoking employees to quit smoking. [The company medical department or work site wellness program offers a number of services for employees who want to quit.] Smoking cessation information is available from the New York Smokers' Quit Line at 1-866 NY QUITS (1-866-697-8487).

**Questions**. Any questions regarding the smoke-free workplace policy should be directed to [company department and phone number handling inquiries].

- A written policy is easier to explain to stakeholders.
- Putting the policy in writing helps stakeholders concentrate on important policy information.

## Developing a Health Promotion Policy

The policy development process guides the creation, writing, revision, and adoption of policies. It can also identify outdated policies for archiving health promotion goals and objectives, and it can identify gaps in policy. The process for developing and implementing a health promotion policy is as follows:

1. Generate support from organization leaders and stakeholders.
   - *Leaders*. Provide leaders with a rationale for establishing a policy. Offer them data that emphasize cost-effectiveness and benefits. Ask for representatives to serve on the advisory committee.
   - *Stakeholders*. Provide stakeholders with knowledge about health concerns (for example, passive smoking, cardiovascular disease, cancer, or personal hygiene). Select representatives from different stakeholder groups to serve on the advisory committee that will set policies. Stress individual, family, and community benefits.
2. Organize a cooperative process for policy development.
   - Form an advisory committee to develop the policy. Designate one person as chair. Include representatives from all segments of the setting (for example, school, workplace, health care organization, or community).
   - Review policy options.
   - Disseminate reports on the process, including the results and findings of the needs assessment.
3. Develop policy content.
   - Locate policy samples from other similar organizations or government agencies.
   - Draft the policy that is the best fit for prevention of disease or for health promotion in the specific setting. Incorporate comments from the public and input from stakeholders.
4. Prepare for implementation.
   - Send notification of the policy to those who will be affected well in advance of the date when it takes effect. Notify people individually.
   - Allow time for questions and adjustments during the transition period, and have a contingency plan.
5. Implement the policy.
   - Devise a comprehensive plan, including a process for dealing with grievances.
   - Make enforcement policy operational and consider any unanticipated consequences or problems as learning opportunities to improve the policy and its implementation.

6. Support stakeholders.
   - Support stakeholders—for example, by providing counseling, preventive health care, or social support.
   - Continue to enforce the policy.
7. Evaluate the policy.
   - Periodically review the policy and its effectiveness. Reviewing the policy will provide feedback on how to best implement the policy.

The most important task for every organization is to ensure that its policy meets the needs of its stakeholders and setting. Whether or not laws and regulations apply, the policy should address the key health topics of concern. Organizations can write (or adapt) and organize content on the key topics using whatever language and structure will best communicate the information to their stakeholders. Organizations do not need to start from scratch. They can borrow and adapt information from other organizations and settings. For example, since the Drug-Free Workplace Act was passed, many national, regional, and local programs have been set up to help employers create effective policies. The programs provide free or low-cost information, technical assistance, or model policies that organizations can customize to meet their particular needs. For more information, visit SAMHSA's Workplace Web site and Helpline information at http://workplace.samhsa.gov.

## Basic Elements of an Effective Policy

The effective policy elements presented in this section are examples from workplace policies in city government and small businesses to promote drug-free workplaces. However, the elements can be adapted for schools, health care organizations, and community settings in order to develop health promotion policies across a range of health concerns, problems, and issues.

### Statement of Purpose

*Background*

- How was the policy developed? (For example, was it developed in meetings with union representatives or employees representing different and diverse segments of the workforce, after consultation with other organizations in the same industry, or in collaboration with the organization's legal counsel?)

*Goals*

- What are the drug-free workplace laws and regulations (federal, state, or local) with which the organization must comply?

- What other goals does the organization expect to achieve? (For example, does the organization hope to reduce or eliminate drug-related accidents, illnesses, or absenteeism?)
- Does the organization want to address the issue of preventing and treating workplace drug use and abuse in the context of accomplishing a broader goal of promoting worker health, safety, and productivity?

### *Definitions, Expectations, and Prohibitions*

- How does the organization define substance abuse?
- What employee behaviors are expected?
- Exactly what substances and behaviors are prohibited?
- Who is covered by the policy?
- When will the policy apply? (For example, will it apply during work hours only or during work hours and also during organization-sponsored events after hours?)
- Where will the policy apply? (For example, will it apply in the workplace while workers are on duty, outside the workplace while they are on duty, or in the workplace and in organization-owned vehicles while they are off duty?)
- Who is responsible for carrying out and enforcing the policy?
- Will the policy include any form of testing for alcohol or other drugs?
- Are any employees covered by the terms of a collective bargaining agreement, and if so, how do the terms affect the way the policy will be carried out and enforced for those employees?

## Implementation Approaches

### *Dissemination Strategies*

- How will the organization educate employees about the policy? (For example, the organization could train supervisors, discuss the policy during orientation sessions for new employees, or inform all employees about the policy through a variety of means such as a section in the employee handbook, posters in gathering places at work sites, or information on the organization's intranet system.)

### *Benefits and Assurances*

- How will the organization help employees comply with the policy?
- How will the organization protect employees' confidentiality?
- How will the organization help employees who seek help for drug-related problems?
- How will the organization help employees who are in treatment or recovery?

- How will the organization ensure that all aspects of the policy are implemented fairly and consistently for all employees?

*Consequences and Appeals*

- What are the consequences of violating the policy?
- What are the procedures for determining whether an employee has violated the policy?
- What are the procedures for appealing a determination that an employee has violated the policy?

## Effective Procedures That Support Programs

Program procedures flow from program policies, mission, goal, objectives, and interventions. They support a health promotion program by addressing the health concern within the context of the site and serving as a foundation for the program's day-to-day operation and logistics such as participant recruitment, retention, and recognition. Without clear, concise, culturally appropriate, and sensitive procedures, programs fail. Program procedures are written and shared in a document called *standard operating procedures*. As a program develops and grows so do the standard operating procedures.

In the planning phase of a health promotion program, prepare the procedures for recruitment, retention, and recognition of program participants. It is essential to be clear and consistent about who is eligible to participate (for example, employees, family members, students, faculty); clearances to participate (for example, from insurance, medical personnel, supervisor, parent); precisely what constitutes the program, including all logistics (time, place, costs, length, activities, expected participation levels, attendance); health benefits; health risks; and any incentives. In planning procedures at the participant level, it is important to consider the many reasons why people do and do not participate in programs. The health theories and models discussed in Chapter Three are particularly relevant to understanding program participation. The health belief model, with its emphasis on people's perceived susceptibility to a health problem, perceived severity of the health problem, perceived benefits and barriers to program participation, cues to action and self-efficacy of the target population in participating in the program and changing health-related behavior can all be considered in the procedures for recruiting, retaining, and recognizing people in the program. Likewise, the transtheoretical model stages of change can provide a framework to help identify different groups of individuals (for example, grouping people by behavior-change stage for a particular health concern) within a target population at a setting. Social marketing and the diffusion of innovations model both provide frameworks to guide how procedures are put in place and disseminated.

And attention to producing effective health communications (Chapter Eight) related to the procedures is important.

The procedures shape the climate (Chapter Four) at a setting. They are the public face of the program. One example of effective setting-level procedures is school procedures to create family-friendly schools as a means to engage parents' participation in their children's learning and health. Creating a school climate that is family-friendly eases tension and creates the opportunity for schools and families to partner and collaborate in order to meet the learning and health needs of students. In discussions, parents, teachers, counselors, social workers, and principals have suggested procedures that lend support to efforts to build good school and family relationships to promote learning and health (Fertman, 2004):

- **Be flexible and creative**. Focus on procedures that encourage staff to take time to build relationships with parents and to involve them in meaningful activities and conversations. Providing flexibility in times for meeting with parents and talking on the telephone or having impromptu feedback sessions when parents and family members are available helps to build trust and rapport.

- **Assess and respect the needs of the families**. Develop procedures to encourage ongoing assessment of families' needs. Focus on regular conversations about their needs and goals with the families individually and in small groups.

- **Provide resources for families**. Make families and parents feel welcome in the school. Simple procedures for offering a beverage and snack when family members visit the school are helpful.

- **Establish a family feedback loop**. Establish procedures for asking parents, family members, and students directly about their health concerns and needs. Ask school-based community health providers to assess families' satisfaction with the school health services. Establish a procedure with the school-based community health providers for conducting feedback and brainstorming sessions on how to improve services and eliminate service gaps.

- **Give clear and consistent messages about health**. Establish a procedure for communicating with students, parents, and family members in order to convey the following messages: (1) every child's health is important; (2) many children have health problems; (3) some problems are real and painful and can be severe; (4) health problems can be recognized and treated; and (5) working together, caring families and communities can help.

- **Create a welcoming, culturally competent school**. Establish procedures that focus on staff training, community outreach, culturally diverse staff, community liaisons recruited from the community, and respect for the diversity of the student population.

## TRANSITIONING TO PROGRAM IMPLEMENTATION

Once program staff, stakeholders, and participants have decided on a program's mission, goals, objectives, interventions, outcomes, policies, and procedures, a transition to program implementation occurs. Program implementation is a process, not an event. It happens over time (maybe over a number of years). Implementation will not happen all at once and probably will not proceed smoothly, at least not at first. In the most effective health promotion programs, staff, stakeholders, and participants are aware of how the program changes and develops over time as it is implemented. According to Fixsen, Naoom, Blase, Friedman, and Wallace (2005), program implementation has six stages:

1. **Exploration and adoption** is program planning, including needs assessments and programmatic decisions about mission, goals, objectives, interventions, outcomes, policies, and procedures. Achieving acceptance and support for the program in the setting is part of this stage.

2. **Program installation** focuses on the structural supports necessary to initiate a program. A capacity assessment (discussed in Chapter Four) is the basis of program installation. A capacity assessment includes ensuring the availability of funding streams, human resource strategies, and supportive policy as well as creating referral mechanisms, reporting frameworks, and outcome expectations. Additional resources may be needed to realign current staff, hire and train new staff members, secure appropriate space, or purchase needed technology (for example, cell phones or computers). These activities and their associated start-up costs are necessary first steps in beginning a new program in any setting (for example, a school, workplace, health care organization, or community).

3. **Initial implementation** means operating a program for the first time with the target population in the setting. No amount of planning and discussion can account for all the complexities involved when staff members run a program with the program participants; there are too many unknowns until a program has been operating for some period of time. During initial implementation, the compelling forces of fear of change, inertia, and investment in the status quo combine with the inherently difficult and complex work of implementing something new at a time when the program is struggling to begin and when confidence in the decision to do the program is being tested. Learning from this initial experience and in particular from unanticipated consequences (both good and bad) is important to meeting the target population's needs. Surprises and challenges may change the trajectory of the

program but hopefully will not derail its work to address peoples' health needs. The strength of many programs can be traced to what is learned during the initial implementation about program participants' needs, critical staff skills, program policies and procedures, and the match between the program interventions and participant needs.

4. **Full operation** occurs when a program is operating with full staffing complements and full client loads, and all of the realities of doing business are impinging on the newly implemented program. Once an implemented program is fully operational, referrals are flowing according to the agreed-on inclusion or exclusion criteria, practitioners are carrying out the evidence-based practice or program with proficiency and skill, managers and administrators are supporting and facilitating the new practices, and the setting has adapted to the presence of the program. Over time, the program becomes accepted practice and a new operationalization of "business as usual" takes place in the setting (see, for example, Faggin, 1985). At this stage, the anticipated benefits are realized as the program staff members become skillful and the procedures and processes become routine.

5. **Innovation** happens over time as staff, stakeholders, and participants learn what works with a target population in a particular setting. Changes in staff, feedback from evaluations, and new conditions present opportunities to refine and expand the program. Ensuring cultural competence of the program is an important part of program innovation.

6. **Sustainability** is about long-term program operation. Skilled practitioners and other well-trained staff leave and must be replaced with other skilled practitioners and well-trained staff. Leaders, funding streams, and program requirements change. New social problems arise; partners come and go. External systems change with some frequency; political alliances are only temporary, and champions move on to other causes. And in spite of all these changes, program staff, stakeholders, and participants adjust without losing the functional components of the program or letting the program die from a lack of essential financial and stakeholder support. The goal during this stage is the long-term survival and continued effectiveness of the implementation site in the context of a changing environment.

## SUMMARY

Planning a health promotion program requires that staff, stakeholders, and participants all know what a program seeks to accomplish and how it will go about trying to accomplish it. As part of planning, decisions are made about the program's mission statement, and goals and objectives are set. Questions about using existing interventions, creating new interventions, or adapting and modifying interventions to achieve program goals are all explored. Increasingly, health promotion programs use evidence-based interventions drawn from health theory, paying attention to the balance between fidelity to the core functions of an intervention and adaptation to meet specific needs in a particular setting, in order to maximize a program's success in achieving its goals and objectives. Cultural sensitivity and appropriateness of the interventions are critical considerations at this point in the planning process if the program is to eliminate health disparities among the target population.

Another part of planning for a successful program is reviewing, creating, or refining policies in order to clearly state the health values and priorities of the organization or community in ways that are tailored to the unique requirements and needs of the setting, staff, stakeholders, and participants. Procedures support a program by addressing the health concerns within the context of the site as well as by serving as a foundation for the program's day-to-day operation and logistics.

With all of the decisions about mission, goals, objectives, interventions, policies, and procedures made, the staff can move forward with implementing the program.

## FOR PRACTICE AND DISCUSSION

1. Review the health theories in Chapter Three (Table 3.10). Select a theory and discuss its potential impact on decisions about program goals, objectives, and interventions. How might it affect what policies and procedures are emphasized in the planning process? Compare and contrast the theories. How do they help you to understand the decision-making process in planning a health promotion program?

2. Identify the main differences between mission statement, goals, and objectives in planning a health promotion program. How are these statements related to each other?

3. Have you heard of the SMART approach to writing program objectives? What does SMART stand for? Write a clear objective statement using the SMART approach, including the four W's rule.

4. In your opinion, what are the key factors in selecting different types of interventions to achieve program objectives? What are the differences between universal preventive interventions, selective preventive interventions, and indicated preventive interventions?

5. Explain the critical components in designing a health promotion intervention for HIV/AIDS prevention among college students. What theory, method, and materials would you select? What Web site might provide evidence-based programs? If the materials are from the Internet, how would you determine their appropriateness?

6. What would be the process for developing policies for a drug-free campus? Who would be the leaders, stakeholders, and enforcer? Where can you find sample policies? What elements do you need to consider in developing the policy?

7. You have been hired by a business to plan, implement, and evaluate a program to promote physical activity among its 450 employees in Reading, Pennsylvania. Fully one-third of the employees are Latino, and one-quarter of the employees are African American. The plan is to offer various physical activities (for example, walking, aerobics, biking, and yoga) to employees at varied times and locations. Using the transtheoretical model stages of change and the health belief model, develop a set of questions to explain and help people understand potential issues pertaining to employees' participation, and propose questions to assess employees' health beliefs. Explain how the employees' responses can be used to recruit participants for the program.

## KEY TERMS

Action objectives

Adaptation

Evidence-based
  interventions

Fidelity

Goal

Health promotion policies

Implementation stages

Indicated preventive
  interventions

Intervention

Institute of Medicine's
  model of preventive
  intervention

Mission

National Registry of
  Evidence-Based Programs
  and Practices (NREPP)

Objectives

Outcome objectives

Policies

Process objectives

Program procedures

Research-Tested Inter-
  vention Programs (RTIPs)

Selective preventive
  interventions

SMART

Standard operating
  procedures

Universal preventive
  interventions

Zone of drastic mutation

# REFERENCES

Doak, C. C., Doak, L. G., & Root, J. H. (1996). *Teaching patients with low literacy skills* (2nd ed.). Philadelphia: Lippincott.

Faggin, F. (1985). The challenge of bringing new ideas to market. *High Technology, 2,* 35–39.

Fertman, C. (2004). Schools and families of students with an emotional disturbance: Allies and partners. In D. Hiatt-Michael (Ed.), *Promising practices to connect schools and families of children with special needs.* Greenwich, CT: Information Age.

Fixsen, D. L., Naoom, S. F., Blase, K. A., Friedman, R. M., & Wallace, F. (2005). *Implementation research: A synthesis of the literature* (FMHI Publication No. 231). Tampa: University of South Florida, Louis de la Parte Florida Mental Health Institute, National Implementation Research Network.

Gilbert, G. G., & Sawyer, R. G. (2000). *Health education: Creating strategies for school and community health* (2nd ed.). Sudbury, MA: Jones & Bartlett.

Hall, G. E., & Loucks, S. F. (1978). Teacher concerns as a basis for facilitating staff development. *Teachers College Record, 80*(l), 36–53.

Institute of Medicine. (1994). *Reducing risks for mental disorders: Frontiers for preventive intervention research.* Washington, DC: National Academies Press.

McKenzie, J. F., Neiger, B. L., & Thackeray, R. (2009). *Planning, implementing, and evaluating health promotion programs: A primer* (5th ed.). San Francisco: Pearson Benjamin Cummings.

Schinke, S., Brounstein, P., & Gardner, S. (2002). *Science-based prevention programs and principles.* Rockville, MD: U.S. Department of Health and Human Services.

Swerissen, H., & Crisp, B. R. (2004). The sustainability of health promotion interventions for different levels of social organization. *Health Promotion International, 19*(1), 123–130.

U.S. Department of Health and Human Services. (1997). *Developing objectives for Healthy People 2010.* Washington, DC: U.S. Government Printing Office.

Weisz, J. R., Sandler, I. N., Durlak, J. A., & Anton, B. S. (2005). Promoting and protecting youth mental health through evidence-based prevention and treatment. *American Psychologist, 60*(6), 628–648.

# PART THREE

# IMPLEMENTING HEALTH PROMOTION PROGRAMS

# CHAPTER SIX

# IMPLEMENTATION TOOLS, PROGRAM STAFF, AND BUDGETS

JEAN M. BRENY BONTEMPI

MICHAEL C. FAGEN

KATHLEEN M. ROE

## LEARNING OBJECTIVES

- Compare action plans, logic models, and timelines and describe their application to program implementation

- Discuss approaches to recruiting, hiring, and retaining program staff with the necessary skills, commitment, and ability to work effectively with a variety of stakeholders

- Suggest methods of advertising program staff openings to attract highly qualified applicants

- Describe the relationship between income and expenses as it pertains to the sound fiscal management of programs

- Describe the role of program staff, their rights, and their responsibilities to program funders

**E**FFECTIVE PLANNING results in a program design that is evidence-based, innovative, and informed by promising practices from the field; that eliminates health disparities; and that is so well organized that—at least on paper—the program is poised for success. This chapter and the subsequent chapters in Part Three (Chapters Seven, Eight, and Nine) discuss the critical link between design and results: implementation. Using the theories and models for developing health promotion programs that were discussed in Chapter Three (Table 3.12), the chapters in Part Three focus on a new phase in the process of creating, operating, and sustaining a health promotion program. According to the PRECEDE-PROCEED model, these chapters focus on phase 5, implementation. Implementation is a process that happens over time, not an event that occurs at a specific moment. This chapter begins with the importance of action plans in guiding staff and stakeholders through the program's planned goals, objectives, and interventions as well as all of the behind-the-scenes activities they will need to do in order to make the program unfold as planned. Several practical implementation tools, including logic models and Gantt charts that will help an organization move from program design to live action, are explained. Next, the role of program staff and stakeholders in following the action plans is discussed, as well as practical strategies for hiring, training, managing, and evaluating staff. The chapter concludes with a discussion of budgeting and fiscal management, which ensure that the resources that will be needed throughout the program are available.

## FROM PROGRAM PLANNING TO ACTION PLANNING

Program goals and objectives have been written, desired outcomes determined, and interventions planned, so now what? Well, now the program that was so painstakingly planned must be implemented as the staff and stakeholders intended if goals are to be achieved. In this important stage, the staff and stakeholders move from program planning to action planning.

One of the most critical steps in the health promotion planning process is the creation of practical and specific *action plans*. These practical documents are based on the program's goals, objectives, and interventions. A good action plan provides a summary of how the program needs to progress. The plan links the specific activities that will be undertaken with the outcomes desired. Once developed, the action plan helps staff members track progress, adapt to changes, and document accountability as the program unfolds. Because the action plan shows what is planned, it can also serve as a key document in process evaluation—ongoing review of the process by which the program is implemented and of the impact that the process has on the outcomes. Process evaluation, an important part of program evaluation, is discussed in detail in Chapter Ten.

Exhibit 6.1 provides an abbreviated example of how goals, objectives, interventions, and activities can be written into an action plan that ensures that all the steps needed to accomplish each intervention are identified and assigned to a staff member to be completed by a certain date. In the example in Exhibit 6.1, one of the goals of the school is to maintain the number of children who are within their healthy weight zone as they progress through school. Another goal is to reduce the number of children who are overweight or at risk of being overweight. Five objectives are provided that address both goals. Objectives 2 and 3 both require a similar strategy: an improved or enhanced physical education program. Objective 1 will also benefit from an enhanced physical education program that increases the amount of time that students engage in vigorous physical activity during physical education classes. In addition, the plan for objective 1 includes an intervention of promoting physical activity as a way to take "brain breaks" within the classroom, an intervention that is facilitated by the regular teachers, thus increasing the number of minutes that students are actively involved in aerobics, strength building, or flexibility exercises. (Only the activities for the first intervention in objective 1 [scheduling classroom breaks] are identified in the abbreviated action plan.)

In the following sections, two additional useful tools for moving from planning to implementation—a logic model and a Gantt chart—will be introduced. A logic model helps communicate the relationships between program elements to stakeholders and potential partners as well as the target population (Erwin et al., 2003; McKenzie, Neiger, & Smeltzer, 2005). Gantt charts help put program elements into a specific timeline in an at-a-glance format that allows staff and stakeholders to better manage the program (Timmreck, 2003). While the action plan also identifies a time when each activity should be accomplished, the Gantt chart displays this information in the most useful format. Both logic models and Gantt charts are dynamic tools that can be revised and updated at regular intervals to reflect program development and growth.

## PREPARING A LOGIC MODEL

As its name suggests, a logic model is a visual depiction of the underlying *logic* of a planned initiative. It shows the relationship between the program's resources (*inputs*), its planned activities (*outputs*), and the changes that are expected as a result (*outcomes*). Logic models can take many forms, but they all are designed to provide a simple graphic illustration of the relationships assumed between

## EXHIBIT 6.1
## Constructing an Action Plan That Documents Activities Needed to Execute Strategies

**Goal:** Decrease the number of students who are overweight and at risk of being overweight in Adams County Middle Schools while maintaining the number of students who are at their correct weight for their height and age.

**Objective 1.** Increase the number of students who are physically active for sixty minutes each day from 30 percent to 55 percent by the end of the school year.

**Objective 2.** Increase the number of students who can achieve the Healthy Fitness Zone on all components of the FITNESSGRAM from 15 percent to 30 percent by the end of the school year.

**Objective 3.** Increase the number of students who can identify and describe the components of fitness from 65 percent to 85 percent by the end of the school year.

**Objective 4.** Increase the number of students who choose to eat five fruits and vegetables each day from 15 percent to 35 percent by the end of the school year.

**Objective 5.** Decrease the number of students who daily eat high-fat, high-salt, low-nutrient foods from 80 percent to 65 percent by the end of the school year.

| Interventions (What will facilitate achieving the specific objective?) | Activities (What are the action steps to implement the intervention strategy?) | Personnel (Who will ensure that each action step is completed?) | Time Frame (By what date does the action step need to be completed?) |
|---|---|---|---|
| Interventions for Objective 1: | | | |
| 1.1. Purchase evidence-based physical activity program that promotes physical activity | 1.1.1. Schedule professional development for elementary teachers. | 1.1.1. Project director | 1.1.1. January 30 |

the actions that will be initiated and the results anticipated. Figure 6.1 shows how to set up a logic model. A logic model reads from left to right. Each column flows into the next, indicating that what is in each column depends on the column before it in order to be successful. The logic model thus shows what the planners are assuming will happen as the program progresses. It also allows the staff and stakeholders to track any changes from what was assumed and analyze the impact of those changes on program outcomes. Logic models

| | | | |
|---|---|---|---|
| breaks within the classroom as a means to improve academic achievement as well as increase daily physical activity. | 1.1.2. Identify and secure needed resources. | 1.1.2. Project administrative assistant | 1.1.2. January 30 |
| | 1.1.3. Provide professional development. | 1.1.3. Project director | 1.1.3. February 10 |
| | 1.1.4. Start sixth-grade program. | 1.1.4. Sixth-grade team | 1.1.4. March 1 |
| | 1.1.5. Start seventh-grade program. | 1.1.5. Seventh-grade team | 1.1.5. March 15 |
| | 1.1.6. Implement coaching initiative to reinforce the implementation of classroom activities. | 1.1.6. Project director | 1.1.6. March 15 |
| | 1.1.7. Evaluate the implementation of classroom activities. | 1.1.7. Project evaluator | 1.1.7. April 20 |
| 1.2. Add program components to increase amount of time students engage in moderate to vigorous activity while in physical education classes. | | | |
| 1.3. Implement fitness testing followed by development of individualized self-improvement fitness action plans by each student. | | | |

are useful for program staff and stakeholders, helping them to succinctly communicate and agree on the overall plan (MacDonald et al., 2001; Gilmore & Campbell, 2005). A clear and simple logic model will explain in a single page how what is planned will make a difference in the health behavior or health status of a population.

Figure 6.2 is an example of a logic model for a program to prevent the initiation of tobacco use among young people (MacDonald et al., 2001).

FIGURE 6.1  Schematic Logic Model

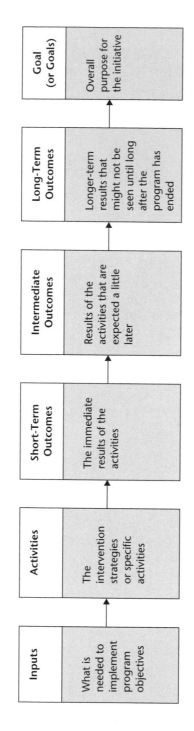

| Inputs | Activities | Short-Term Outcomes | Intermediate Outcomes | Long-Term Outcomes | Goal (or Goals) |
|--------|-----------|---------------------|-----------------------|--------------------|-----------------|
| What is needed to implement program objectives | The intervention strategies or specific activities | The immediate results of the activities | Results of the activities that are expected a little later | Longer-term results that might not be seen until long after the program has ended | Overall purpose for the initiative |

*Source:* Adapted from W. K. Kellogg Foundation, 2004.

FIGURE 6.2  Logic Model for Preventing the Initiation of Tobacco Use Among Young People

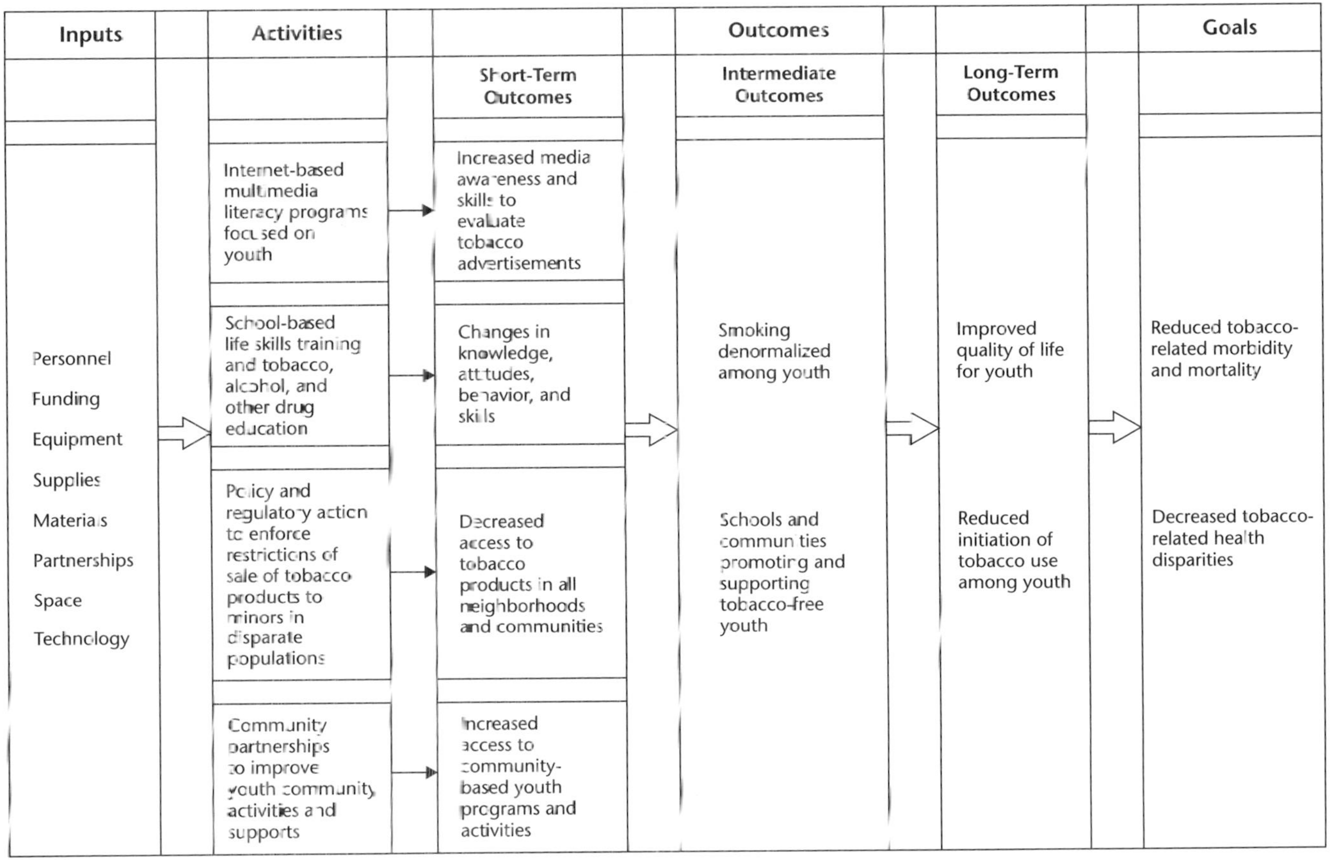

| Inputs | Activities | Outcomes | | | Goals |
|---|---|---|---|---|---|
| | | Short-Term Outcomes | Intermediate Outcomes | Long-Term Outcomes | |
| Personnel | Internet-based multimedia literacy programs focused on youth | Increased media awareness and skills to evaluate tobacco advertisements | | | |
| Funding | School-based life skills training and tobacco, alcohol, and other drug education | Changes in knowledge, attitudes, behavior, and skills | Smoking denormalized among youth | Improved quality of life for youth | Reduced tobacco-related morbidity and mortality |
| Equipment | | | | | |
| Supplies | Policy and regulatory action to enforce restrictions of sale of tobacco products to minors in disparate populations | Decreased access to tobacco products in all neighborhoods and communities | Schools and communities promoting and supporting tobacco-free youth | Reduced initiation of tobacco use among youth | Decreased tobacco-related health disparities |
| Materials | | | | | |
| Partnerships | | | | | |
| Space | Community partnerships to improve youth community activities and supports | Increased access to community-based youth programs and activities | | | |
| Technology | | | | | |

The program's long-term goals are to reduce tobacco-related morbidity and mortality and to decrease tobacco-related health disparities.

## Program Inputs and Activities

The first two columns in the logic model in Figure 6.2 contain information generated during the program planning process when the planners developed the goals, objectives, and strategies. In the first column (*Inputs*), the major resources from the state public health department, along with its partners, are represented. These resources could include funding and staff from the health department's office of tobacco use prevention, the program staff of the health department's bureau of drug and alcohol education, and the staff and resources of various community agencies, as well as the staff and resources of the local education authorities (superintendent, principals, school health council or school health teams, school health coordinator). The shorthand notation of the logic model is used so that the entire plan can be reduced to one page that identifies all the critical elements that are needed to implement the program as well as their relationship to each other. Resources could be staff, locations to hold program events, organizational resources, appropriate supplies, equipment, technology, curricula, or instructional resources.

Moving to the right from *Inputs* to *Activities* brings into focus the specific strategies and interventions that were selected during the planning process on the basis of the staff and stakeholders' understanding of the underlying problem, its context, the program's theoretical framework, and the desired outcomes. In this second column, the key strategies specified in this plan are Internet-based multimedia literacy programs focused on youth; school-based life skills and tobacco, alcohol, and other drug education; policy and regulatory action; and community partnerships focused on youth community activities and supports.

## Outcomes

Moving from what is planned to what is hoped will happen, we arrive at the three *Outcomes* columns on the right side of the logic model. The *Short-Term Outcomes* column lists the things that we expect will happen as an immediate result of each of the planned activities. For example, the media literacy program, school-based prevention, policy initiatives, and the community activities and supports should increase students' knowledge, awareness, and skills, as well as produce changes in students' attitudes. The key is making sure that there is a logical link between the items that are specified in the *Activities* column and what is assumed will happen if these are properly implemented (specified in the *Short-Term Outcomes* column).

The *Intermediate Outcomes* column is next; it refers to results that may not be seen after a single activity but can be measured or verified at some future point. In the example, the planners are hoping to denormalize tobacco use. This intermediate outcome could be assessed by doing student surveys at school or within the community after the instructional programs have been delivered for several years.

The column *Long-Term Outcomes* depicts the ultimate extension of the program's impact. If the activities are effective and the planners achieve both the short-term and the intermediate outcomes, the logic model specifies that the related long-term results that could be reasonably expected are reduced initiation of tobacco use among youths and improvement in youths' quality of life. In this case, the program manager might think that the program has been successful if measurements completed each year of the program and for three years after the program is terminated demonstrate a steady decline in youth tobacco use.

Most health promotion programs are designed to achieve a very long-term outcome that is health- or disease-related. The ultimate very long-term outcomes that are envisioned are the program's *goals*. In this case, as shown in the *Goals* column, a reasonable long term outcome for the program to set as a goal might be a 20 percent reduction in tobacco-related morbidity and mortality twenty to forty years later, when the youths who received the intervention are adults. Another very long-term result (goal) for the program to strive for is a decrease in tobacco-related health disparities.

Not all programs achieve their desired outcomes; others achieve the outcomes but not at the levels anticipated. If, in the example shown in Figure 6.2, participants gain the intended knowledge by the end of the exposure to the lessons but do not demonstrate any change in attitudes or behavioral intention, the project manager will be able to identify the point in the logical chain that needs reinforcement. Working backward and forward within a logic model throughout the action phase of a program provides valuable checks that can greatly enhance the program's effectiveness if the project manager is able to learn through analyzing what has happened and why.

## USING A GANTT CHART TO GUIDE IMPLEMENTATION

A logic model, as was just illustrated, provides a visual picture of the underlying logic of a program and how its key components rely on and build on each other. However, it does not provide one very important thing—a timeline. This is where a Gantt chart comes in handy.

A Gantt chart is a visual depiction of a schedule for completing a program's objectives. This particular method of charting project activities and phases over time was developed in the early 1900s by a mechanical engineer, Henry Gantt. Originally drawn by hand on graph paper, Gantt charts and other project management planning tools are now easily developed with software such as Microsoft's Excel or Project. Ideally, a Gantt chart should be no more than a single page, even for a complex project. The goal is to show in clean and simple lines the development of the project across time and on time. (Remember that the action plan has the details of who will do what by when in order to implement each strategy.) A Gantt chart will help program staff to organize all of those people and activities across the time that is available to complete the program (McKenzie, Neiger, & Thackeray, 2009). It will also help communicate this calendar to all of the program staff and stakeholders. A good Gantt chart can quickly become one of the most useful tools available to program staff.

While an action plan lists everything that must be accomplished by date and by the person responsible, the items are presented in order of the program's goals and objectives. The action plan does provide the staff with useful information, but completing a Gantt chart that puts all activities on a common calendar allows the staff to make sure that nothing is overlooked and to see at a glance what activities need to be accomplished—and by when. In order to move from an action plan to a program timeline (a Gantt chart), the following questions need to be answered:

- Which activities need to be done before others?
- What are the critical deadlines for each activity?
- How much time will be needed for each activity?
- Are there any scheduled holidays, vacations, or other predictable periods in which less work might get accomplished or activities won't be successful?
- When are our evaluation and progress reports due?

In the example in Figure 6.3, the intervention is a set of educational activities: a workshop series, including a skill-building session, and a follow-up workshop.

The Gantt chart in Figure 6.3 identifies all of the things needed in order to complete one full cycle of the educational intervention. For example, if program funding begins January 1, staff need to be hired and trained immediately. If it is assumed that it will take eight weeks to get the staff on board and ready, the first workshop series can begin in late March and conclude by late April, if the workshop is going to use instructional materials that have already been developed. If the staff is to construct or adapt the lessons, additional time for curricula development

FIGURE 6.3    Abbreviated Gantt Chart of Educational Activities

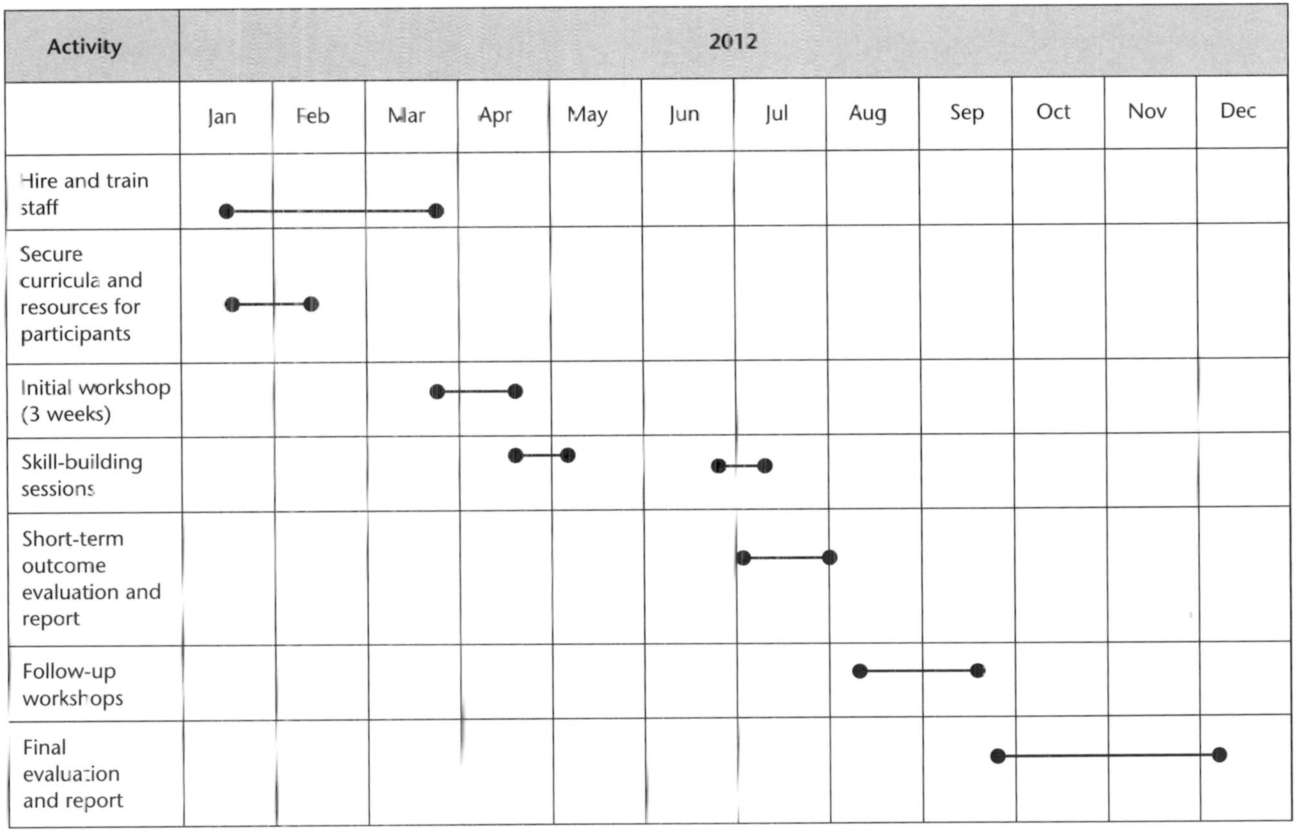

2012

| Activity | Jan | Feb | Mar | Apr | May | Jun | Jul | Aug | Sep | Oct | Nov | Dec |
|---|---|---|---|---|---|---|---|---|---|---|---|---|
| Hire and train staff | ● | | ● | | | | | | | | | |
| Secure curricula and resources for participants | ● | ● | | | | | | | | | | |
| Initial workshop (3 weeks) | | | ● | ● | | | | | | | | |
| Skill-building sessions | | | | ● | ● | ● | ● | | | | | |
| Short-term outcome evaluation and report | | | | | | | ● | ● | | | | |
| Follow-up workshops | | | | | | | | ● | ● | | | |
| Final evaluation and report | | | | | | | | | ● | | | ● |

would need to be built into the Gantt chart. Continuing to plot the activities across actual time, it becomes evident that the first full set of educational activities—and evaluation data collection and reporting—will be completed by the end of July. But what if the teaching staff assigned to the project typically take vacation in July? Or what if staff are ready to start the workshops in February but the weather is typically so harsh or unpredictable at that time of year that participants might have trouble attending? These kinds of considerations stemming from the organizational or community context are crucial when moving from planning to action. A carefully designed and updated Gantt chart helps the manager plan ahead, adjust, and stay on top of the program as the specifics of implementation unfold.

A good Gantt chart also includes critical evaluation and reporting deadlines. Figure 6.3 shows the evaluation data collection periods associated with each component of the educational intervention. Each period concludes with an evaluation report. However, the funder or stakeholders may require progress reports on a regular basis. If so, these need to be added to the Gantt chart. If the process evaluation plans call for ongoing monitoring of program activities for fidelity to the original design, that monitoring also needs to be added to the chart.

## PLANNING FOR IMPLEMENTATION CHALLENGES

There are no right or wrong formats for an action plan, logic model, or Gantt chart. All should be thoughtful, living documents that help the program staff and stakeholders accomplish the program objectives on time and in the way intended. They are tools that program staff and stakeholders (and even participants) can use to build and shape a program. Ideally, they also reflect the energy, passion, and excitement of the program stakeholders for addressing health problems by proactively promoting health and eliminating disparities.

Program staff should be prepared for changes and challenges during a program's implementation period; programs may be planned on paper, but they take place in schools, workplaces, health care organizations, and communities, where change and challenge are to be expected. Talking about a program is very different from actually implementing it. Chapter Five discusses the transition from planning to implementation and the six stages of implementation (Fixsen, Naoom, Blase, Friedman, & Wallace, 2005): exploration and adoption, program installation, initial implementation, full operation, innovation, and sustainability. In the remainder of this section, we discuss some common challenges that are often encountered when moving through the stages, particularly program installation, initial implementation, and full operation.

**Lack of attention to details is hampering execution of the program**. Attention to the details at the start of a program's operation is necessary and important. As the first day of program operation approaches, brainstorm a list of details to attend to, down to "open the doors and let people into the program." Anticipating how staff members will get to know participants' names and contact information, establishing how participants will arrive at the program (for example, taking a bus, being dropped off by parents, walking from their offices), having room door keys and equipment ready to use, and having computer access are small details that, if not attended to, will disrupt the flow and progress of a program. Tending to these details establishes staff and participant relationships that are trusting, supportive, and caring, which is important because good staff-participant relationships are fundamental to an effective health promotion program. It also has the wider effect throughout the organization or setting on the program's image and creditability as a competent and caring resource that is an asset to the organization.

**The realities of actual program operations are more difficult than program planners anticipated**. Rarely do programs function as planned, at least initially. There are too many unknowns and variables to permit program staff to plan for everything. Some typical problems are confusion on the part of participants about start and finish times (for example, date, day of the week, time) or location (for example, street address, building, room number), equipment problems, technology failures, program schedule conflicts caused by allotted times being either too long or too short, too few or too many participants, and erratic attendance (for example, some participants come late, others miss parts of the program, and some have to drop out). All of these initial problems have the potential to derail operations. These situations require staff members to troubleshoot by quickly assessing problem areas and what actions are needed to address them. When problems arise, it is essential to avoid blaming the participants or the organization. Focus on what is being learned, and incorporate it into the operation of the program.

**Staff and stakeholders do not follow the action plan or Gantt chart as closely as they should**. Staff and stakeholders often need to make decisions as the program is developing, particularly in response to participants' needs. Adherence to the plan and schedule may be viewed as no big deal by a staff member but have real consequences if future program segments depend on sequential completion of activities and tasks. Not everyone has to agree on every detail in the plan during program implementation; however, staff knowledge of what is actually occurring is critical to problem solving when programs struggle. Sharing the timeline and routinely referring back to it helps everyone see the way in which their responsibilities contribute to the integrity and ultimate success of the project. It also helps people realize in advance what the consequences will be for the entire program if they make independent decisions about the program without communicating them to the entire staff. Having frank and honest discussions of progress to date on a regular basis and adjusting the timeline as needed can help keep everyone on track. The Gantt chart will also help make expectations about timelines very clear for staff, which is helpful in both program process evaluation and staff performance evaluation.

**Conflicts occur**. Conflict and struggles are natural parts of program implementation. Each staff member and stakeholder will have his or her own work style, priorities, and level of commitment. For some, working with the health promotion program may be only one of their responsibilities. Complicating staff and stakeholders' concerns is the fact that participants will each have their own reasons and motivations for participating in the program. All of these personal concerns can lead to conflicts in the daily operations and delivery of a program. Agreed-on deadlines may be missed. Conflicts are opportunities for program staff and stakeholders to learn how best to move from theory to practice, from plan to action. Most adults are shy about engaging in conflicts, yet conflicts and struggles are hard to avoid, given the nature of the work and of working with people and organizations who may have very different agendas and needs. It is best to talk about the struggles. Creative problem-solving and conflict resolution strategies can be used in these situations. It may be difficult and awkward to deal with the conflicts and struggles, but there is a lot to be learned from them.

**Unanticipated staff turnover leaves vacancies in positions that are critical to accomplishing the plan**. Hiring, training, and retaining staff is an integral part of program implementation, as we will discuss later in this chapter. The person who was hired to provide instruction in the planned workshops may leave for another position or may be reassigned to another department, or the process evaluation may indicate that this staff member is not capable of delivering the instruction and must be assigned to other responsibilities. When such emergencies occur, the Gantt chart will help prioritize the next steps by identifying how much time is available before the vacancy seriously disrupts the program. If the disruption is for more than a very short time, updating the Gantt chart to reflect the time spent dealing with the situation and getting back on track will help guarantee that subsequent activities are completed on time. It will also document what really happened during implementation—a critical data element for the process evaluation.

**Crisis occurs in the organization or community, and the program has to be put on hold**. Despite the best planning, events sometimes require staff or participants to focus their efforts in another area for short or long periods of time. Deadlines for new proposals, year-end reports, and emergencies can all interfere with health promotion programs. If a program needs to be placed on hold, the Gantt chart will be very helpful in getting back on track once the crisis is resolved.

**The timeline is unrealistic**. This also happens. The process of moving from an action plan to a Gantt chart timeline helps identify whether this might be the case as all the necessary activities are placed on one calendar. If the timeline turns out to be unrealistic, the staff may need to "rightsize" the plan. Discussing the situation with a supervisor or funder may be helpful; it may be possible to get an extension or additional support in order to bring the program to completion on time and as planned.

**Staff members are unhappy with their job**. Unhappy staff members typically do not perform to their capabilities and contribute to turbulent work environments. The best way to promote staff satisfaction is through systematic hiring decisions followed by quality training, management, and evaluation. Despite managers' best efforts, however, some staff members may become dissatisfied with their job. In these instances, it is important to help the staff member find work in a different program or organization.

**Staff members are challenged by working in teams**. Working in teams has become a common approach to implementing health promotion programs. While some staff members naturally work well in these types of small groups, others are challenged in a variety of ways, which may include not being able to compromise, share leadership, or make meaningful contributions. Effective leaders engage their staff in a variety of team-building activities that are designed to maximize overall team performance, ensure contributions from each team member, and minimize conflict. However, even effective leaders sometimes need to reorganize staff teams when teams are not performing near their capacity.

Planning is analytical, but implementation is an art. The more experience that a program's staff and stakeholders have with program implementation, the better they will be able to anticipate, deal with, and adjust to the many challenges that can happen once a program is under way. Each experience in implementing a health promotion program provides insight and information for the next time. Clear and current action plans, logic models, and Gantt charts can be critical tools that facilitate the open and proactive communication with the program's stakeholders, staff, and participants that keeps a program moving forward, even when change happens. Regularly updating and modifying the action plans, logic model, and Gantt chart can create a visual record of a program's growth and development. These tools can tell the story of how the planned program was implemented in real time with real people, reflecting the actual changes and challenges.

# HIRING AND MANAGING HIGH-QUALITY PROGRAM STAFF

Hiring staff is one of the most important program leadership functions. Quality hiring decisions contribute to effective programs and positive work environments. Conversely, hiring mistakes can lead to program implementation problems and turbulent work environments. Thus, investing time, energy, and resources in making effective hiring decisions is critical for producing successful programs (Hunt, 2007).

## Hiring Considerations

A number of strategies can be used in order to make effective hiring decisions. In general, seek to hire staff who

- **Have skills and experience that are specifically matched to program goals**. If a youth development program is to be implemented, seek staff who have experience in working with young people.
- **Have interpersonal qualities that are desirable for the program**. If the program's work is highly collaborative, seek staff who value compromise and working in teams.
- **Are culturally competent**. Cultural competence should be a requirement for program staff. Staff diversity and cultural competence contribute to supportive and caring relationships with stakeholders and participants as well as among the staff members. These relationships are critical to participants' participation in a program and their motivation to address a health concern.
- **Have an interest in the organizational mission**. If the organization's mission is to help eliminate health disparities, seek staff who are committed to this work.

In addition, use the following techniques to improve the hiring process:

- **Create high-quality job announcements**. An effective job announcement will describe the organization, program, minimum qualifications, and desired skills and experiences in an easy-to-understand and attractive format. Interested candidates will know how to apply, to whom, and by what deadline.
- **Distribute job announcements widely**. Circulate the job announcement in multiple formats and places, including Internet career sites, electronic

TABLE 6.1    Applicant Screening Grid

| Applicant | Desired Trait | | | |
| --- | --- | --- | --- | --- |
| | Suitable Educational Background | Ability to Design Program Materials | Ability to Work in Collaborative Teams | Experience with Similar Programs |
| Applicant 1 | 5 | 2 | 3 | 3 |
| Applicant 2 | 4 | 4 | 4 | 4 |
| Applicant 3 | 5 | 3 | 4 | 2 |
| Applicant 4 | 3 | 4 | 2 | 5 |

mailing lists, professional journals, and local bulletin boards. The object is to generate the largest possible pool of qualified applicants.

- **Screen applicants systematically**. Identify leading candidates by using a grid that rates each applicant on qualifications, skills, and experience. Table 6.1 shows a sample grid in which applicants' attributes are rated on a scale of 1 (lowest) to 5 (highest). Such grids help clarify which traits are applicants' strengths and which are most important to the project. Augment this rating process with brief telephone interviews of ten to fifteen minutes as necessary. The object is to create a short list of three to five candidates who will be interviewed.

## Interview Leading Candidates

Conduct in-person interviews with the short list of candidates. Ask interview questions that will help clarify candidates' relevant skills, experiences, and potential fit with the rest of the program staff and your organization's mission (Camp, Vielhaber, & Simonetti, 2001). One way to identify the best candidates is by asking them to describe potential approaches to program-specific scenarios. Exhibit 6.2 provides a list of sample interview questions. You might also ask applicants to perform some appropriate skill—for example, teaching an abbreviated sample lesson or constructing a letter to a specific group of program participants. If you keep your hiring considerations in mind as you interview the candidates, the chance that the staff member hired will be a good fit for your program and your organization increases.

## Training, Coaching, Managing, and Evaluating Staff

After making good hiring decisions, effective leaders retain qualified staff by investing in staff development: training, coaching, management, and evaluation

## EXHIBIT 6.2
## Sample Interview Questions

- Describe your previous work experience that is relevant to this position.
- Describe a needs assessment you performed as part of planning a health promotion program.
- How have you applied health theories and planning models in your work?
- How have you adapted an evidence-based health promotion intervention to fit a population in a setting different from the intervention's intended use while maintaining the intervention's fidelity?
- Provide a logic model or Gantt chart you have prepared as part of a grant application.
- How have you addressed challenges during a health promotion program implementation in a school, workplace, health care organization, or community setting?
- How do you engage and support program participants and stakeholders?
- Describe how you have used program evaluations to improve a health promotion program.

(Barbazette, 2007; Fixsen, Naoom, Blase, Friedman & Wallace, 2005). Staff development focuses on supporting staff so that they can (1) perform their work effectively, (2) contribute meaningfully to the organization's mission, (3) achieve high levels of satisfaction with their job, and (4) continue to expand the depth and breadth of their knowledge of health promotion.

The best staff development programs are concrete, tailored to staff needs, and ongoing. Initial sessions cover the organization's mission, policies, and procedures. Orientation sessions often match new staff members with more experienced ones in a shadowing or mentoring relationship. The new staff member learns from the established staffer through a series of observations, initial implementation efforts, and debriefing sessions. Ideally, the relationship develops on a basis of trust, understanding, and mutual respect. If so, the new staffer then has a person to consult for discussion and support about implementation challenges as they are encountered. The initial sessions will be followed closely by training sessions on the program and its implementation.

Professional development does not stop once staff members are grounded in program implementation. Rather, training includes ongoing supervision. In most program structures, staff members report to a specific program director. The best programs provide time and space for these directors to meet regularly with their staff in supervisory meetings that focus on problem solving. The process of learning from a mentor continues with supervisors, who coach their staff members, using the same process (observations, debriefing, discussion). Supervisors may also demonstrate skills and work directly with staff members on tasks, helping to strengthen and refine staff skills. Furthermore, good supervisors will help their staff identify areas for additional training, which may include technical skills (such as techniques for designing program materials) or process skills (such as techniques for motivational interviewing). These training sessions might be provided by the organization or via external professional development opportunities.

Effectively trained staff should be pleasant to manage because they understand their job responsibilities, have the skills to fulfill them, and are supported through mentoring and supervision. Strong leaders are effective managers who understand the importance of structuring programs so that staff members will be poised for success. Preparing staff members for success means matching staff skills and experience with job functions while providing opportunities for growth and learning. Staff members must feel comfortable approaching their managers with concerns and requests for additional professional development opportunities. In turn, managers must create work environments that allow these requests while ensuring that all staff members perform in ways that are beneficial to both the program and the organization.

The primary method that effective leaders use to manage for staff success is performance evaluation. Workplace performance evaluation is often thought to mean year-end reviews that determine raises, bonuses, or even job cuts. While annual reviews play a role in performance evaluation, the best leaders evaluate their staff on a continual basis. Such ongoing evaluation starts with staff goals that are formulated in partnership with supervisors and that meet staff, program, and organizational needs. These goals provide the blueprint for staff work, are discussed in regularly scheduled meetings with the primary supervisor, and are adjusted as necessary on the basis of changes at the staff, program, or organizational level. In this manner, the year-end review becomes a culminating event that synthesizes and summarizes staff performance instead of providing a single high-stakes, make-or-break performance rating (McDavid & Hawthorn, 2005).

## BUDGETING AND FISCAL MANAGEMENT

The extent to which staff members of a health promotion program need specialized training in finance, accounting, and funding and resource development depends, to some degree, on the size and complexity of the health promotion program for which they work. Generally, the larger or more complex the organization, the greater the likelihood that the program will use specialized financial management expertise. For example, the norm for major health promotion organizations with large health promotion programs (for example, the American Heart Association or the Centers for Disease Control and Prevention) is to appoint senior staff members as the chief financial officer and business manager. These individuals assume primary responsibility for coordinating the organization's cash and credit, financial planning, accounting, budgeting, funding development, and management information services.

Despite the increased presence of trained financial specialists in organizations that operate health promotion programs, it is important to understand that almost all decisions made by program directors and program staff—no matter what their role in the organization—have financial implications. Even in organizations in which staff members take on specialized roles in direct services (for example, health educators, social workers, physical therapists, physicians, or nurses), it is critical for those individuals to understand how their decisions affect and are affected by available funds, cash flow considerations, project revenue streams, and budget constraints. Therefore, it is extremely important for any person who is working or aspires to work in a health promotion program and organization to develop skills in basic accounting, financial analysis and planning, funding and resource development, and budgeting.

At the minimum, a well-prepared health promotion staff member should have the ability to interpret three basic financial documents: balance sheet, income statement, and cash flow statement. A balance sheet shows what an organization owns and how it is financed. An income statement shows the financial performance of an organization over a specified time period—typically, a year. Finally, a cash flow statement shows how an organization's operations have affected its cash position. Effective interpretation of these three documents is crucial to making sound business decisions. These documents equip health educators with information that is essential to analyzing, controlling, and improving their organization's day-to-day operations and long-term prospects. In addition to acquiring basic skills in financial and managerial accounting, students who are contemplating senior executive roles in health promotion organizations should gain knowledge of the fundamental concepts of corporate and public sector finance.

During the planning process, a budget needs to be developed for the program that is to be implemented. Effective program implementation requires careful adherence to the budget and timely reporting of any variation between what was planned and what actually happens. Effective leadership establishes a tone of honesty, problem solving, and transparency in every aspect of the program, but particularly in regard to budget and resources. An effective program leader is a good steward of the trust that comes with the position and the resources of the organization.

## Budget Basics

A budget is simply a detailed statement of the resources available to a program (income) and what it costs to implement it (expenses). In the planning phase, the budget is a reasoned prediction; in the implementation phase, the budget is a living document, changing as resources come in and funds are spent. Budgets for small programs are simple and fairly straightforward; they often have a limited number of expense categories and a single funding source. More complex health promotion programs may have more complicated budgets, with multiple funding streams, varied expenses, and anticipated changes in both expenses and income at various program stages. Whether the budget is large or small, complex or simple, the principles of sound financial management are the same (KU Work Group for Community Health and Development, 2007).

## Resources

Some health promotion programs have fixed incomes. They are funded at a certain level to implement a set of activities over a given period of time. In the case of multiple year funding, annual reports that show how the resources for one year have been used may be required before funds are released for the next year. Careful spending of resources according to the approved categories and within the approved limits makes this kind of fiscal management relatively easy.

In contrast, some health promotion program budgets are based on variable factors, such as the number of people who enroll, the number of clients who complete a series of program activities, matching funds, revenue from services, fundraising, or in-kind contributions from other sources. Luckily, when a program has this many moving parts in its resource base, it is usually housed in an organization that has professionals who can help program staff and program leaders understand, manage, and utilize their resources to ensure their program's viability (Johnson & Breckon, 2007).

## Expenses

Most program budgets have four primary expense categories:

- **Personnel**: the compensation to the paid staff of the program. In most cases, the personnel category is actually divided into two categories: wages and benefits. Personnel who work more than 50 percent of full time on the program usually have associated benefit costs, including health insurance and retirement benefits. Benefits can add 15 to 30 percent to the amount allocated for wages.

- **Supplies**: items that are needed to implement the program. Standard supply categories include printing and copying, postage, office supplies, telephone, and equipment. Depending on the program plan and the rules of the organization or funder, it may be possible also to include reasonable costs for entertainment or incentives in supply categories (for example, lunch for an advisory group, food and music for a volunteer thank-you reception, grocery store gift cards for participants).

- **Services**: specific skills, talent, or expertise that must be hired—usually for a short period of time. Examples might include kitchen staff for two nights to supervise a school-based family health night, translators to adapt or create materials, or transportation for a youth group's field trip. These services are usually priced by the hour and do not include benefits. A funder or organization may place limits on the hourly rate or number of hours allowed.

- **Travel, training, and dissemination of results**: the travel and professional development costs needed to train staff or participants and the costs of sharing what the program has done with others. This expense category may include modest compensation for local or regional travel required for site visits or program delivery in remote areas, usually calculated as cost per mile. Some funders who require grantees or staff to attend an annual meeting include the associated costs in the program's travel budget. Some funders even encourage program staff or leadership to present program findings at regional or national conferences in order to disseminate results in the field. If so, full or partial travel costs may be funded as a program expense.

It is very important that program staff understand in advance what can and cannot be claimed against the expense projections in the budget. For example, organizations may require proof of defensive driving instruction prior to authorizing travel reimbursement. Some funders will fund meal expenses, but most will not fund alcohol. Reviewing the expenses in the program budget and the rules and procedures of both the funder and the fiscal agent in their own organization will help program staff manage the budget, pay the bills, and keep their program running smoothly—at least on the financial end.

## Monitoring the Budget

Program resources and expenses can be monitored with simple spreadsheet software such as Microsoft Excel or Apple's Numbers. It is very important to monitor the budget on a regular basis in order to make sure that expenses and income are within the projected range (Dropkin, Halpin, & La Touche, 2007). It is also important to make sure that program staff, stakeholders, and participants understand the rules and procedures for spending money and obtaining reimbursement for program-related expenses. Submitting requests for reimbursement without appropriate receipts, submitting requests too late, or expecting reimbursement for items that are not approved by the funder wastes time and resources and disappoints everyone.

The program director is responsible for making sure that the allocated funds are spent by the end of the time periods designated by the funder. For example, a three-year grant for $60,000 may require that $20,000 be spent each year. Underspending in year 1 will not benefit the program if the funder cannot allow funds for year 1 to be spent in year 2 (called *carryover* or *roll-forward*). The program director needs to make sure that everyone involved is aware of the key deadlines for each reporting period and does his or her part to make sure that the resources are used for the intended purpose within the designated time frame.

## Budget Challenges

A budget lays out what is expected to happen with program resources and expenses and then tells the story of what actually happened. Ideally, the two scenarios are identical. However, even the best-planned program may deviate from its budget during the implementation phase (Johnson & Breckon, 2007). Two common budget challenges are presented here, along with strategies for overcoming them.

First, what if there's not enough money in the budget? Sometimes this happens despite careful planning. If a resource shortfall is identified during the planning phase, the program staff can search for funding or resources that will cover the additional expenses. For example, some federal grants cannot pay for food at program-related events. If this is known, yet the plan involves training or events at which the staff would like food to be served, donations (for example, from local stores) could be requested, a small grant (from a local organization or foundation) could be solicited, or resources from another source could be explored. Perhaps another resource stream within the agency that is running the program could be tapped to cover the expenses not included in the base funding.

If the staff are not successful in obtaining additional funds to cover providing lunch at the training event, the implementation plan will need to be adjusted so that program activities stay within budget. Overspending without prior approval from the funder might result in fewer resources for the next phase of the program. Even worse, overspending might jeopardize the program's continued or future funding, the project manager's position as a program leader, or the ability of the agency to successfully seek future support from this funder. These are serious consequences, but they can be avoided by carefully planning and monitoring the program budget.

Second, what if money is left over? This is a good problem to have, and it can happen for several reasons. Sometimes an expense item ends up costing less than anticipated or personnel costs are reduced through in-kind contributions of staff time from other sources. Careful monitoring of the budget on at least a monthly basis should help staff members to identify places where savings are occurring in plenty of time to make wise decisions about what to do with the extra money.

Minor changes within budget categories (for example, spending money saved on printing costs to upgrade the cover of a training manual) usually only need careful accounting in the next budget report. More significant changes within categories (for example, using money saved on printing volunteer manuals to print banners promoting program events) should probably be raised with the funder or at least the grant or fund manager within the host agency prior to investing the resources. Changes across budget categories (for example, using the money saved on printing to fund travel for an additional staff person to the national conference where program results are being presented) must be cleared with the funder in advance. Remember that money left over at the end of a project year may not be allowed to roll forward into the next year. Similarly, unspent funds that were awarded to an agency in order to carry out a particular program may need to be repaid if they are not spent within the designated period. So watch the budget carefully, process expenses and reimbursements on time, and maintain open communication with the funder so that there are no surprises for anyone at year's end.

And when exactly does a project year end? That depends. The term *fiscal year* refers to the dates of the funding year. Some grants or contracts begin on January 1 and end on December 31, so the funding cycle follows the calendar year. Other funding, particularly that associated with schools or universities, begins on July 1 and ends on June 30. Still other funds may have a start date based on the day the award was made—March 1, October 1, or any other month in the year. It can be challenging for managers to handle grants with different fiscal years. However, it is manageable, given careful planning, organized files, and someone who can help with questions. Never be afraid to ask questions about managing a program's budget; both one's supervisor and the funder will appreciate proactive attention to the responsibilities of budget management. Good stewardship shows commitment to the program participants, the organization, and the funder. It also communicates to potential funders that the agency is a good investment for future funding.

## SUMMARY

At some point in time, a health promotion program moves from planning to action. Action plans, logic models, and Gantt charts are tools that program staff and stakeholders can use to implement a program and reach the desired program objectives and goals. All should be thoughtful, living documents that help program staff and stakeholders accomplish the program's objectives on time and as intended.

Program staff and stakeholders should be prepared for changes and challenges during a program's implementation period; programs take place in schools, workplaces, health care organizations, and communities, where change and challenge are to be expected. While it can be anticipated that challenges and struggles will arise, what they will be for any one specific program is unknown until the program is operating. It may be difficult and awkward to deal with challenges and struggles, but there is a lot to be learned from them.

During implementation, staff and stakeholders also need to attend to managing the program's human and fiscal resources. Recruiting, selecting, developing, and supporting a skilled, motivated, diverse, and culturally competent staff contributes to caring and supportive relationships between and among program staff, stakeholders, and participants. A program's finances are a shared responsibility; everyone involved in the program should be made aware of his or her role in maintaining good fiscal practices that will contribute to long-term program growth and sustainability.

By using tools such as action plans, logic models, Gantt charts, budgets, and staff resources, the challenges of program implementation can be made manageable and often turned into learning opportunities.

## FOR PRACTICE AND DISCUSSION

1. Review the planning models for developing health programs in Chapter Three (Table 3.12). Select a model and discuss its approach to program implementation. Compare and contrast the models. How do they help you to understand how to implement a health promotion program?
2. A middle school is implementing a program to promote students' eating healthy lunches that include fresh vegetables and fruit, healthy beverages, whole grains, and low-fat choices. Program components include increasing healthy school lunch selections and providing classroom education and personal nutrition counseling for children, parents, and guardians. What challenges might be expected as the program moves from installation to initial implementation and full operation (stages discussed in Chapter Five)?
3. Have you ever had to plan anything big, like a wedding, a Thanksgiving dinner, or a graduation party? Discuss how you planned it to make sure that all the elements were done on time and under budget. Did you use any kind

of timeline? Budget? Develop a budget and timeline for this event or for an event you would like to plan.

4. What have your experiences been with on-the-job training? Has any job you have worked at provided training for you? Describe how the training was helpful, how it could have been improved, and what it entailed. Next, design a training program for a health promotion staff working in a school-based health clinic. What do they need to know in order to do their job? In what areas do you thinking coaching by program supervisors will be effective?

5. What tools do you use for your personal financial record keeping and financial planning? Do you use computer programs like Quicken or Excel? Or do you use paper-based products? How might any of these tools help you implement your program's budget? Complete a tutorial for Microsoft Excel. What makes this a useful budgeting tool for health promotion professionals?

6. Draw a logic model based on the academic program in which you are enrolled. Start with the program's resources, then its objectives, and finally its long-term goals. Discuss whether you see the program activities being able to reach the program goals.

## KEY TERMS

Action plan

Balance sheet

Budget

Cash flow statement

Fiscal management

Fiscal year

Gantt chart

Implementation challenges

Income statement

Intermediate outcomes

Logic model

Long-term outcomes

Performance evaluation

Short-term outcomes

Staff management

Staff training

## REFERENCES

Barbazette, J. (2007). *Managing the training function for bottom line results: Tools, models and best practices*. San Francisco: Pfeiffer.

Camp, R., Vielhaber, M., & Simonetti, J. L. (2001). *Strategic interviewing: How to hire good people*. Hoboken, NJ: Wiley.

Dropkin, M., Halpin, J., & La Touche, B. (2007). *The budget-building book for nonprofits: A step-by-step guide for managers and boards* (2nd ed.). San Francisco: Jossey-Bass.

Erwin, D. P., Ivory, J., Stayton, C., Willis, M., Jandorf, L., Thompson, H., et al. (2003). Replication and dissemination of a cancer education model for African American women. *Cancer Control, 10*, 13–21.

Fixsen, D. L., Naoom, S. F., Blase, K. A., Friedman, R. M., & Wallace, F. (2005). *Implementation research: A synthesis of the literature* (FMHI Publication No. 231). Tampa: University of South Florida, Louis de la Parte Florida Mental Health Institute, National Implementation Research Network.

Gilmore, G. D., & Campbell, D. (2005). *Needs and capacity assessment strategies for health education and health promotion* (3rd ed.). Boston: Jones & Bartlett.

Hunt, S. (2007). *Hiring success: The art and science of staffing assessment and employee selection.* Alexandria, VA: Society for Human Resource Management.

Johnson, J. A., & Breckon, D. J. (2007). *Managing health education and health promotion programs: Leadership skills for the 21st century* (2nd ed.). Sudbury, MA: Jones & Bartlett.

KU Work Group for Community Health and Development. (2007). *Managing finances.* Lawrence: University of Kansas. Retrieved January 30, 2008, from http://ctb.ku.edu/en/tablecontents/chapter_1043.htm.

MacDonald, G., Starr, G., Schooley, M., Yee, S., Klimowski, K., & Turner, K. (2001). *Introduction to program evaluation for comprehensive tobacco control programs.* Atlanta, GA: Centers for Disease Control and Prevention, Office on Smoking and Health.

McDavid, J. C., & Hawthorn, L.R.L. (2005). *Program evaluation and performance measurement: An introduction to practice.* Thousand Oaks, CA: Sage.

McKenzie, J. F., Neiger, B. L., & Smeltzer, J. L. (2005). *Planning, implementing, and evaluating health promotion programs* (4th ed.). San Francisco: Pearson Benjamin Cummings.

McKenzie, J. F., Neiger, B. L., & Thackeray, R. (2009) *Planning, implementing, and evaluating health promotion programs: A primer* (5th ed.). San Francisco: Pearson Benjamin Cummings.

Timmreck, T. C. (2003). *Planning, program development, and evaluation* (2nd ed.). Boston: Jones & Bartlett.

W. K. Kellogg Foundation. (2004). *Using logic models to bring together planning, evaluation, and action: Logic model development guide.* Retrieved January 30, 2008, from http://www.wkkf.org/Pubs/Tools/Evaluation/Pub3669.pdf.

# CHAPTER SEVEN

# ADVOCACY

REGINA A. GALER-UNTI

KELLY BISHOP ALLEY

REGINA MCCOY PULLIAM

## LEARNING OBJECTIVES

- Compare and contrast the perspectives of health educators and health promoters on the role of advocacy in health programs

- Describe the essential elements of a successful health advocacy effort and the relative importance of each element

- Define the roles played by advocacy, media advocacy, community engagement, and mobilization in moving a health agenda forward

- Describe the key methods of gaining support from elected officials for a health promotion agenda

- Identify the ways that 501(c)(3) status affects agency efforts

A**DVOCACY** is action in support of a cause or proposal. It can be political, as in lobbying for specific legislation, or social, as in speaking out on behalf of those without a voice. Broadly, advocacy is part of being a professional in a health field. At the same time, from the narrow perspective of a staff member, stakeholder, or participant in a health promotion program, advocacy is championing the program, fighting for funding, and engaging others in order to sustain the program, address a specific health problem, and eliminate health disparities. Health promotion programs live with the tension that on any given day, changes may happen: funding may be cut for political reasons, regardless of program performance; legislation may divert funding to new, higher-priority initiatives; changes in program participants' eligibility criteria may affect the priority population's access to a program; economic factors such as recession might make money tight; or a new national (or state, local, school, business, hospital, or community) health priority might usurp a program's place in funders' and people's consciousness, leaving the program and its staff, stakeholders, and participants vulnerable to program closure.

Advocacy is a thread that runs through all the phases of health promotion planning, implementation and evaluation. During planning, advocacy is about being a champion of a specific health concern and fighting to have it addressed. The money, time, materials, and people that support the needs assessment and program design come from the efforts of these champions. During implementation in each setting, program staff and stakeholders work to engage and serve participants and at the same time compete for funding and resources. Clearly, if there were unlimited resources, all health needs would be met, but given limited resources of time, materials, knowledge of what works best, and people's energy, advocacy is one tool that health promotion programs staff, stakeholders, and participants need to use in implementing programs. In the evaluation phase of a program, advocates use evaluation data and reports to communicate a program's effectiveness and sustain program growth and development. Without advocacy, programs disappear, even if they are effective. The vulnerability of health promotion programs to negative consequences due to changes in the larger environment or particular setting and their dependence on others for support makes it essential to pursue an advocacy agenda as part of program implementation.

## CREATING AN ADVOCACY AGENDA FOR A PROGRAM

Advocating for a health promotion program based on health theory that eliminates health disparities and uses evidence-based interventions requires calling on someone with power to take action. That power can derive from different sources—from an elected or legal mandate or from popular support and the power of numbers. In a particular setting (for example, a school, workplace, health care organization, or community) power is held, for example, by owners, stockholders, chief executive officers, boards of directors, superintendents, program directors, foundation staff members, government workers, and politicians such as local, state, and federal legislators.

Advocacy during implementation is not about a specific health promotion program. (Chapter Eleven talks about sustainability, which is about championing a specific program in a particular setting.) Advocacy is about affecting the larger environment of public policy, and raising awareness of a single program is insufficient to create lasting social change. Public policy must be shaped in a way that will sustain change across institutions. For example, advocates might aim for passage of a public policy that creates safe housing through testing and removal of lead-based paint, but advocates might also make the point that community members need to get informed about safe housing issues and lead paint poisoning prevention, communicate with elected officials, and vote.

Advocacy during program implementation has roots in a number of the health theories discussed in Chapter Three. Community mobilization theory supports advocacy through its focus on individuals' taking action organized around specific health issues at a site. Social network and social support theory, with its emphasis on relationship building based on mutual support and shared interest, reinforces for advocates the importance of building social support and networks when advocating. The more people involved with advocacy the better. Furthermore, communication theory, the diffusion of innovations model, and social marketing all help to shape how and with whom program staff, stakeholders, and participants talk in order to champion a program.

As part of implementing a health promotion program, the program staff may develop an advocacy agenda and strategy. The agenda is part of the program's action plan, just as an evidence-based health intervention is. One of the most important parts of effective advocacy is having a clear vision of the big issue the program addresses, what has to change, and a plausible plan of action for making the changes. Five key questions can help show the way:

1. **What action—one that is feasible—will actually solve the health problem?** What action needs to happen? Is it a new law, regulation, funding, service, or research initiative? The action needs to be compelling in order to get people interested in working for it. It also needs to be small enough that the program can achieve at least part of the action within a year or two, to keep people interested. Whatever the action, state it clearly and succinctly. Often such a statement is thought of as a program action (or behavioral)

objective (discussed in Chapter Five) which directs and shapes a program's advocacy. It would be titled the *advocacy action objective*.

2. **Who needs to take action?** Who actually has the authority to make the change? For example, can a mayor, city council, or state or federal agency or legislature effect the desired change? Who needs to be wooed because they can influence those with authority? For example, can members of the media or specific citizen groups help advance the cause?

3. **What does your audience need to hear?** What advocacy message will move all those people to make the change? An effective advocacy message has two parts: an appeal on the merits ("This bill is important because . . . ") and an appeal to self-interest ("Hundreds of voters want to know how you'll vote on . . . ").

4. **Whom does your audience need to hear the message from?** What messengers can be recruited, and who will be most persuasive? An advocacy campaign needs a mix of messengers—people who can speak from personal experience, people with recognized authority, and others who might have some special pull with the people you are trying to reach.

5. **What actions will you use to make your point?** What will people be asked to do to deliver the message? The options are many: people can be asked to lobby officials politely or protest in front of their offices, get an article in the newspaper, or attend a town meeting. Generally, the best actions to advocate are those that require the least effort and confrontation but still get the job done.

## ADVOCACY AS A PROFESSIONAL RESPONSIBILITY

Advocacy for funding, legislation, regulations, governmental infrastructure, services, or research ensures successful health promotion programs. Researchers assert the importance of combining programs and advocacy in order to best serve the needs of the public (Christoffel, 2000; Howze & Redman, 1992; Roe, Minkler, & Saunders, 1995). Clearly, the importance of advocacy to health promotion programs is profound. Health advocacy is defined as "the processes by which the actions of individuals or groups attempt to bring about social and/or organizational change on behalf of a particular health goal, program, interest, or population" (2000 Joint Committee on Health Education and Promotion Terminology, 2002). In short, health advocacy creates environments in which health promotion programs can be successful.

Engagement in advocacy has long been suggested as a professional responsibility of health professionals (Freudenberg, 1982; Ogden, 1986; Steckler &

Dawson, 1982). The Institute of Medicine report *Who Will Keep the Public Healthy?* contains a call to action for advocacy around health policy issues (Institute of Medicine, 2003). *Healthy People 2020* stresses the importance of developing policies that aid in achieving the goals and objectives of the Healthy People 2020 initiative (U.S. Department of Health and Human Services, 2009). The Galway Consensus Conference Statement lists advocacy as one of the areas of core competency necessary for engaging in successful health promotion practice (Allegrante et al., 2009). Health promotion practitioners clearly need to be effective advocates for a piece of the resource pie for their profession and for the people they work to help.

For many people working in health promotion programs, the acquisition of advocacy skills seems difficult and just one more thing among many that they need to know. Health promotion specialists are busy with the daily reality of implementing interventions, mobilizing and organizing stakeholders, and writing and revising policies. They often feel that the extra time and energy to advocate for their program just is not there. However, this view is shortsighted. Health promotion programs require supportive and receptive environments in order to achieve long-term sustainability. Focusing only on health promotion interventions and policies leaves out part of the work involved in the planning, implementation, and evaluation of successful health promotion programs; advocacy is part of the work.

## EXAMPLES OF SUCCESSFUL HEALTH POLICY ADVOCACY

Public health measures such as improvements in clean air and water, proper sanitation, and adequate and nutritious food have significantly increased longevity and lessened human suffering. In 1999, the Centers for Disease Control and Prevention listed the top ten advances in public health in the twentieth century (Centers for Disease Control and Prevention, 1999). It is safe to say that many of these advances, including vaccinations, improvements in motor vehicle safety, safer workplaces, better food safety, and recognition of tobacco as a health hazard are attributable not only to scientific discoveries but to advocacy for education and policy change. In the following examples, note how advocacy was used to contribute to these advances.

Mothers Against Drunk Driving (MADD) was founded by Candy Lightner after her daughter was killed by a drunk driver. The driver of the automobile was a repeat offender, and MADD used a media advocacy campaign to educate the public about the dangers of drunk driving. This advocacy raised public consciousness about the threat of drunk driving and spurred lawmakers to initiate more legislation to curb this danger. MADD's media advocacy has been recognized as the impetus that inspired action that decreased fatalities resulting from drunk driving (DeJong, 1996).

The March of Dimes (originally known as the National Foundation for Infantile Paralysis) is an example of a voluntary health organization that achieved its goal. Founded in 1938 by President Franklin D. Roosevelt, it began as a campaign to collect money toward research to find a cure for polio and toward care for those suffering from the disease. All individuals residing in the United States were asked to voluntarily give one dime toward the effort. In 1958, three years after the Salk vaccine was introduced to the general public, the March of Dimes changed its focus, becoming an organization dedicated to preventing birth defects, premature birth, and infant mortality (March of Dimes, n.d.); the March of Dimes had achieved its goal of finding a vaccine for polio. As times have changed, many organizations such as the March of Dimes have applied their efforts not just toward soliciting donations for research but also toward advocacy for more funding for research in their chosen areas. Today's March of Dimes works in the areas of research, education, community services, and advocacy (March of Dimes, n.d.).

The strides made in legislation to control tobacco use can be credited largely to the advocacy of researchers, activists, health practitioners, and nonprofit organizations. Long-term efforts to educate and heighten awareness about the harmful effects of tobacco have resulted in increased legislative activity in the area of tobacco control. It is interesting to note that these efforts have been accentuated by researchers' and advocates' efforts to heighten awareness about not only the health impact but also the economic costs of tobacco use (Givel & Glantz, 2004). As a result, significant legislation has been passed that limits tobacco manufacturers' contact with children, confines the use of tobacco products in public settings, and protects the worker from the health consequences of secondhand smoke. Advocacy techniques coupled with researchers' conclusions and recommendations have been used to decrease smoking in the United States (Chaney, Jones, & Galer-Unti, 2003).

Not all advocacy efforts are as well documented or as noticeable as the ones we have just described. Nutrition advocates have been responsible for a fair amount of legislation designed to protect and strengthen the healthful food supply in the United States. These advocacy efforts led to sweeping reforms in federal policy such as Public Law (P.L.) 101-535, commonly known as the Nutrition Labeling and Education Act of 1990, which mandates nutrition labels on packaged foods. This law represented a major victory for dietitians and consumers who had heavily advocated for the addition of this educational tool.

Some policy advocacy results in changes at state and local levels. Tip O'Neill, former Speaker of the U.S. House of Representatives, has been credited with stating, "All politics is local." That is also true for many types of health policy, as one can see in the wide variance, for example, in ordinances that restrict the purchase of guns in municipalities, designate speed limits in states, direct alcohol sales, and ensure swimming pool safety.

At times, ordinances formulated for use in one area rise to the state or national level. This frequently occurs when a local news story gets attention in the national media (for example, through an article in a national newspaper or a story on cable television or National Public Radio). Increasingly, a news story will catch the fancy of a legislator, a legislative body, or the constituents of another state. In this age of rapid media transfer and multiple media outlets, news of unusual or important ordinances is quickly disseminated to other municipalities.

## BECOMING FLUENT IN THE LANGUAGE OF ADVOCACY

In order to build skills in advocacy, it is necessary to learn the terminology of advocacy. Table 7.1 lists some key advocacy terms. The terms reflect the interactions of organized political and government structures in the making and administering of public decisions for a society. Advocates and lobbyists have the task of getting the public involved in the decision-making and administration processes and influencing the decisions made within them.

Legislative advocacy is, essentially, advocating for or against bills, ordinances, and laws. A bill is a piece of legislation that has been introduced as a proposed law. At the federal level, when a bill has been approved by the Senate and the House, it is signed into law by the president. Information about the process through which bills are formulated and processed through Congress can be found at the House of Representatives Web site (see Table 7.2). The Library of Congress has created a Web site (http://thomas.loc.gov) to aid in tracking legislation. States vary widely in their processes of passing a bill to create a law. Use the state and local government Web site given in Table 7.2 in order to find information about state legislative processes. Table 7.2 lists some useful Web sites that pertain to advocacy for health promotion programs.

Municipalities typically pass ordinances, which are enforced within the confines of the city. So an ordinance that applies within the confines of one town may not exist in the next town over. This is often confusing to people. One town may allow drivers to use cell phones while an adjacent community requires a hands-free device. Driving across the city limit, then, while talking on a cell phone, might result in a fine.

Two types of legislative processes are of significant interest to us. An authorization is a law that authorizes a program. An example of this, as previously discussed, is P.L. 101-535. The legislative history of the bill is available at

TABLE 7.1   Key Advocacy Terms

| Term | Definition |
|---|---|
| Advocacy | The processes by which individuals or groups attempt to bring about social or organizational change on behalf of a particular health goal, program, interest, or population |
| Appropriations | Legislation that designates or appropriates funding to a program |
| Authorizations | Legislation that sets policies or programs |
| Bill | A proposed law presented for approval to a legislative body |
| Direct lobbying | Communication with a legislator or a member of a legislator's staff that gives a viewpoint on a specific piece of legislation |
| Electioneering | Persuasion of voters in a political campaign |
| Grassroots lobbying | Any attempt to indirectly influence legislators by motivating members of the public to express specific views to legislators and legislative aides |
| Law | A local, state, or federal bill that has been passed by a legislative process (for example, a federal law passed by the U.S. Senate and the House of Representatives and signed by the president) |
| Lobbyist | An individual hired to represent the legislative interests of an organization (or related group of organizations) to members of a legislature |
| Media advocacy | Strategic use of news media and, when appropriate, paid advertising to support community organizing to advance a public policy initiative |
| Ordinance | A statute or regulation, usually enacted by a city government |

http://thomas.loc.gov. Knowing the numbering system for public laws is helpful in gaining a clearer understanding of them. Congress meets in two-year terms. The first number in the P.L. number is the number of the Congressional session. Thus, the 101 means that the bill was enacted during the 101st Congress. The second number is the number of the law passed in that two-year session. In our example, 535 is the number of the law.

Appropriations differ from authorizations in their emphasis. Whereas authorizations set policy or programs, appropriations designate money for specific purposes. The federal government and state legislatures have clear deadlines for their

TABLE 7.2 Advocacy Organizations and Web Sites

| Organization | URL | Brief Description |
|---|---|---|
| American Public Health Association | http://www.apha.org/advocacy/tips | Provides advocacy tips and instructions for carrying out advocacy work |
| Centers for Disease Control and Prevention—The Community Guide | http://www.thecommunityguide.org | Encourages the use of evidence-based research for policy decisions, program planning, and research design |
| Coalition of National Health Education Organizations—Health Education Advocate | http://www.healtheducationadvocate.org | Site dedicated to advocacy for legislation and funding for health education and health promotion |
| Library of Congress | http://thomas.loc.gov | Provides access to bill histories, resolutions, House and Senate committee reports, and the Congressional Record |
| Midwest Academy | http://www.midwestacademy.com | Provides online training and information for activism |
| Research America | http://www.researchamerica.org | Provides links to sites on advocating for health research |
| State and Local Government on the Net | http://www.statelocalgov.net | Provides links to official sites of states and municipalities |
| University of Kansas—The Community Toolbox | http://ctb.ku.edu/en | Provides information on community building and advocacy; maintained by the Work Group for Community Health and Development at the University of Kansas |
| U.S. House of Representatives | http://www.house.gov | Official site of the U.S. House of Representatives: provides information about House members, leadership, committees, and how a bill becomes a law |
| U.S. Senate | http://www.senate.gov | Official site of the U.S. Senate: provides information about Senate members, leadership, committees, and how a bill becomes a law |

budget approvals. Unlike bills, which can be debated throughout the legislative calendar, appropriations occur at a set point in the legislative calendar. It is a good idea to keep an eye on these funding cycles in order to know when arguments for funding for health promotion programs will be most effective.

Influencing the legislative process occurs in a variety of ways. Different types of lobbying might be used to influence passage of a bill or approval of an appropriation. In the following section, the legal and employment ramifications of participation in lobbying are discussed.

## Legalities of Health Advocacy

Advocacy and lobbying involve some legal issues. Health advocacy might take the form of delivery of general information and educating the public about a topic. For instance, an opinion piece about the dangers of hepatitis C and how it is transmitted is an important form of advocacy. Such an opinion piece might be written, for example, if there is a current attempt by a local governing body to enact an ordinance regulating tattoo parlors in the community. The piece is not written either for or against the ordinance; instead, the piece advocates for healthy and safe practices. There are no restrictions on this type of advocacy behavior.

U.S. tax code exempts certain types of organizations from federal taxation of income. All of these organization types appear in Section 501(c)(3) of the Internal Revenue Code. Organizations must apply for tax-exempt status; if they receive this status, they are often referred to as 501(c)(3) organizations. Organizations receiving tax-exempt status are primarily schools, colleges, universities, religious organizations, and charitable organizations (for example, community health organizations as discussed in Chapter One). Many health promotion programs are initiated by 501(c)(3) organizations or government agencies.

The IRS is very clear about banning the involvement of tax-exempt organizations in electioneering. *Electioneering* is defined as any attempt to persuade voters in a political campaign. For instance, making telephone calls that actively try to persuade people to vote a particular way on Election Day is electioneering. Organizations with 501(c)(3) status are barred from electioneering activity by tax law, and they cannot actively work for a candidate or a political party, nor can they support or oppose a candidate for political office (Vernick, 1999) or intervene in partisan elections. This regulation covers all houses of worship in America. Thus the law is clear that tax-exempt institutions cannot engage in electioneering; however, their ability to legally participate in lobbying is a little less clear.

*Lobbying* occurs when an attempt is made to influence legislation. The tax status of an employer determines whether employees may lobby and to what extent employees may engage in specific activities.

Basically, there are two types of lobbying: direct lobbying and grassroots lobbying. These distinctions are important; definitions for both are provided in Table 7.1. In direct lobbying, individuals make contact with a legislator, a member of the staff of a legislator, or a government official who is involved in formulating legislation. A request may be made, for instance, that a senator vote yes on a bill. This request is direct lobbying because it is an attempt to directly influence legislation (Vernick, 1999). In grassroots lobbying, the public is encouraged to approach legislators about a piece of legislation—for example, when members of an organization contact members of the public through a call to action that urges them to ask a government official to vote in a certain manner (Vernick, 1999). There is a complicated formula for the percentage of time that employees of a tax-exempt organization can spend on lobbying. Organizations need to be certain that they are in compliance with lobbying restrictions. Failure to comply may result in extra taxes or loss of tax-exempt status. Employees of tax-exempt organizations should consult their employer about the policies of their organization.

## Advocating While Maintaining One's Job

Advocacy activities on the part of employees may be encouraged or discouraged, depending on the employer. Government employees must be exceedingly careful about advocacy work because of the need for employees of the government to avoid any appearance of bias. Employees of 501(c)(3) organizations should be careful to stay in compliance with IRS rules that their organization must follow in order to maintain tax-exempt status. If you are encouraged as an employee and even as a private citizen to engage in advocacy activities, be certain to stay within your employer's guidelines.

Supervisors need to be informed when employees are engaging in advocacy efforts outside of regular work duties. Although the First Amendment to the U.S. Constitution ensures individuals' right to advocate (the right to free speech), there are no protections from firing if these activities put the employing agency at risk or harm the functioning of the agency.

Once the employer has been informed about the employee's intention to engage in advocacy work, care should be taken to be certain that work and after-work advocacy activities are kept separate. When speaking in public, making a phone call, or sending a written communication, be certain that everyone is informed that advocacy work is being performed by you as private citizen. For example, if you are speaking before the city council on restricting the sale of alcohol, you might say, "My name is _____. Some of you may know me as the head of the student health center. Today, however, I am expressing my personal views on the subject of bar hours." Note that in general, as a person's visibility increases, people will increasingly tend to see that person's private remarks as opinions of the employing agency. There may come a point at which the public is unable to differentiate between an individual's personal remarks and his or her position in the agency. Take this factor into account and be pragmatic when making decisions about engaging in advocacy work.

Additional precautions should be taken when engaging in advocacy work outside of an employing agency: do not use work titles, work stationery, work phones or fax machines, work e-mail or Internet systems, your work address, or a work cell phone, pager, or BlackBerry when you are acting as a private citizen. In the event that someone sends an e-mail to you at work, for instance, asking that recipients of the e-mail contact a legislator to urge passage of a bill, do not respond from the work account. Forward the e-mail to a home account, and use your home account and home computer for private advocacy efforts. If a local reporter calls to ask questions about your involvement in a local campaign, call her back on a private cell phone while on a break from work. Think twice before using your work facilities, workplace communication devices, or your work title.

## FORMING ALLIANCES AND PARTNERSHIPS FOR ADVOCACY

Successful advocacy efforts do not happen in isolation; they are the result of coordinated, collaborative efforts by individuals and organizations working to achieve common goals. Effective partnerships rely on the strengths each individual or organization brings to the group. One partner may have more financial resources; another may have an established network that can be easily mobilized. One may have more clout and thus be able to bring attention to the cause.

In addition, each organization's ability to advocate must be considered. As we noted earlier, employees of government agencies are restricted in how much and what types of advocacy and lobbying they are allowed to do. Nonprofit organizations (for example, community health organizations) tend to have fewer restrictions on advocacy and lobbying, and many for-profit organizations have paid lobbyists on staff or under contract.

When recruiting partners to advocate for health, examine what types of resources are needed, identify who or what organizations can bring those resources to the group, and then actively recruit the individuals or organizations. Consider all sectors of the community. Each sector can and perhaps should take an active role in advocating for health. Consider all traditional health allies, but also consider nontraditional partners: businesses, schools, faith-based organizations, youths, health care providers, elected officials, and community leaders. Be sure that partnerships represent the diversity of the community.

Establishing effective partnerships is a lot like establishing an effective relationship with a significant other. Individuals find each other and then spend time learning more about each other, including compatibility issues, commonality of goals, likes and dislikes, what each brings to the relationship (including excess baggage), and the amount of energy each is willing to expend to make the relationship successful and lasting. And like relationships, effective partnerships require care and maintenance.

Many effective public health advocacy campaigns are collaborations between national, state, and local partners. A good example of such a campaign began in 1991 when public health practitioners were encouraged to advocate for policy change as part of the National Cancer Institute's American Stop Smoking Intervention Study for Cancer Prevention (ASSIST) (National Cancer Institute, 2005). ASSIST was a demonstration project designed to bring public and private partners together to advocate for policies to prevent tobacco use and for tobacco control policies. On the national level, ASSIST was a joint effort of the National Cancer Institute (NCI) and the American Cancer Society (ACS). Both organizations had a common goal: to prevent cancer. NCI contracted with seventeen state health departments (SHDs) to hire staff and fund interventions, including advocating for policies that had shown promise in reducing and preventing tobacco use. ACS committed resources (time, dollars, and staff) to ASSIST at national, state, and local levels.

As in any relationship, dynamics and challenges had to be recognized and addressed. From the beginning, ASSIST was beset with challenges that may not have been anticipated. The project required two structurally and functionally different types of organizations (SHDs and ACS) to work together. Funding the SHDs and not the ACS units was perceived by some to cause inequity in power. Despite these and other challenges, effective ASSIST partnerships at national, state, and local levels were successful, and today, ASSIST is considered a best practice model for effecting policy change to reduce disease and death.

C. Everett Koop, then U.S. Surgeon General, believed ASSIST was successful in advancing his goal for a smoke-free society. In NCI's monograph *ASSIST: Shaping the Future of Tobacco Prevention and Control*, Koop states, "I have seen the important role that ASSIST leaders and coalitions played in advancing smoking cessation efforts and tobacco containment. They were in the vanguard of these efforts and helped to fashion the next phase of comprehensive tobacco control interventions." He further states, "In my estimation, several key points stand out as legacies of ASSIST," including "the strong emphasis on policy and media strategies to shift the focus from the individual to population-based interventions has had a long-lasting impact on behavioral health . . . and the lessons of ASSIST are broadly applicable to many public health disciplines." Koop goes on to say, "The lessons of ASSIST are essential to the tobacco prevention and control movement and, perhaps even more important, to the entire field of public health" (National Cancer Institute, 2005).

Since the end of ASSIST in 1999, the national tobacco control movement has grown to include all fifty states; territories; municipalities; numerous public and private for-profit and nonprofit organizations; and individuals—paid staff and volunteers from all walks of life—and has been successful in advocating for local, state, and national policies to prevent tobacco use, eliminate exposure to environmental tobacco smoke, and help people quit using tobacco.

## ADVOCACY METHODS

There are many advocacy methods, and new ways of advocating are being developed as times, technologies, and communication styles change. Only a few years ago, e-mail was not available to the masses, but it is now of tremendous use in advocacy efforts. Podcasts, blogs, and the move to more rapid transfer of information offer a host of opportunities for empowerment through advocacy.

### Talking Points

One of the first things that should be developed is a list of *talking points*, which can then be used in a variety of advocacy efforts such as a meeting with a legislator, developing a public service announcement, or writing a letter to the editor.

Talking points should be succinct, should stay on the topic, and should be developed with a specific message in mind. Collect and assemble facts on the health problem or issue. Concentrate on short, understandable, manageable facts that will aid a reader or listener in understanding the importance of the problem on a personal or local level. For example, when speaking about lung cancer in Alabama, pull out the figures on cancer in Alabama. Find the percentage of cancer deaths per annum in Alabama, the cost to Alabama for treatment of cancer and loss of revenue due to cancer, the figures that show the impact of cancer on the ability of Alabama facilities to handle all of their patients, and other relevant statistics.

Different points might be accentuated for different groups. The development of talking points can actually aid in the development of a strategy for an advocacy campaign. Once the list of talking points is developed, use them in developing the other advocacy methods.

### Newspaper Editorial Pages

Newspapers' editorial pages include letters to the editor and op-ed articles. Typically, these appear in both print and online versions of most papers, allowing them to be e-mailed to a person, which is a plus. Writing either a letter to the editor or an op-ed requires preparation. Use the talking points in writing your piece. A letter to the editor employs the principles of persuasive letter writing in that it has three basic parts. In the first portion, or introduction, the writer introduces the reader to the problem and provides a *hook* that will encourage the reader to continue reading. The second portion guides the reader through an understanding of the problem or issue. Here, it is wise to use a couple of facts, which can be taken from the talking points that have already been developed. The third portion of the letter may be a call to action or a suggestion for resolution of the problem. Good guidelines for writing letters to the editor can be found on the Web sites of the American Public Health Association (APHA) and the University of Kansas's Community Toolbox (see Table 7.2).

Letters to the editor are regularly read by staffers of legislators. These letters are considered key items in helping federal and state representatives to understand activities in their home district. Be aware that letters to the editor are important forms of advocacy to policymakers. The editorial page (where the letters are found) is also read by the features editors and news editors of the publishing paper and other newspapers. Media coverage is frequently generated as a result of a letter to the editor. Finally, average citizens read letters to the editor.

Another way to reach the audience of the editorial page is an op-ed. An op-ed is a short article that expresses the views of the writer on a topic. An op-ed is typically 750 words and may contradict remarks that have been made by the editor. Sometimes opposing views are sought and run on the same editorial page. These persuasive arguments are often written by subject matter experts or well-known writers. Spend a little time perusing the editorial pages of major newspapers to get a sense of the importance of op-eds.

## Letters, E-Mails, and Phone Calls

A letter to a key policymaker has elements of persuasion similar to those of a letter to the editor or an op-ed piece, but a few additional tips may prove useful. First, be certain to properly address the letter to a congressperson—use *The Honorable* rather than *Mr.* or *Ms.* Second, the letter should be short and to the point. Examine your talking points for ideas about how to address concerns and spark the interest of the policymaker or her aide. Third, look at the preceding paragraphs about writing a letter to the editor to aid you in thinking about the construction of a letter to a legislator. The APHA Web site (see Table 7.2) provides sample letters to congresspersons.

Sometimes it is necessary to send a letter to a policymaker through the U.S. mail. Seek permission to use your organization's letterhead (if appropriate).

However, keep in mind that since the anthrax attacks of 2001, U.S. mail is delayed by thorough inspections, so e-mails, faxes, and phone calls are preferred and are more quickly received by staffers.

## Public Service Announcements

Public service announcements (PSAs) are part of the public relations toolbox of health educators. PSAs aid in advertising events but may also advocate a specific perspective or action in regard to a health problem. Some PSAs are used to heighten awareness of a health problem. Radio and television airwaves are owned by the public, and television and radio stations must pay for their use of the airwaves by giving back a certain amount of public service time. So, if there is upcoming legislation that would positively affect HIV funding, for example, it makes sense to write a PSA that will heighten awareness about the issue. It is indirect advertising, and the legislation cannot be discussed, but heightened awareness will be helpful in passage.

PSAs are discussed at various points in the training process for health educators. Remember that all good news articles, feature articles, and PSAs tell some kind of story. All good news stories address the five W's (*who, what, where, when, why*) and *how*. Some individuals would add *wow* to that list. Use one of the statistics pulled from the talking points to punctuate the wow factor of the PSA.

## Press Conferences

Press conferences begin with a short statement, which is then followed by a series of questions from the press. The short statement should contain information about the health issue, some facts that will be of immediate interest to the press, and a sound bite for the evening news. Keep in mind that the sound bite that will be the hook for viewers frames the issue and increases the chances that people will discuss it in appropriate terms. The purpose of a press conference is to raise public awareness about a topic, so make the issue relevant to the viewers of the show or the listeners of the radio station.

All members of the press should be provided with a press packet that contains a copy of the prepared statement, fact sheets, other relevant materials, and a business card or contact information. Keep a cell phone close by, check e-mail, and promptly answer all questions over the course of the days following a press conference. Be available, reliable, and ready with answers to questions, and stay on message.

## Blogs

*Blog* is an abbreviation of *weblog*. A blog is an online diary or journal, but many are rapidly evolving to more sophisticated journals that include vlogs (video logs), podcasts, and other video items. Blogs tend to provide commentary or news on a particular subject. Many blogs allow the interactive feature of receiving commentary from readers. More and more journalists have blogs, which creates an interesting blurring of the line between objective journalism and subjective chronicling of the issues of the day. Many people read blogs and accept these diary postings as factually correct. Blogs can be most effective for communicating with advocates and supporters about current information and resources important to the health-related change and action being sought through the advocacy efforts.

## Meetings with Legislators

The classic advocacy method is meeting in person with legislators in their offices. Many believe it is the most effective method. In preparing to meet with a legislator, there are a few things to keep in mind: Consider that dozens of visitors may be coming in to ask for a favor, a vote, or some other action. Everyone has an argument, a cause, and a reason why their request trumps all others. The other visitors may have long-standing connections with the official. (Tips on how to forge such a connection are provided later in the chapter.)

The four P's of marketing (see Chapter Three) provide the basic elements of a marketing campaign. Similarly, we have developed a basic approach to meetings that we call the four P's of advocacy: preparation, prioritization, punctuality, and politeness:

1. **Preparation**. Preparation for meetings with legislators should be as thorough as preparation for a job interview. Prepare a set of talking points to inform your conversation. Prioritize the talking points, and leave a list of facts with the government official. Remember to begin the conversation with the most salient point. During the preparation phase, information about the policymaker's viewpoints and personal background may come to light. If you are advocating for an increase in cancer education funding, it may be advantageous to know that the senator's mother has cancer. The best preparation for the meeting, however, occurs far in advance of the actual appointment. Over time, it is wise to aid the policymaker with fact checking and with education and information, by sending him news on triumphs of local and state health programs and apprising him of changes in health activities in the community. The policymaker will view this help as the work of a trusted friend and expert on health.

2. **Prioritization**. Earlier, we mentioned that talking points should be prioritized. Change the order of the discussion of the talking points depending on the elected official. The prioritization of talking points in a meeting may be informed by viewing the voting record of the elected official. The APHA

advocacy Web site provides the voting records of Congressional leaders on health issues (see Table 7.2). Choose the order of talking points to address in your meeting on the basis of research on the official's voting record and personal interests. In persuasive argument, it is wise to consider the audience receiving the message.

3. **Punctuality**. First, be punctual. Arrive early and check in with the assistant. Use this punctuality principle during the meeting. Stay on task; don't overstay your welcome; and be certain to use time to your advantage in advancing your goal. If you are asking for increased funding for school health programs, don't waste time complaining about the potholes in the roads. Talking about the potholes is off point, wastes the elected official's time, and will give the official the option of solving the problem of the potholes rather than increasing funding for school health programs.

4. **Politeness**. An air of politeness should underlie all proceedings of the day. Citizens do pay the salaries of elected officials, but that does not mean that employees should be treated rudely. Don't react in a rude manner if the official does not respond in the desired manner. Make all your points in a dignified, forthright manner, and provide statistics the policymaker may be able to use in the decision-making process. It may not appear that the elected official is listening, but that observation may be in error. This meeting may not achieve its desired outcome, but it may aid subsequent successful dealings with this government worker. President Ronald Reagan was known for arguing with Democratic leaders during the day and having friendly dinners with them at night. Holding a grudge rarely helps in any interaction with others, and this is particularly true in politics. When the meeting ends, thank the elected official or aide, send a follow-up thank-you note, and provide promised materials immediately.

## Building Relationships with the Media

The best time to begin advocacy efforts is prior to any kind of crisis. It is better to begin building a team of journalists, legislators, and stalwart supporters long before the problem is the issue of the day. Wallack, Dorfman, Jernigan, and Themba (1993), writing about media advocacy, inform readers that their advocacy efforts will not be taken seriously unless they take the media seriously. One way to do that is by applying the four P's to interactions with members of the media: be prepared, prioritize all remarks, be punctual, and be polite.

Be certain to contact and compliment a reporter when a good health story appears in the newspaper. When an error is noted, be polite in making the necessary correction, and volunteer to be a fact checker in the future. Make a list of reporters who are friendly to health issues, and work to keep up a relationship with each of those reporters. If contacted by someone in the media, respond immediately. Let reporters know about emerging health issues, and help them to see the local angle. This preparation and politeness will help in future advocacy efforts. Media advocacy will aid in promoting local health programs and in advancing an advocacy agenda (Wallack & Dorfman, 1996).

Whenever possible, give reporters (and legislators) a local peg. What percentage of the local population is affected by cancer? Use *social math* to help people to conceptualize problems in real terms, although it does have a somewhat sensational element. For example, instead of saying that 400,000 people will die of tobacco-related disorders each year, the fact sheet on the APHA Web site states that this is the equivalent of losing the population of a number of towns. Use a list of the populations of nearby towns to formulate a local example.

It is helpful to think like a journalist. Be aware of their need to sell the story to an editor and to the public. Be aware of deadlines, keep the focus of the story on the journalist's priority population, and conform to guidelines. When pitching a story to local media, imagine a fifteen-second elevator ride in which the health problem or cause must be explained to a stranger. This exercise will help narrow the topic because it will force you to choose your words very carefully. Think about the hook for the story, and succinctly deliver the most important parts of the message. Writing the elevator speech will also serve the purpose of framing the issue. Framing the issue, according to Wallack, Woodruff, Dorfman, and Diaz (1999), helps to construct the delivery of the message around the message for delivery.

## ADVOCACY AND TECHNOLOGY

Rapid technology advances and changes in forms of communication have resulted in the use of new techniques that provide opportunities for advocacy and political action that move far beyond the opportunities in print media. The Internet has opened up ways to communicate with diverse audiences (Temple, 1999). This tremendous ability to communicate with large numbers of people can be seen in today's large-scale organizing efforts. Although a great deal of these efforts appear to be top-down organizing (for example, political campaigns), there are signs of grassroots organizing efforts that use the Internet.

Blogs, vlogs, e-mails, blog carnivals (blog articles with links pointing to more blog articles on a particular topic), Twitter, social networking sites (for example, Facebook, LinkedIn), and podcasts are ways to reach large numbers of people very quickly. Smart phone platforms and other handheld communication devices are causing an uptick in cyber-activism. Advocacy alerts and activities can be introduced so quickly after a news event that it is increasingly difficult to discern which came first—the advocacy effort or the issue itself. The next changes in communication technology are for the omniscient to predict. Irrespective of the latest technology, efforts in health advocacy must be led by a skilled, educated, and enthusiastic group of health promotion program staff, stakeholders, and participants.

## SUMMARY

Advocacy is a set of actions used by individuals and groups to create supportive environments for health promotion programs through organizational or legislative change. Advocacy for funding, legislation, regulations, governmental infrastructure, services, or research aids in ensuring successful health promotion programs. Advocacy is an important part of implementation for a health promotion program and, thus, an important skill in health promotion. When advocacy efforts are successful, awareness of a disease or risk behavior is heightened, funding for health promotion programs is increased, or legislation that creates an environment in which good health can be attained is created.

It is important to engage in advocacy activities that are acceptable to one's employer. Understanding the difference between advocacy and lobbying and what is acceptable to different employers is critical in protecting employers from difficulties due to tax code violations.

Effective communication and organizing at the program site are fundamental skills of health advocacy. Communicating with large groups of people can be accomplished, for example, through letters to the editor, public service announcements, or blogs. Mobilizing individuals for change is based on communicating with people but also on helping individuals see the relevance of a health topic to their own life. Successful advocacy efforts have education, motivation, and action as critical components of the work.

## FOR PRACTICE AND DISCUSSION

1. Go to the Web site of a community health organization (a 501(c)(3) organization) and locate the mission of the organization. Has the organization defined an advocacy agenda? If the answer is yes, does the advocacy agenda have clear underpinnings in the mission statement of the organization? Have action steps (or activities) been assigned to the advocacy agenda? If the organization does not have an advocacy agenda create one. For both situations (with and without an advocacy agenda) discuss strategies and action steps that will help with the advocacy agenda of the organization.

2. Several of the health theories from Chapter Three (Table 3.10) were mentioned early in this chapter. How might these be used to shape and influence the advocacy agenda of a health promotion program during the implementation phase?

3. Have you, a family member, or friend ever participated in advocacy work? If so, describe what these advocacy efforts were. Were the efforts successful? How was success evaluated? What observations or tips would you give to others who are interested in performing advocacy work?

4. Do you agree that people working in health promotion programs have an ethical responsibility to engage in advocacy work? What is the role of health researchers in advocacy work? Are there ethical considerations for health researchers who want to become involved in advocacy work?

5. Define (using reliable sources) the word *activism*. Can you describe differences between advocacy work and activism? Give examples of different types of advocacy and activism initiatives. Would participation in any of these affect your job security? If so, describe how this work would affect your employment.

6. Consider a health problem in your local community. How would you frame the issue in such a way as to gain maximum media attention? Outline a media advocacy campaign with a timeline. What benchmarks would you use to measure success, and how would successes or failures affect your advocacy strategy?

## KEY TERMS

Advocacy

Advocacy agenda

Appropriations

Authorizations

Bill

Direct lobbying

Electioneering

Elevator speech

501(c)(3)

Grassroots lobbying

Hook

Law

Letter to the editor

Media advocacy

Mothers Against Drunk
  Driving (MADD)

Op-ed

Ordinance

Public service announce-
  ments (PSAs)

Talking points

## REFERENCES

Allegrante, J. P., Barry, M. M., Airhihenbuwa, C. O., Auld, M. E., Collins, J. L., Lamarre, M., et al. (2009). Domains of core competency standards and quality assurance for building global capacity in health promotion: The Galway Consensus Conference Statement. *Health Education & Behavior, 6*(3), 476–482.

Centers for Disease Control and Prevention. (1999). Ten great public health achievements—United States, 1900–1999. *Morbidity and Mortality Weekly Reports, 48*(12), 241–243.

Chaney, J. D., Jones, E., & Galer-Unti, R. A. (2003). Using technology in advocacy efforts to aid in tobacco policy and politics. *Health Promotion Practice, 4,* 218–224.

Christoffel, K. K. (2000). Public health advocacy: Process and product. *American Journal of Public Health, 90,* 722–726.

DeJong, W. (1996). MADD Massachusetts versus Senator Burke: A media advocacy case study. *Health Education Quarterly, 23,* 318–329.

Freudenberg, N. (1982). Health education for social change: A strategy for public health in the U.S. *International Journal of Health Education, 24,* 138–145.

Givel, M., & Glantz, S. A. (2004). The "global settlement" with the tobacco industry: 6 years later. *American Journal of Public Health, 94,* 218–224.

Howze, E. H., & Redman, L. J. (1992). The uses of theory in health advocacy: Policies and programs. *Health Education Quarterly, 19,* 369–383.

Institute of Medicine. (2003). *Who will keep the public healthy? Educating public health professionals for the 21st century.* Washington, DC: National Academies Press.

March of Dimes. (n.d.). *About us.* Retrieved May 25, 2009, from http://www.marchofdimes.com/789_821.asp.

National Cancer Institute. (2005). *ASSIST: Shaping the future of tobacco prevention and control* (Tobacco Control Monograph No. 16; NIH Publication No. 05-5645.). Bethesda, MD: U.S. Department of Health and Human Services, National Institutes of Health, National Cancer Institute.

Ogden, H. G. (1986). The politics of health education: Do we constrain ourselves? *Health Education Quarterly, 13,* 1–7.

Roe, K. M., Minkler, M., & Saunders, F. F. (1995). Combining research, advocacy, and education: The methods of the Grandparent Caregiver Study. *Health Education Quarterly, 22,* 458–475.

Steckler, A., & Dawson, L. (1982). The role of health education in public policy development. *Health Education Quarterly, 9,* 275–292.

Temple, M. (1999). How to effectively use the Internet for advocacy. *Health Education Monograph Series, 17*(2), 32–35.

2000 Joint Committee on Health Education and Promotion Terminology. (2002). Report of the 2000 Joint Committee on Health Education and Promotion Terminology. *Journal of School Health, 72,* 3–7.

U.S. Department of Health and Human Services. (2009). *Healthy People.* Retrieved November 11, 2009, from www.healthypeople.gov.

Vernick, J. S. (1999). Lobbying and advocacy for the public's health: What are the limits for nonprofit organizations? *American Journal of Public Health, 89,* 1425–1429.

Wallack, L., & Dorfman, L. (1996). Media advocacy: A strategy for advancing policy and promoting health. *Health Education Quarterly, 23,* 293–317.

Wallack, L., Dorfman, L., Jernigan, D., & Themba, M. (1993). *Media advocacy and public health: Power for prevention.* Thousand Oaks, CA: Sage.

Wallack, L., Woodruff, K., Dorfman, L., & Diaz, I. (1999). *News for a change: An advocate's guide to working with the media.* Thousand Oaks, CA: Sage.

# CHAPTER EIGHT

# COMMUNICATING HEALTH INFORMATION EFFECTIVELY

NEYAL J. AMMARY-RISCH

ALLISON ZAMBON

KELLI MCCORMACK BROWN

## LEARNING OBJECTIVES

- Discuss the importance of various modes of health communication in the adoption, cessation, and maintenance of individual health behavior

- Describe health literacy in terms of contributing factors, vulnerable populations, message construction and format, and media considerations

- Describe the components of an effective health communication plan from development through implementation

- Explain why pretesting concepts and materials is important to health information campaign implementation

THE OPTIONS for communicating health information through a health promotion program are changing with each new wave of technological advances. Instant messaging has been replaced by texting, which in turn may be eclipsed by tweeting. Social networking sites (for example, Facebook, Yahoo groups, LinkedIn) have expanded beyond individuals in their twenties and thirties to include elementary school students, business users, and senior citizens well into their eighties and nineties. However, with all the advances in the ways that people communicate, the concerns and challenges of effective health communication have grown greater. Decisions about health are personal. Often, individuals make health decisions on the basis of critical small pieces of information communicated to them by a health professional (for example, health promotion program staff) either personally or through some type of media (for example, a brochure, information sheet, video, podcast, or Web site).

Effective health communication, similar to advocacy (discussed in the preceding chapter), is a thread that runs through all the phases of a program. In the planning phases, needs assessment reports and ways of sharing program decisions about mission, goals, objectives, interventions, policies, and procedures shape people's perceptions of a program before it even starts. During program implementation, effectively communicating health information to program participants, stakeholders, and staff is an important part of a health promotion program. In the evaluation phases, effective health communication is critical to dissemination of program evaluation results and findings in order to build program sustainability. In addition, effective, culturally appropriate health communications are an essential component of health promotion programs that seek to eliminate health disparities. Culturally appropriate communication includes assessing participants' health information needs and learning from them the most appropriate and meaningful way (channel) of communicating health information to them. Being proactive in attending to program participants' health information needs and health literacy level, implementing an overall communication plan for the program, and paying particular attention to the development of communication materials (for example, through pretesting) are three actions that will help program staff to ensure the delivery of effective health communications to program participants, staff, and stakeholders.

## COMMUNICATION IN HEALTH PROMOTION PROGRAMS

Health communication has its roots in the communication theory that was discussed in Chapter Three (Table 3.10). *Health communication* is defined as the art and technique of informing, influencing, and motivating individual, institutional, and public audiences about important health issues (U.S. Department of Health and Human

Services, Steps to a Healthier US, 2004). It has been described further as "a multifaceted and multidisciplinary approach to reach different audiences and share health-related information with the goal of influencing, engaging and supporting individuals, communities, health professionals, special groups, policy makers and the public to champion, introduce, adopt, or sustain a behavior, practice or policy that will ultimately improve health outcomes" (Schiavo, 2007). Exhibit 8.1 lists the attributes of effective health communication that were identified in *Healthy People 2010*.

Understanding and using principles of health communication, program staff can craft and deliver health messages in a way that is meaningful and appropriate for the audience the program is trying to reach. All too often, well-intended and seemingly clear health communications leave unanswered questions that may have unintended negative consequences (see Exhibit 8.2). Knowing that people are frequently making important and complicated health decisions with only the written or oral instructions of a health professional has added urgency to the creation of effective health communications.

The practice of effective health communication contributes to health promotion and disease prevention. For example, through the training of health promotion staff and program participants in effective communication skills, the interpersonal and group interactions in a program can be improved. Collaborative relationships are enhanced when all parties are capable of good communication. Likewise, the dissemination of health messages through health promotion programs and campaigns can create awareness of an issue, change attitudes toward a health behavior, and encourage and motivate individuals to follow recommended health behaviors. While health communication alone cannot change behavior, understanding its role and how its principles can be used in a health promotion program will increase the likelihood that a program will succeed.

## What Is Health Literacy?

The U.S. health care system forces people to be active consumers of health care. People are increasingly responsible for making their own decisions about their health. They are challenged with seeking and understanding health information, communicating with their providers, managing and monitoring their own diseases, maintaining good health, navigating the health care system, filling out insurance forms, signing informed consent forms, seeking out options of and access to care, acting as caregivers, comprehending medications and correct dosages, advocating for their health or the health of loved ones—and the list goes on.

With these many challenges, health literacy skills become a major factor in determining a successful outcome. Although experts are still debating the single

**EXHIBIT 8.1**
**Attributes of Effective Health Communication**

**Accuracy:** The content is valid and without errors of fact, interpretation, or judgment.

**Availability:** The content (whether targeted message or other information) is delivered or placed where the audience can access it. Placement varies according to audience, message complexity, and purpose, ranging from interpersonal and social networks to billboards and mass transit signs to prime-time TV or radio, to public kiosks (print or electronic), to the Internet.

**Balance:** Where appropriate, the content presents the benefits and risks of potential actions or recognizes different and valid perspectives on the issue.

**Consistency:** The content remains internally consistent over time and also is consistent with information from other sources (the latter is a problem when other widely available content is not accurate or reliable).

**Cultural competence:** The design, implementation, and evaluation process that accounts for special issues for select population groups (for example, ethnic, racial, and linguistic) and also educational levels and disability.

**Evidence base:** Relevant scientific evidence that has undergone comprehensive review and rigorous analysis to formulate practice guidelines, performance measures, review criteria, and technology assessments for telehealth applications.

**Reach:** The content gets to or is available to the largest possible number of people in the target population.

**Reliability:** The source of the content is credible, and the content itself is kept up to date.

**Repetition:** The delivery of/access to the content is continued or repeated over time, both to reinforce the impact with a given audience and to reach new generations.

**Timeliness:** The content is provided or available when the audience is most receptive to, or in need of, the specific information.

**Understandability:** The reading or language level and format (including multimedia) are appropriate for the specific audience.

*Source:* U.S. Department of Health and Human Services, 2000.

definition of *health literacy*, the most commonly accepted definition is the degree to which individuals have the capacity to obtain, process, and understand basic health information and services needed to make appropriate health decisions (Selden, Zorn, Ratzan, & Parker, 2000; U.S. Department of Health and Human

**EXHIBIT 8.2**
Example of the Need for Plain but Comprehensive
Health Communication

A two-year-old is diagnosed with an inner ear infection and prescribed an antibiotic. Her mother understands that her daughter should take the prescribed medication twice a day. After carefully studying the label on the bottle and deciding that it doesn't tell how to take the medicine, she fills a teaspoon and pours the antibiotic into her daughter's painful ear.

*Source:* Parker, Ratzan, & Lurie, 2003.

Services, 2000). Because the word *literacy* is included in the phrase, people often mistakenly think that health literacy is an issue of concern only for those who cannot read or write. However, health literacy expands beyond reading and writing skills to include the ability to comprehend and assess health information in order to make informed decisions about healthy behaviors, self-care, and disease management (U.S. Department of Health and Human Services, Steps to a Healthier US, 2004; Zarcadoolas, Pleasant, & Greer, 2003).

A range of factors contribute to health literacy. They include social and individual factors such as cultural and conceptual knowledge and listening, speaking, arithmetical, writing, and reading skills (Nielsen-Bohlman, Panzer, & Kindig, 2004). Studies have shown that individuals with inadequate health literacy report less knowledge about their medical conditions and treatment, worse health status, less understanding and use of preventive services, and a higher rate of hospitalization than those with marginal or adequate health literacy (Nielsen-Bohlman, Panzer, & Kindig, 2004; Berkman et al., 2004).

Health literacy is often talked about in terms of the individual. However, health care providers, public health professionals, policymakers, and health care and public health systems are also responsible for health literacy. Although individuals' health literacy skills and capacities can be linked to their own education level, culture, or language, it is also important to acknowledge the role of the communication and assessment skills of those whom people interact with in regard to their health, as well as the ability of the media, the marketplace, and the government to provide health information in a manner appropriate to the audience (Nielsen-Bohlman, Panzer, & Kindig, 2004).

## Who Is Most Likely to Have Low Health Literacy?

People most likely to experience low health literacy fall into the following groups (Nielsen-Bohlman, Panzer, & Kindig, 2004):

- Older adults
- Racial and ethnic minorities
- People with low education levels
- People with low income levels
- Non-native speakers of English
- People with compromised health status

These populations often have the greatest health care needs and the highest rates of chronic diseases, but low health literacy can limit their ability to comprehend health information, navigate the health care system, or manage their own diseases and conditions.

Low health literacy is particularly common among older adults. The high prevalence of low health literacy in older adults is of particular concern because they are the most likely to have chronic conditions such as diabetes, cardiovascular disease, or cancer. Approximately 80 percent of Americans aged 65+ in 2005 have at least one chronic condition, and 50 percent have at least two (He, Sengupta, Velkoff, & DeBarrow, 2005).

Although low health literacy predominantly affects more vulnerable populations, it continues to grow as a problem for all Americans as our health care system becomes increasingly complex and technologically advanced. Even well-educated individuals can have difficulty understanding or acting on health information, for reasons that vary. A person's age, race, ethnicity, language, disability, or even emotional state when hearing or reading health information can affect health literacy.

## Literacy and Health Literacy in the United States

The scope of the health literacy problem is far reaching. The National Adult Literacy Survey (NALS) found that approximately 90 million adults, half of the U.S. population, lack the literacy skills necessary to effectively use the U.S. health system (Kirsch, Jungeblut, Jenkins, & Kolstad, 1993). Health literacy issues can affect people of all backgrounds, but it is particularly burdensome for those with low literacy to try to read and understand health-related information. Most health information is written at or above the tenth-grade reading level, yet the average reading level of people in the United States is eighth grade, and 20 percent of the population reads at or below the fifth-grade level (Kirsch, Jungeblut, Jenkins, & Kolstad, 1993). The NALS also discovered that 50 percent of African Americans and Hispanics read at or below the fifth-grade level. Given the disproportionate rates of chronic diseases in these populations, the need for clear, easy-to-read health information is evident.

The 2003 National Assessment of Adult Literacy (NAAL) included the first-ever national assessment of health literacy of adults in the United States, based on this definition of health literacy: "the ability to use printed and written information associated with a broad range of goals at home, in the workplace, and in the community (including healthcare settings)" (Kutner, Greenberg, Jin, & Paulsen, 2006). Results were reported in terms of four literacy levels: below basic, basic, intermediate, and proficient. *Below basic* means that the person has, at most, only the most simple and concrete health literacy skills. *Basic* means that the person has the skills necessary to perform simple and everyday health literacy activities. *Intermediate* means that the person has the skills necessary to perform moderately challenging health literacy activities. *Proficient* means that the person has the skills necessary to perform more complex and challenging health literacy activities. Findings indicated that the majority of adults (53 percent) had intermediate health literacy, meaning that they could do things like determine the healthy weight range for a person of a specific height on a body mass index chart or determine the times when it would be correct for a person to take a prescribed medication after reading the label. About 22 percent had basic health literacy, meaning that they could do things like read a clearly written brochure and then identify reasons that a person with no symptoms of a specific disease should be tested for it anyway. And 14 percent had below basic health literacy, meaning that they were able to do things like circle the date on a medical appointment slip or identify how often a person should have a specific medical test after reading a clearly written pamphlet (Kutner, Greenberg, Jin, & Paulsen, 2006).

The 2003 NAAL also examined where adults get information about health issues. Kutner, Greenberg, Jin, and Paulsen (2006) found that adults with below basic or basic health literacy were less likely than adults with higher health literacy to get information about health issues from written sources (newspapers, magazines, books, brochures, or the Internet) and more likely than adults with higher health literacy to get a lot of information about health issues from radio and television. These findings are important because they can help to determine the best communication channels to use in reaching out to a specific target audience. Written brochures or pamphlets are often not the best way to provide people with health information, particularly those who are more likely to have low health literacy.

## Plain Language and Other Strategies to Improve Health Literacy

Presenting information in plain language (or plain English) is an integral component of improving health literacy. *Plain language* has many definitions, but it is fundamentally defined as communication that the audience can understand the first time they read or hear it. Written material in plain language means that the members of an audience can

- Find what they need
- Understand what they find
- Use what they find to meet their needs

While definitions vary, the essence of plain language is a focus on the audience, clarity, and comprehension. Using clear and concrete words in a straightforward manner is the best way to organize information, particularly health content. Take, for example, the messages in Exhibit 8.3, which shows how information about exercise was rewritten, using clear, concise words.

All people can benefit from information in plain language, but it is especially important when communicating with people with low health literacy. *Plain language* refers not only to the specific words that are used but also to *how* information is presented. Figure 8.1 is an example of a health education resource for people with diabetes that uses plain language techniques. Here are a few of the techniques the

---

### EXHIBIT 8.3
### Example of Text Before and After Rewriting in Plain Language

**Before**

The Dietary Guidelines for Americans recommends a half hour or more of moderate physical activity on most days, preferably every day. The activity can include brisk walking, calisthenics, home care, gardening, moderate sports exercise, and dancing.

**After**

Do at least 30 minutes of exercise, like brisk walking, most days of the week.

--------

*Source*: PlainLanguage.gov, n.d.

FIGURE 8.1   Health Education Resource for People with
Diabetes That Uses Plain Language Techniques

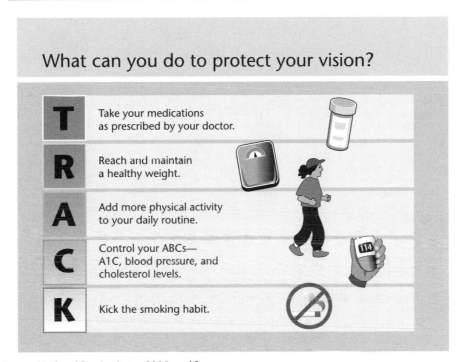

## What can you do to protect your vision?

**T** Take your medications
as prescribed by your doctor.

**R** Reach and maintain
a healthy weight.

**A** Add more physical activity
to your daily routine.

**C** Control your ABCs—
A1C, blood pressure, and
cholesterol levels.

**K** Kick the smoking habit.

*Source*: National Eye Institute, 2005, p. 18.

figure uses to present information that is visually appealing, logically organized, and comprehensible:

- Use ample white space. Break up dense amounts of text. Keep sentences short.
- Use clear headings and bullets. Try using question-and-answer formats with straightforward answers.
- Use the active voice and strong verbs.
- Avoid medical jargon, and use conversational language.
- Use a design that increases comprehension. Include pictures or graphics that are visually appealing to illustrate examples or important points.
- Supplement written materials with audiovisual materials or conversation.

For many more examples and tips on using plain language and improving communication, visit PlainLanguage.gov: *Improving Communication from the Federal Government to the Public* (www.PlainLanguage.gov).

Many other strategies can be effective in communicating with people with low health literacy, particularly people with chronic conditions, whose health relies heavily on their self-care skills and abilities. For example, successful strategies for communicating with people with diabetes have included selecting critical behaviors to focus on; reducing the complexity of information given; using clear, concrete examples; concentrating on single topics at a time; avoiding medical jargon; and using teach-back methods (Rothman et al., 2004). Using teach-back methods in the health care setting can be particularly helpful in identifying any misunderstandings a patient may have. In this technique, after patients are given instructions, they are asked to explain back how they'll take a particular medication or follow other instructions. Similar strategies can be used in teaching self-care skills for a variety of diseases and conditions in which individuals play a central role. When people are able to fully understand and act on health information, they are better able to manage their conditions and make healthy decisions.

## DEVELOPING A COMMUNICATION PLAN FOR A SITE

Health communication is an integral part of health promotion programs. It is recommended that each program have a communication plan to guide and develop information exchange between and among the program staff, stakeholders, and participants as the program is implemented. Program staff need to take responsibility for addressing issues of health literacy by communicating with intention and clarity in order to ensure that the program message is received and acted on in a manner that is consistent with the program's goals and objectives. Simply stated, program staff need to make sure that participants are hearing the messages and information that the program wants them to hear and that the information is being understood.

Plans can be formal or informal, but the important element is that a health promotion program has a consistent strategy for what information is communicated and how that communication will occur. Here are nine steps to follow in creating effective communication:

### Step 1: Understand the Problem

The needs assessment discussed in Chapter Four is the foundation for the communication plan. It provides a clear picture of the health problem or concern, the program's stakeholders and participants, and the program's priorities (National Cancer Institute, 2001). Likewise, the program's mission, goals, and interventions (see Chapter Five) provide a context and framework for developing materials and deciding what is to be communicated. The final part of this step is a review of existing materials and identification of any gaps in the type of media or communication activities used, intended audiences targeted, or messages conveyed. All of these factors should be considered and included as part of the communication plan.

## Step 2: Define Communication Objectives

Communication objectives define what the staff hope to articulate in a program's health communications. Defining the objectives assists with setting priorities. As Chapter Five discusses, it is important to set objectives that are measurable and achievable. Exhibit 8.4 provides some examples of well-written communication objectives. In many instances, it is unrealistic to expect a complete change as the result of one program. Objectives should be

- Aligned with the program's goals
- Realistic and reasonable
- Specific to the change desired, the population to be affected, and the time period during which change should occur
- Measurable, in order to track progress
- Prioritized, to aid in allocation of resources (National Cancer Institute, 2001)

**Exhibit 8.4**
**Sample Communication Objectives**

- By the end of the stress management program, 90 percent of participants at this work site will have received stress reduction brochures and one-page tip sheets.
- After this campaign, 90 percent of the families with children younger than age three in Montgomery County will have received information on childhood immunization.
- By the end of the school year, two public service announcements on physical activity will be developed and viewed in at least three physical education classes at ten different middle schools in the county.
- After attending a three-session course on self-management of diabetes, 75 percent of the participants will be able to report their daily blood sugar results via the Web site of the health promotion program.

## Step 3: Learn About the Intended Audiences

The audience may already be defined by the location of the health promotion program, or there may be several audiences. The goal in this step is to learn as much as possible about the individuals who make up the target audience in order to tailor the program most effectively. Audience segmentation and formative research can help in this process.

*Audience segmentation* is the division of priority populations into subgroups that share similar qualities or characteristics (Thackeray & Brown, 2005). Populations can be divided into segments according to multiple factors, including geography, demographics, psychographic traits (for example, attitudes, beliefs, self-efficacy), behaviors, and readiness to change (National Cancer Institute, 2001). The goal is to segment the intended population on characteristics that are relevant to the health behavior to be changed and to organize the program's efforts around these groups of similar individuals (National Cancer Institute, 2001; Slater, Kelly, & Thackeray, 2006). In an example reported by Thackeray and Brown (2005), the audience for the national 5 A Day campaign to encourage people to eat more vegetables and fruits was segmented into the following groups: between the ages of twenty-five and fifty-five, have a busy and hectic lifestyle, cut corners in meal preparation, value convenience, are concerned about losing weight, or view cancer as the health problem to be most concerned about. The 5 A Day campaign was then tailored to these audience segments.

The goal of formative research is to describe the intended audience: who they are, what is important to them, what influences their behavior, and what would enable them to engage in the desired behavior (Thackeray & Brown, 2005). Formative research can also be used to determine how ready the intended audience is to change; what social or cultural factors may affect the program; when and where the audience can best be reached; what communication channels are preferred by the audience; and what learning styles, language, and tone the intended audience prefers (National Cancer Institute, 2001).

## Step 4: Select Communication Channels and Activities

To reach your program's intended audience, consider the settings, times, places, and states of mind in which they may be receptive to and able to act on the program's key message (National Cancer Institute, 2001). Then identify the *channels* (routes of message delivery) through which the program's message will be delivered and the activities that can be used to deliver it (National Cancer Institute, 2001). The following channel categories should be considered:

- *Interpersonal channels* are more likely to be trusted and put the message into a personal context. These channels include physicians and other health professionals, friends, family, and counselors. Examples of activities or methods for delivering the message within interpersonal channels are one-on-one counseling, telephone hotlines, informal discussions, and personal coaching and instruction. Interpersonal channels are the most effective for teaching and can be very influential, but they can also be time-consuming and expensive to use and can have a limited reach.

- *Group channels* can reach more of the intended audience while still retaining many of the positive aspects of interpersonal channels. Group channels include neighborhood groups, workplaces, churches, or clubs. The activities associated with these channels are classroom instructions, large and small group discussions, recreational and sporting events, and public meetings. As with communicating through interpersonal channels, working with groups requires significant levels of effort and can be time-consuming and expensive.

- *Community channels* involve working with community groups to conduct activities such as meetings, conferences, and other events to disseminate the program's message. Community channels can reach a large intended audience, may be familiar to the audience, may have influence with the audience, and can offer shared experiences. Community channels can also be time-consuming to establish. Another negative aspect is the possibility of losing control of the message if it has to be adapted to fit organizational needs.

- *Mass media campaigns* are a tried-and-true approach that has been used to spotlight many health promotion topics (National Cancer Institute, 2001). Mass media channels include but are not limited to newspapers, magazines, newsletters, radio, and television (Glanz, Rimer, & Lewis, 2002). These channels offer many opportunities for dissemination of a program's message.

- *Education entertainment* (a form of health communication in which educational content and information is intentionally incorporated into an entertainment format) is another powerful way to engage an audience, and studies have demonstrated that exposure to health information and behaviors through entertainment media can have strong effects (National Cancer Institute, 2001).

- *Interactive media* are communication technologies that can be used to reach multiple audiences. These technologies extend both the reach and depth of mass media (Glanz, Rimer, & Lewis, 2002). They include interactive CD-ROMs, webinars, online courses, electronic bulletin boards, newsgroups, chat rooms, blogs, e-mail, text messages, Listservs, podcasts, online videos and social networking sites (for example, Facebook and Twitter). The types of channels in this category are constantly changing and evolving. These technologies provide opportunities to overcome barriers such as low literacy by using audio and video to demonstrate desired health behavior or action, and they also offer a venue for more tailored communications such as videos produced for viewing at specific locations (for example, patient information videos shown at a health care organization) (Freimuth & Quinn, 2004). The technologies also allow outreach to large numbers of people, can be quickly updated with new information, and can provide health information in a graphically appealing and exciting way. Exhibit 8.5 details the VERB campaign's use of interactive media. Disadvantages of interactive media include expense (for example, the cost of individual electronic devices, user fees such as monthly telephone service charges), unsuitability if the intended audience lacks access to the Internet, and the fact that the intended audience must sign up or search for information on the program in order to receive the message.

## Exhibit 8.5
## VERB: An Example of the Use of Interactive Media

VERB was a media campaign that was run by the Centers for Disease Control and Prevention from 2002 to 2006. VERB used social marketing techniques to take action against the problem of sedentary lifestyles among youth. The VERB campaign used a mix of media strategies to become a presence in the lives of its audience ("tweens": kids aged nine to thirteen) at school, at home, and in the community. Television and radio spots, posters, print advertising, and a Web site where tweens could interact with celebrities and win prizes for being active were employed. During the summer of 2005, the VERB campaign added promotion via text messaging on cell phones. This segment of the campaign was called 8372, which spells *VERB* on a cell phone keypad. The goal of this campaign was similar to the original VERB goal but was more tailored to specific geographic locations; 8372 aimed to connect tweens in innovative ways with specific places and events in their local area where they could be physically active. The campaign used TV, the Internet, and cell phones:

- **TV:** Three commercials encouraged tweens to visit the Web site at www .8372.com.
- **Internet:** Once on the 8372 Web site, tweens could download an application in order to receive instant messages about local activities, participate in live webcasts with athletes, play games, enter contests, and win prizes.
- **Cell phones:** Tweens could sign up to receive text messages on their cell phone about campaign-sponsored promotions, tours, contests, and events in their zip code.

*Source:* Kaiser Family Foundation, 2006.

## Step 5: Develop Partnerships

Employing other organizations as partners is a useful and cost-effective method to broaden the reach of a program. Maibach, Van Duyn, & Bloodgood, (2006) explain that partners can serve as a "powerful and sustainable distribution channel." The foundation of the partnership approach is the value of collaboration between organizations that share common interests and reach diverse audiences in order to achieve outcomes that neither could achieve alone (Hasnain-Wynia, Margolina, & Bazzoli, 2001). Many organizations work with partners or intermediaries in order to reach their intended audience. In addition, partnerships can

- Provide more credibility for a program's message because the partner organization might be considered a trusted source for the intended audience.
- Increase the number of messages the program can share with the intended audience.
- Provide additional resources.
- Expand support for an organization's high-priority activities (National Cancer Institute, 2001).

Potential partner organizations should be identified and included in the health communication plan. Determine the roles that potential partners might play in the program, and include this information as well. Roles might include promoting and disseminating messages and materials, sponsoring publicity and promotion, advertising the program, providing use of communication materials, or evaluating the program.

## Step 6: Conduct Market Research to Refine Your Message and Materials

This step includes conducting market research and pretesting in order to determine the activities for each intended audience, messages for each market, and materials to be developed. The next section will go into greater detail on how to develop and test messages and materials.

## Step 7: Implement the Communication Plan

In this step, communication activities are integrated into the overall implementation of the health promotion program. At this time, it is important to ensure that all materials and communications that program stakeholders and participants receive are consistent with their health literacy. Likewise, it is important that all channels of communication be accessible, supported, and utilized. For example, if cell phone technology such as text messaging is to be used, all program participants need to have a cell phone or access to a cell phone and know how to receive and send text messages.

### Step 8: Review Tasks and Timeline

The timeline of the communication plan specifies what needs to be accomplished when. Detailing the tasks enables the work to be assigned and kept on schedule and allows resources to be allocated for each task. The timeline should be reviewed and adjusted as the program progresses. The communication plan timeline can be incorporated into the Gantt chart for the entire program (see Chapter Six).

### Step 9: Evaluate the Plan

Evaluation of the communication plan is part of the evaluation of a health promotion program (see Chapter Ten). Evaluation of a communication plan can focus on a number of issues—for example, utilization and penetration of the program communications (brochures, posters, activity materials, videos, and so on), satisfaction with the communications, or recommendations on how to improve the program materials and information. Table 8.1 provides an overview of communication plans for different sites, including their evaluation.

## DEVELOPING AND PRETESTING CONCEPTS, MESSAGES, AND MATERIALS

In the preceding section, the steps in developing and implementing a communication plan were explained. The topic of this section is step 6 of the process: conducting market research in order to develop effective messages and materials.

Communicating effectively to an audience (for example, program participants) is a key factor in developing successful health promotion programs. In communicating with the program participants, it is essential to know how the audience members view their health and what they are being asked to do (or not do). One way to understand different audiences and create programs, materials, and messages that resonate with them is to develop and pretest concepts, messages, and materials to see which ones have the most meaning for them and motivate them to take action.

TABLE 8.1  Examples of the Process of Planning Health Communication in Various Settings

| | School | Workplace | Health Care Organization | Community |
|---|---|---|---|---|
| Problem assessment | Data from the Youth Risk Behavior Survey suggest that bullying is an increasing problem in middle schools. | Human resource data suggest an increase in days off due to stress-related illness. | A local health care clinic in south Florida recently surveyed its clients and found that people with diabetes did not understand the importance of glucose control to their overall health. | Recent school data suggest that more children are entering school without the appropriate immunizations. |
| Objective | Decrease the incidence of bullying among sixth, seventh, and eighth graders by 30 percent, 25 percent, and 15 percent, respectively, within the next school year. | Decrease stress-related sick days by 10 percent over the next two years. | 75 percent of the clinic's patients with diabetes will attend a diabetes self-management class within the next twelve months. | By the beginning of the 2011 school year, 90 percent of the children entering public schools in Montgomery County, Maryland, will be appropriately immunized. |
| Intended audience | Middle school youths. | Secretarial workers. | Patients with diabetes. | Parents of children aged three and younger. |
| Channels and activities | School-wide posters. Safe Internet venues. Articles in PTA or PTO newsletter (targeting parents as secondary audience). School-wide curriculum on preventing bullying. | Tailored information sheets on stress. On-site yoga, Pilates, and meditation classes at no cost to employees. Peer-led brown bag lunches and forums to talk about how to overcome stress. | Posters in clinics. Personalized invitations to attend workshop. Workshop with child care provided and food provided for patient and family. Posters and written materials in three languages: English, Spanish, and Creole. | Newspaper articles and ads in national newspapers and community newspapers. Information sheets at pediatricians' offices and clinics that service children. Tray cover at McDonald's during key months. |

(Continued)

TABLE 8.1   Examples of the Process of Planning Health Communication in Various Settings (Continued)

| | School | Workplace | Health Care Organization | Community |
|---|---|---|---|---|
| Partners | Community youth development agencies.<br><br>After-school programs.<br><br>PTAs and PTOs.<br><br>High school and middle school students.<br><br>Feeder elementary schools. | Managerial staff.<br><br>Human resources. | All health care providers and staff in clinic.<br><br>Local grocery store chain.<br><br>Glucose monitor company's local representative. | Pediatricians.<br><br>Clinics that serve children.<br><br>Local McDonald's franchises. |
| Development and implementation | Create a plan that includes activities across all three grade levels and feeder schools. | Create a staff advisory committee to develop a series of fact sheets and workshops for staff over a twelve-month period. | Develop and deliver interactive workshops.<br><br>Deliver workshops on a variety of days and times, and offer some in Spanish and Creole. | Work with local pediatrician association, and inform members of places where children can receive free or reduced-cost immunizations. |
| Evaluation | By the start of the third grading period:<br><br>Posters developed, tested, and distributed at school and community sites.<br><br>Two articles in PTA newsletter.<br><br>Bullying information sheet distributed to 100 percent of students. | By January 15:<br><br>Stress reduction tip sheets available.<br><br>Class brochures developed, tested, and distributed.<br><br>Announcement template for lunch forum developed. | By March 1:<br><br>Trilingual posters developed, tested, and distributed.<br><br>Template for personalized invitation developed, tested, and used. | By the first day of school in fall:<br><br>All materials (articles, ads, fact sheets, and tray covers) developed and tested.<br><br>By Thanksgiving: All materials distributed in the fall months. |

## What Is Pretesting?

Knowing which messages are most salient to the intended audience is one critical component of a successful intervention or program. Pretesting should be used in developing new materials, revising existing materials, and developing messages and concepts. Pretesting materials and messages can assist in discovering how the audience members will respond to a message, whether they will read the materials and act appropriately, and how the messages will be received.

## Why Pretest?

Before describing the steps in detail, it is important to understand why pretesting is important and to consider some challenges or resistant attitudes that might occur when one is advocating for pretesting (National Cancer Institute, 2001). Some may say that pretesting takes too much time and money. But it's just the opposite: if the materials or messages are not pretested, valuable time and financial resources will be wasted on materials or messages that do not resonate with the target audience. Taking some extra time can actually save time and money in the end. Some say, "I know what a good brochure is and what a bad brochure is, so I do not need to pretest." Because most health promotion implementers are not a part of the target audience, it is essential to pretest messages and materials to ensure that they will meet communication objectives when they are received by people in the intended audience who may have very different issues and concerns from members of the program staff. Another situation that may arise is that a supervisor might suggest using materials that have been used successfully elsewhere. Again, consider the intended audience. Are there similarities between this audience and the one the materials were created for? More than likely they are different, and because they are different, it is very important to pretest previously developed materials with members of the intended audience.

## Pretesting Process

Pretesting is an iterative, data-driven process (Brown, Lindenberger, & Bryant, 2008). The health communication plan can be used as a guide through the pretesting process. The purpose of the communication plan is to define the intended audience, the tone of the messages, and the types of materials that will be used. Use the communication plan to help you ensure that pretesting remains on strategy.

The basic iterative steps in pretesting are

1. Review existing materials.
2. Develop and test message concepts.
3. Decide what materials to develop.

4. Develop messages and materials.
5. Pretest messages and materials.
6. Revise the materials, then produce and distribute them (National Cancer Institute, 2001).

## 1. Review Existing Materials

Developing materials can be costly and time-consuming, so it is best to begin by reviewing all the materials that are currently available. There are many places to look for existing materials, including local and state health departments, professional and voluntary health associations, and federal agencies such as the Centers for Disease Prevention and Control and the National Institutes of Health. Materials produced by federal agencies are in the public domain and are free for anyone to use. To determine the relevance of materials, ask the following questions:

- Are the materials appropriate for the intended audience? Are they culturally appropriate?
- Are the messages consistent with the health communication plan?
- Will the materials meet the communication objectives? (National Cancer Institute, 2001)

When deciding whether to use existing materials, talk with those who developed the materials and determine what permissions would be required for their use or modification, whether they were evaluated for effectiveness, and how effective they were. The answers to these questions will aid in determining whether to use the materials as they are, revise them, or develop new materials.

## 2. Develop and Test Message Concepts

Concept development is the process of using the health communication plan (which is often part of the health program's marketing plan) and formative research to generate ideas that can be tested and used in developing materials. Message concepts are messages in general form and are intended to present ideas to the audience. Message concepts are not the final messages.

*Working with a Creative Team.*  In developing a concept, the opportunity to work with a creative team may arise. A creative team is a group of graphic artists and multimedia professionals (for example, videographers or filmmakers). The creative team may consist of external consultants, staff members internal to the organization that is creating the program, or both. The key to working with a creative team is making sure to stay on strategy as outlined in the health communication plan. When managing the creative team, it is important to keep in mind the following suggestions:

- Develop a good working relationship with the team, and determine the point person.
- Explain to the team the health communication strategy, including who the intended audience is and what they value.
- Talk about pretesting and how all concepts and materials must be pretested. Explain that you will assist with arranging access to the intended audience for pretesting.
- Ensure that the creative team understands the importance of developing culturally appropriate concepts and materials (National Cancer Institute, 2001).

*Concept Testing.* Once several concepts have been developed, test these concepts with the intended audience to ensure that the message appeals to them, that they understand the message, and that they are willing to act on the message. Include the creative team in developing at least two message concepts, but three may be best. It is best to test concepts using a variety of data collection methods, for no one method is optimal (National Cancer Institute, 2001; Salazar, Bryant, & Kent, 1997; Salazar, 2004). Focus groups, in-depth interviews, or one-on-one interviews are often used.

Prior to testing the concepts or materials, develop a list of questions for the intended audience. Although every project is different, ask questions that generally help determine the following:

- Comprehension of the behavioral recommendation or call to action
- The ability of the message or materials to attract attention
- The intended audience's ability to recognize the message as relevant
- Cultural appropriateness for the intended audience
- Believability
- Credibility
- Persuasiveness
- Usefulness
- General attractiveness
- Acceptability (Brown, Lindenberger, & Bryant, 2008)

When developing concepts, remember not only the primary audience, but the stakeholder audience as well. In Florida Cares for Women, a screening program for breast and cervical cancer (Brown et al., 2000), the primary audience was women over the age of fifty who lacked health insurance to cover mammograms and who had been screened irregularly in the past. The stakeholders or gatekeepers in this program were program partners who distributed the materials and determined whether or not to use them; these partners were usually cancer prevention professionals (Brown, Lindenberger, & Bryant, 2008). Given this scenario, the message concepts needed to be tested with not just the primary audience (women over fifty) but also the stakeholder audience, because no matter how on target the message was for the intended audience, if the program partners were not involved from the beginning, they were less likely to distribute the final materials.

### 3. Decide What Materials to Develop

After determining an effective message for the intended audience, begin to consider what format to use to present the message. Some of the decision about format may come from formative research in which audience members reveal which formats they are most likely to look at, read, or listen to. As we discussed earlier, materials can be presented in many formats via interpersonal channels, organizational channels, community channels, mass media channels, or interactive channels.

### 4. Develop Messages and Materials

The following guidelines will help ensure that program materials are understood, accepted, and used by the intended audience (National Cancer Institute, 2001).

- **Ensure that the message is accurate**. Make sure that the information provided is factual. It is always good to have the materials reviewed by experts on the topic.
- **Be consistent**. Consistency is critical to a program's success and, ultimately, to its identity. Make sure that the messages in all materials are consistent not only with the communication strategy but also with one another.
- **Be clear**. Keep the message simple and clear. Do not use a lot of technical terms. Make sure that the intended audience's tasks are clear and understandable.
- **Make sure that materials are relevant**. Talk about the program's benefits. The formative or consumer research will provide insight into what the intended audience values.
- **Ensure that materials are credible**. Again, use formative research to guide the decision about whom to use as a spokesperson.
- **Create appealing materials**. Ensure that materials are appealing and eye-catching, so they grab the attention of the intended audience.

## 5. Pretest Messages and Materials

Much like pretesting concepts, it is necessary to pretest draft materials with the intended audience. Some people believe they can skip this step because they have tested the concept and have had professionals review the health content, so to expedite the process, they go from draft material to final production with no review or input from the intended audience. This is a big mistake because one never knows what detail in a finished piece might be problematic to the target audience. In the long run, this round of pretesting will save valuable time and money. Many health education professionals can recall a close call when they were about to skip this step but decided at the last minute to test with the intended audience and found out that they would have had a major flaw in the final material had they not tested the draft first. Testing draft materials is not a step to skip.

## 6. Revise and Produce the Materials

After revising the materials and testing them with the audience, send the materials to press and put them to use for the program. Eventually, you will find that developing a set of materials is only the beginning, because as the audience changes, the materials will need to change as well. Thus the process of testing the materials with the audience and making appropriate changes will begin again.

## Using Pretesting to Its Fullest

Pretesting is one way to ensure that the intended audience will understand the materials developed and act on their message. It is important to remember that pretesting is not a popularity contest to see which message or type of material the intended audience members like the most or what color they like the best. It is determining what message or what material best fulfills the health marketing and communication plan. Testing at this stage permits you to identify flaws before spending money on final production. To test materials in draft form, use a facsimile version of a poster or pamphlet, a video version of a television PSA, or a prototype of text materials like a booklet. Test these materials with members of the intended audience to accomplish the following:

- **Assess comprehensibility**—Does the intended audience understand the message?
- **Identify strong and weak points**—What parts of the materials are doing their job best—for example, attract attention, inform, or motivate to act? What parts are not doing their job?

- **Determine personal relevance**—Does the intended audience identify with the materials?
- **Gauge confusing, sensitive, or controversial elements**—Does the treatment of particular topics make the intended audience uncomfortable?

## Pretesting Example

For Believe in All Your Possibilities, a community-based program to prevent the initiation of smoking and alcohol consumption among middle school students, formative research was collected (Zapata et al., 2004; Eaton et al., 2004) and a social marketing and health communication plan was developed (Florida Prevention Research Center, n.d.).

The marketing and health communication plan guided the concept development. The primary audience was middle school youths, and as is the case for many community-based projects with limited funds, the messages also had to resonate with secondary audiences—community organizations and parents. The community, working with a social marketing firm, tested four concepts, shown in Figure 8.2. These four concepts were tested with middle school youths, parents,

**FIGURE 8.2   Four Test Concepts for a Community Program**

| Overall Concept | Graphic Depiction of Concept |
|---|---|
| **Believe in all possibilities.** *Believe* says faith in oneself, in one's family, and in the power of the community to solve problems by working together. | believe IN ALL POSSIBILITIES |
| **Stand.** *Stand* grabs the audience at the emotional level. Stand up for what you believe in, and be strong in your resolve. | STAND UP \| OUT \| TOGETHER |
| **Take Charge Sarasota.** Solutions to community issues require assertive, positive action by community members. This message reflects a community already dedicated to and working for the health and well-being of all its members. | TAKE CHARGE SARASOTA IT'S EVERYONES JOB |
| **Trust: it carries us through the day.** Conventional wisdom is wrong; trust is the next logical step. This message connects with the national and statewide Truth™ campaign. | tRUSt it carries us through the Day |

and community partners. For the middle school youths and parents, interviews were used. For community leaders, appointments were made in order to share the concepts and obtain their feedback. The pretesting data suggested that Take Charge Sarasota seemed like an environmental program, not a tobacco and alcohol program, and that the graphic for Stand resembled a national hotel logo. Believe and Trust were well received by all three audiences; however, the Believe logo looked too religious and audience members wondered, "Whose possibilities?" Audience members liked the people in the Trust logo and suggested that it have more family members. Using the audience feedback, the Believe and Trust concepts were revised in two different formats (see Figure 8.3) and tested again with audience members.

After a second round of pretesting the revised Believe and Trust concepts and comparing audience reactions with the goals of the marketing and communication plan, the Believe concept was determined to be the best concept to meet the health marketing and communication plan's objectives. Using this concept, all materials developed for middle school youths, parents, and community members, including brochures, fact sheets, videos, teen theater, stickers, and a Web site, had a consistent message, look, and feel that were based on the theme of Believe in All Your Possibilities.

**FIGURE 8.3    Revisions of Two Concepts for a Community
Program After Audience Testing**

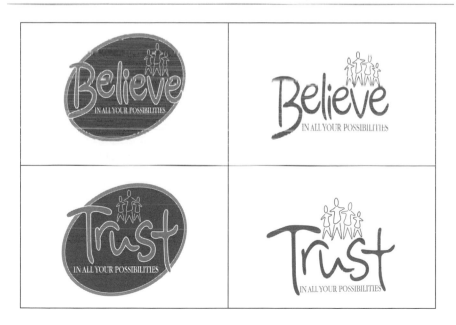

## SUMMARY

What and how a health promotion program communicates with its participants and other stakeholders are critical to its success. Plain language is a strategy for developing health promotion resources and materials that are clear, attractive, and easy to understand. Considering the information needs of the program participants and how they prefer to give and receive as well as process health information enhances program effectiveness.

Having a communication plan strengthens a health promotion program. Developing and pretesting concepts, messages, and materials with the intended audience is a critical step in the communication process. Pretesting processes includes developing and testing concepts, deciding what types of materials need to be developed, testing the materials with the target audience, revising them as necessary, and implementing them. Understanding the role that health communication plays in health promotion will help staff develop effective programs in any setting by understanding the audiences' needs and ensuring that information is provided in a meaningful and appropriate manner.

Health communication alone cannot change systemic problems related to health, such as poverty, environmental degradation, or lack of access to health care, but health communication as part of a health promotion program should include a systematic exploration of all the factors that contribute to health and the strategies that could be used to influence these factors. Well-designed health communications help individuals better understand their own needs so that they can take appropriate actions to maximize their health.

## FOR PRACTICE AND DISCUSSION

1.  Visit a local market where you shop for food and health supplies (such as prescription drugs, toiletries, vitamins, and over-the-counter medications). Read the labels and instructions on both food and health items. Find an example of an item that uses Plain English well to communicate how to prepare and use the item. What makes this a good example? Find an example of an item that communicates poorly about how to prepare and use the item. How can these instructions be improved?
2.  You are implementing a new driver safety program to encourage seat belt use by drivers and passengers. You work with the state Bureau of Motor Vehicles and will implement the program in high schools in partnerships with driver education teachers. Describe the approach you will take and how you will develop a health communication plan.

3. Have you ever pretested a message or concept for a health promotion program? If so, describe how you did it. What was the message or concept? Who was the target audience? How did you go about the pretesting process? What did you learn from the audience? What changes did you make?

4. How would a program's health communication plan differ for, on the one hand, a rural community of 5,000 people (including adults, children, and senior citizens) and, on the other hand, a large urban hospital with 1,500 employees working seven days a week, twenty-four hours a day or a school district with 4,000 students in grades from kindergarten to twelfth grade? How might the audience segments for each program differ?

5. A manufacturing company is implementing a program to promote physical activity among its 1,000 adult employees at a company site. Prepare a fifty-word statement on the importance of physical activity for adults, using plain language.

6. You are implementing a nutritional health program for incoming freshmen at the University of Texas at El Paso. What steps will you take to implement and ensure effective, culturally appropriate health communications?

## KEY TERMS

Audience segmentation

Channels

Communication objectives

Concept development

Education entertainment

Formative research (or consumer research)

Health communication

Health communication plan

Health literacy

Intended audience

Message concepts

Plain language

Pretesting

## REFERENCES

Berkman, N. D., DeWalt, D. A., Pignone, M. P., Sheridan, S. L., Lohr, K. N., Lux, L., et al. (2004). *Literacy and health outcomes* (Evidence Report/Technology Assessment No. 87; AHRQ Publication No. 04-E007-2). Rockville, MD: Agency for Healthcare Research and Quality.

Brown, K. M., Bryant, C., Forthofer, M. S., Perrin, K., Quinn, G., Wolper, M., et al. (2000). *Florida Cares for Women* social marketing campaign: A case study. *American Journal of Health Behavior, 24*(1), 44–52.

Brown, K. M., Lindenberger, J. H., & Bryant, C. A., (2008). Using pretesting to ensure messages and materials are on strategy. *Health Promotion Practice, 9*(2), 116–122.

Eaton, D. K., Forthofer, M. S., Zapata, L. B., McCormack Brown, K. R., Bryant, B. A., Reynolds, S. T., et al. (2004). Factors related to alcohol use among 6th through 10th graders: The Sarasota County Demonstration Project. *Journal of School Health, 74*(3), 95–104.

Florida Prevention Research Center. (n.d.) *Tobacco and alcohol prevention.* Retrieved November 8, 2009, from http://health.usf.edu/publichealth/prc/sarasota_tap/index.html.

Freimuth, V. S., & Quinn, S. C. (2004). The contributions of health communication to eliminating health disparities. *American Journal of Public Health, 94,* 2053–2055.

Glanz, K., Rimer, B. K., & Lewis, F. M. (Eds.). (2002). *Health behavior and health education: Theory, research, and practice* (3rd ed.). San Francisco: Jossey-Bass.

Hasnain-Wynia, R., Margolina, F. S., & Bazzoli, G. J. (2001). Models for community health partnerships. *Health Forum Journal, 44,* 29–33.

He, W., Sengupta, M., Velkoff, V. A., & DeBarrow, K. A. (2005). *65+ in the United States: 2005* (U.S. Census Bureau, Current Population Reports, P23-209). Washington, DC: U.S. Government Printing Office. Retrieved November 8, 2009, from http://www.census.gov/prod/2006pubs/p23-209.pdf.

Kaiser Family Foundation. (2006, March). *New media and the future of public service advertising: Case studies.* Washington, DC: Author.

Kirsch, I., Jungeblut, A., Jenkins, L., & Kolstad, A. (1993). *Adult literacy in America: A first look at the National Adult Literacy Survey.* Retrieved November 8, 2009, from http://nces.ed.gov/pubs93/93275.pdf.

Kutner, M., Greenberg, E., Jin, Y., & Paulsen, C. (2006). *The health literacy of America's adults: Results from the 2003 National Assessment of Adult Literacy* (NCES 2006-483). Washington, DC: U.S. Department of Education, National Center for Education Statistics.

Maibach, E. W., Van Duyn, M.A.S., Bloodgood, B. (2006). A marketing perspective on disseminating evidence-based approaches to disease prevention and health promotion. *Preventing Chronic Disease* [serial online]. Retrieved November 8, 2009, from http://www.cdc.gov/pcd/issues/2006.

National Cancer Institute. (2001). *Making health communications programs work* (NIH Publication No. 02-5145). Retrieved November 8, 2009, from www.cancer.gov/pinkbook.

National Eye Institute. (2005). *Diabetic eye disease: An educator's guide* (NIH Publication No. 2642). Washington, DC: National Institutes of Health. Retrieved November 8, 2009, from http://www.nei.nih.gov/diabeteseducation/materials/DED_Flipchart_ENGLISH.pdf.

Nielsen-Bohlman, L., Panzer, A. M., & Kindig, D. A. (Eds.). (2004). *Health literacy: A prescription to end confusion.* Washington, DC: National Academies Press.

Parker, R. M., Ratzan, S. C., & Lurie, N. (2003). Health literacy: A policy challenge for advancing high-quality health care. *Health Affairs, 22*(4), 147–153.

PlainLanguage.gov. (n.d.). *Examples: Public Health Service, Department of Health and Human Services, Brochure.* Retrieved November 8, 2009, from http://plainlanguage.gov/examples/before_after/pub_hhs_losewgt.cfm.

Rothman, R. L., DeWalt, D. A., Malone, R., Bryant, B., Shintani, A., Crigler, B., et al. (2004). Influence of patient literacy on the effectiveness of a primary care-based diabetes disease management program. *Journal of the American Medical Association, 292*(14), 1711–1716.

Salazar, B. P. (2004). Practical applications of pretesting health education concepts and materials. *Health Education Monograph Series, 21*(1), 6–12.

Salazar, B. P., Bryant, C. A., & Kent, E. B. (1997). Applications of materials pretesting to Florida's Healthy Start program. *Journal of Health Education, 28*(6), 357–363.

Schiavo, R. (2007). *Health communication: From theory to practice.* San Francisco: Jossey-Bass.

Selden, C. R., Zorn, M., Ratzan, S. C., & Parker, R. M. (2000). *National Library of Medicine current bibliographies in medicine: Health literacy* (NLM Publication No. CBM 2000-1). Bethesda, MD: U.S. Department of Health and Human Services, National Institutes of Health.

Slater, M. D., Kelly, K. J., & Thackeray, R. (2006). Segmentation on a shoestring: Health audience segmentation in limited-budget and local social marketing interventions. *Health Promotion Practice, 7,* 170–173.

Thackeray, R., & Brown, K. M. (2005). Social marketing's unique contributions to health promotion practice. *Health Promotion Practice, 6*(4), 365–368.

U.S. Department of Health and Human Services. (2000). *Healthy People 2010: Understanding and improving health.* Washington, DC: U.S. Government Printing Office.

U.S. Department of Health and Human Services, Steps to a Healthier US. (2004). *Prevention: A blueprint for action.* Retrieved November 8, 2009, from http://aspe.hhs.gov/health/blueprint/blueprint.pdf.

Zapata, L. B., Forthofer, M. S., Eaton, D. K., Brown, K. M., Bryant, C. A., Reynolds, S. T., et al. (2004). Cigarette use in 6th–10th grade youth: The Sarasota County Demonstration Project. *American Journal of Health Behavior, 28*(2), 151–165.

Zarcadoolas, C., Pleasant, A., & Greer, D. S. (2003). Elaborating a definition of health literacy: A commentary. *Journal of Health Communication, 8,* 119–120.

# CHAPTER NINE

# DEVELOPING AND INCREASING PROGRAM FUNDING

CARL I. FERTMAN

KAREN A. SPILLER

ANGELA D. MICKALIDE

## LEARNING OBJECTIVES

- Compare and contrast funding sources in terms of scope, population, and setting

- Compare the perspectives of funder staff and program staff on what matters in a program proposal

- Discuss the factors that motivate funders and how knowing these factors can foster relationships

- Describe opportunities for health promotion specialists to engage in professional fundraising

- Identify the challenges and benefits of working with agency volunteers on fiscal management and development activities

**M**ONEY is the focus of this chapter. Even if program staff have no
interest in or expectation of being involved with the financial aspects of
health promotion programs, it is still critical for staff to understand how
their decisions affect and are affected by a program's fiscal condition. Therefore, it
is extremely important for any individual aspiring to work or working in a health
promotion program and organization to know where and how programs get
money to operate. Earlier, Chapter Six focused on budgeting and fiscal management as part of program implementation. This chapter focuses on getting money
for program operations. Money is also a thread that runs through all of the phases
of planning, implementing, and evaluating a health promotion program.

Americans spend about $1.65 trillion a year on health care (including health
promotion programs). That amount represents 15 percent of the gross domestic
product, the total output of goods and services in the United States. Health care
expenses consume one-fourth of the federal budget—more than defense. Americans
spend large amounts of money on their health. On one hand, there is a lot of money
involved in and available to health promotion programs as part of the health care
industry. On the other hand, there is tremendous competition for the money that is
available. Although the general financial condition of health promotion programs
is good and improving, serious challenges face individuals who are responsible for
the money aspects of programs. And even if staff members are not now responsible
for finding the money, they may be some day. It appears that the financial challenges
facing health promotion program directors and staffs are universal, cutting across
all settings and program types. No matter the setting, the staff (and their programs)
most likely to succeed will have some knowledge and expertise in financial management. This observation holds regardless of the size of the programs; it is true for the
largest national (and international) programs as well as for programs operating on a
shoestring with a few dedicated individuals who donate their time at no cost.

## SOURCES OF PROGRAM FUNDING

Money for health promotion programs comes from the three sectors of the
economy:

*   **Public sector**: federal, state, and local governments that generate money
    through taxes (for example, personal income, property, business, and sales
    taxes). In addition to money, the federal, state, and local governments are also
    sources of legislation, resources, and research. Public schools and colleges
    are part of the public sector. Private and parochial schools and colleges can
    be part of the other sectors.

- **Private sector**: big and small businesses operated to generate profits for owners and shareholders. In the United States, 65 percent of the members of the U.S. workforce have a job in a small or big business. Businesses pay taxes.
- **Nonprofit sector**: organizations that operate for the benefit of the community and meet the federal criteria for exemption from paying taxes. Any money generated from these organizations' operations is directed back to the community rather than to personal gain or profit. Foundations and charitable organizations are included in this sector and are important sources of funding for health promotion programs.

A program's setting determines what its funding options are. Listed here are ten sources of money for health promotion programs. Another term for funding money is *revenue*. Typically, a health promotion program receives money and support from a number of the sources in the following list. Likewise, over the phases of planning, implementing, and evaluating a program, funding from different sources will be sought and used.

1. **Public funds** are tax dollars collected and spent by the government to provide the infrastructure for the systems and organizations that operate state and local health and human services. At the federal level, the main organization that coordinates health services is the U.S. Department of Health and Human Services, which includes the National Institutes of Health and the Centers for Disease Control and Prevention. At state and local levels, services and programs use public funds to provide needed services and address health concerns of the local citizenry (National Institutes of Health, 2007). Schools and many hospitals receive public funds to finance their day-to-day operating costs. For example, many schools get money from property taxes as well as tax dollars from their state. A school health promotion program might have its staff (for example, school nurse and health education teacher) paid for from the public funds while materials and supplies might be from a different source.

2. **Grants** are sums of money awarded to finance a particular activity or program. Generally, these grant awards do not need to be paid back. Federal agencies and other organizations sponsor grant programs for various reasons. Before developing a grant proposal, it is vitally important to understand the goals of the particular federal agency or private organization as well as the goals of the grant program itself (Texas Education Agency, 1999). An understanding of the goals of a grant program can be gained through discussions with the person listed as an information contact in each grant description. Through

these discussions, a potential applicant may find that in order for a particular project to meet the criteria of the grant program and be eligible for funding, the original project concept would need to be modified. In allocating funds, grantmakers base their decisions on the applying organizations' ability to fit their proposed activities within the grantmaker's interest areas.

3. **Foundations** are entities that are established as nonprofit corporations or charitable trusts with a principal purpose of making grants to unrelated organizations or institutions or to individuals for scientific, educational, cultural, religious, or other charitable purposes. This broad definition encompasses two foundation types: private foundations and public foundations. The most common distinguishing characteristic of a private foundation is that most of its funds come from one source, whether an individual, a family, or a corporation. A public foundation, in contrast, normally receives its assets from multiple sources, which may include private foundations, individuals, government agencies, and fees for service. Moreover, a public foundation must continue to seek money from diverse sources in order to retain its public status.

4. **Client fees** (also known as *fees for services*) are the prices that individuals pay to receive or participate in a service. Often, services are offered at no cost to the recipient because the organization collects revenue from other sources to cover the costs of offering the service or program. Increasingly, however, individuals are being asked to pay some fee for their participation. Public and nonprofit organizations with client fees usually have policies that regulate the fee amounts as well as safeguards to ensure that fees are not a barrier to receiving services.

5. **Matching funds**, **cost sharing**, and **in-kind contributions** all refer to monies and resources that are provided by another organization. Matching funds are monies paid concurrently during the expenditure of an organization's funds for the operation of a program. In cost sharing, monies from another organization have to be spent by the time the program concludes. In-kind contributions are non-cash contributions (for example, materials, equipment, vehicles, or food) that are used to operate programs or services.

6. **Collaboration and cooperative agreement** may not directly involve money but rather access and use of resources that are critical to a health promotion program's service delivery and that ultimately save programs money through not having to duplicate the services of another organization. Collaborations and cooperative agreements are formalized with a document (letter of agreement) detailing the resources, staff, and materials each organization will use in program implementation. Typically, this letter will be signed by each organization's director and will have a stated time frame (for example,

six months or one year). Each organization keeps a copy. Often copies of letters of agreement are provided to funders as part of applications for grants and support. In developing agreements, organizations use their complementary strengths and resources to address a health need that otherwise might go unmet.

7. **Infrastructure (operating, core, or hard) funding** are monies that an organization obtains in order to operate its infrastructure before offering any program, activities, or services. Such monies might pay for the director's salary, staff salaries, rent, janitorial services, clerical staff, or bookkeeping and payroll operations. Some schools and colleges have endowments (funding with specific instructions and criteria for how the money can be spent) that can be used for the infrastructure costs of health promotion programs that target particular groups of students.

8. **Fundraising** is the process of soliciting and gathering money or in-kind gifts by requesting donations from individuals, businesses, charitable foundations, or government agencies. Some organizations have dedicated fundraising staff. Many organizations rely on their local United Way to raise funds for them. The United Way, a national network of more than 1,300 locally governed organizations, is the nation's largest community-based fundraiser. Local United Way organizations engage their community in order to identify the underlying causes of the most significant local issues, develop strategies and pull together financial and human resources to address them, and measure the results. In 2006–07, the United Way system raised $4.07 billion (an increase of 2.3 percent over 2005–06), continuing its status as the nation's largest private charity. U.S. tax laws encourage private citizens to make tax-deductible contributions and donations to tax-exempt organizations (for example, human service, faith-based, and arts organizations) (University of Toronto, Division of Business Affairs, 2007).

9. **Volunteers** are individuals who serve an organization or cause. By definition, a volunteer does not get paid or receive compensation for services rendered. In health promotion programs, volunteers perform many tasks from direct service delivery to service on boards of directors or as program advocates. Popular in many schools are service-learning programs, in which students volunteer in community health organizations as part of their course work. Volunteers provide countless hours of services in health promotion programs through community health organizations.

10. **Health insurance** is protection against the costs of hospital and medical care or lost income arising from an illness or injury. Health insurance is sometimes called *accident insurance, sickness insurance, accident and health insurance,* or *disability insurance.* Health promotion programs might be eligible to receive

payment (reimbursement) for their services. Health insurance benefits are defined by an agreement with the health insurance company. Health insurance coverage purchased by an employer is offered to eligible employees of the company (and often to the employees' family members) as a benefit of working for that company. The majority of Americans who have health insurance have it through their employer or the employer of a family member. Health insurance coverage is sometimes available through state and federal government programs—for example, through state workers compensation systems if the care relates to injuries suffered on the job. Government-subsidized or government-provided care includes Medicare for the elderly or disabled, Medicaid (which may be known in different states by different names, such as MediCal in California) for the disadvantaged, CHAMPUS for military dependents, and medically indigent adult (MIA) programs for the indigent poor at the county level. In addition, in many communities, there are private free clinics that are unaffiliated with any insurance company, plan, or government entity.

It is important to explore all available funding options when planning and implementing a health promotion program. Keep in mind that many health promotion programs require funding and resources from more than one source.

## FUNDING VARIES BY PROGRAM PARTICIPANTS AND SETTING

At any specific site or in a particular setting, how the money needed to operate a health promotion program gets to the program varies. Table 9.1 shows funding sources for programs that address specific populations in particular settings. The funding for programs at each site shown in Table 9.1 is discussed in this section.

Health promotion programs for adults at work sites, including small and large businesses, health care organizations, and schools, are increasingly provided as part of their health insurance employee benefits packages. These are negotiated between the insurance company and the organization (for example, a business, school, or hospital). Many people don't realize that health insurance is issued differently for different types of employers and that because insurance is regulated at the state level of government, the laws in regard to health insurance offered by the different types of employers can vary significantly from state to state. Millions of Americans work for small employers, which, for health insurance purposes, are generally those with fifty employees or fewer. Millions of other Americans get their health insurance coverage through large employers. Generally, those are businesses with more than fifty employees. Increasingly, as part of a health insurance benefit, employees at worksites are offered the opportunity to participate in health promotion programs. The range of health interventions varies according to costs and employee needs. Frequently employers provide in-kind support such as access to classrooms, computers, and organizational e-mail lists in order to circulate program announcements. At some sites, employees pay a small fee for individual program sessions or classes (for example, $5 per session for a twelve-session nutrition class held during lunch hour).

Funding for health promotion programs at schools that target children, teenagers, and young adults (K–16) can have a number of sources (Table 9.1). Schools summarize the different funding sources (or streams) in a single public document called the *school budget*. School districts are required by law to adopt a balanced budget each year. Each state has a legally mandated school budget cycle (timeline) with legal deadlines, education code requirements, and a budgeting process that

**TABLE 9.1   Primary Funding Sources for Health Promotion Programs, by Program Participants and Setting**

| Funding Sources | Program Participants and Setting | | |
| --- | --- | --- | --- |
| | **Adults at Work Sites** *(for example, small and large businesses, health care organizations, schools)* | **Children, Teenagers, and Young Adults Attending School and College (K–16)** | **Adults, Children, and Teenagers in Community Settings** *(for example, preschools, senior centers, recreation centers)* |
| Public funds | | ✓✓ | ✓✓ |
| Grants | | ✓✓ | ✓✓ |
| Foundations | | ✓✓ | ✓✓ |
| Client fees (fees for services) | ✓✓ | | ✓✓ |
| Matching funds, cost sharing, and in-kind contributions | ✓✓ | ✓✓ | ✓✓ |
| Collaboration and cooperative agreement | ✓✓ | ✓✓ | ✓✓ |
| Infrastructure (operating, core, or hard) funding | ✓✓ | ✓✓ | ✓✓ |
| Fundraising | | ✓✓ | ✓✓ |
| Volunteers | | ✓✓ | ✓✓ |
| Health insurance | ✓✓ | | |

districts follow. A district's budget is a record of past decisions and a spending plan for its future. It shows a district's priorities, whether they have been clearly articulated or simply occurred by default. And a district budget is a document that can communicate a lot about the district's priorities and goals to its constituents.

A school district's budget can be difficult to understand and even more challenging to describe. Districts have volumes of mandatory reporting forms, accounting procedures, and jargon. School district officials must use responsible fiscal management, make inevitable adjustments to their budget, and comply with the oversight procedures that the states put into place to ensure that districts remain solvent and maintain their financial health. A health promotion program's funding in a school district is found in the district budget. School principals, program directors, and district budget directors are some of the people who are involved in preparing and administering the school budget.

A health promotion program that works in the community and focuses on the community members also involves a number of funding sources. Local health departments, which run some community programs, are funded by public dollars. However, many local health departments will use a mix of funding sources to operate a particular program of local interest and need (for example, programs on pregnancy prevention or smoking cessation). Sometimes state or local governments will receive public funds to operate programs mandated by law that have to operate in every community (for example, child protection or breakfast and lunchtime food programs). Many community health promotion programs are operated by community health organizations. Typically, the organization's president, executive director, or program director is responsible for finding the money to operate a program. Community organizations rely on grants, fundraising, service contracts, and health insurance. In both small and large organizations, members of the organization's board of directors (a group of individuals who oversee an organization's operation and mission) might also be involved. Finally, at large organizations, there probably are dedicated staff people whose full-time job is to raise money. They have jobs with titles such as director of development, grant writer, special activities and events director, and fundraiser.

## WRITING A GRANT PROPOSAL

An important part of getting funding for a health promotion program is sending a grant proposal to a funder. Typically, this occurs in one of two ways: (1) an organization has a great idea for a new program and sends a proposal to a funder in order to pay for it, or (2) a request for a proposal or grant notice has been made available and an organization tries to adapt an existing idea to fit the funder's program. Another reason that organizations write grant proposals is simply to fund the operation of an organization. Whether one is trying to fund programs or operations, the ability to win grants through proposal writing is critical.

Grant funding is highly competitive. For instance, the National Institutes of Health and the National Science Foundation receive nearly 70,000 proposals each year and fund only one-quarter to one-third of them. The proposal selection process differs among organizations. Typically, the proposals are reviewed by the staff of the organization requesting the proposals, experts in the particular program area, and representatives of individuals who might be served by the grant being offered. Proposals are rated and scored according to predetermined criteria.

Even though there are many types of grants available across many different fields, grant seekers all follow a basic process and standards that remain constant across every professional area. Further, many organizations require applications to be submitted online and thus require a certain level of technological skill. To help grant seekers, many organizations, especially national foundations, offer online tutorials for writing a proposal that will fit with their specific goals and objectives in awarding grants. Regardless of the funder, grant seekers must understand how to find funding sources and opportunities, write the grant proposal, deal with the technological aspects of submitting a proposal, and attend to the funder's needs. It is best to embrace the idea that applying for grants involves following a prescribed formula.

## Finding Funding Sources and Opportunities

Finding funding sources and opportunities requires these steps:

1. Clarify the purpose of the health promotion program and write a concise statement (that is, a mission statement). Define the scope of work in order to focus the funding search. Identify exactly what items you are seeking funds for.
2. Identify the right funding sources. Do not limit your search to one resource. Foundation centers, computerized databases, publications, and public libraries are some of the resources available for you to use in a funding search (Foundation Center, 2007). Look at the federal government's Web site on grants (http://www.grants.gov) as well as the *Federal Register* (http://www .gpoaccess.gov/fr). The *Federal Register* is the official daily publication where the rules, proposed rules, and notices of federal agencies and organizations appear. The *Federal Register* also includes the announcements of new federal grants, many of which are health-focused. The goal is to find groups that

are interested in the health problem addressed by your health promotion program.

3. Contact the funders. Think of the funder as a resource and a friend who wants to help, if there is mutual interest. Some funders offer technical assistance; others do not. Ask for technical assistance, including a review of proposal drafts. Try to talk with a staff member about what is currently being funded by the group. Ask for an annual report. Ask for names of organizations that have previously been funded. Talk with people from those organizations.

4. Acquire proposal guidelines. Read the guidelines carefully, and then read them again. Ask the funder to clarify any questions that you have about the guidelines. Pay attention to the technical details (for example, page length, font size, number of copies, instructions for electronic and hard-copy submissions).

5. Know the submission deadline. Plan to submit the proposal on or preferably before the deadline. Be realistic about whether you have the time to prepare a competitive proposal that meets the deadline.

6. Determine personnel needs. Identify required personnel both by function and, if possible, by name. Contact project consultants, trainers, and other personnel to inquire about their availability; acquire permission to include them in the project; and negotiate compensation. Will staff actually be available to implement the program if it is funded?

7. Assess the feasibility of writing and submitting the proposal, of winning funding, and of fully implementing the program if it is funded. Writing proposals is hard work and takes time. There are a lot of unknowns, but going through these steps will help program staff to make an informed decision about which funding opportunities to pursue.

## Writing Process

The time frame for writing a grant proposal varies. For federal grants, it can take three to six months to write a grant proposal, and another nine months or so from the time it is sent until it might get funded. Local community foundations and United Ways might announce funding opportunities and proposal guidelines at the beginning of a month with a due date for a finished proposal one month later and may expect that funded programs will be implemented one or two months after that.

Before writing the grant proposal, form an internal working committee. Key stakeholders and individuals (often members of the advisory board discussed in Chapter One) who will be involved with the funded project are included on the working committee. Next, consider asking objective and experienced individuals who have worked in the particular health area or with the funding organization to share their experiences and recommendations about what would be of interest to the funder. After consulting with these individuals and creating an outline of the agreed-on project details, the committee can draft a short description of the specific aims of the program. Using this strategy will make composition of the proposal easier. And although one or two people may be responsible for writing the proposal, the committee can provide feedback throughout the writing process.

As in any writing assignment, it is important to consider the audience that one is writing for. In grant applications, it is often best to use a balance of technical and nontechnical writing because the reviewers at the grant-making organization may not be familiar with the terminology used in your field. Further, most reviewers will just scan your application, and they may not be familiar with theories and methods used in your field. For these reasons, consider separating technical and nontechnical information in the parts of the application that reviewers will most likely read—the abstract, significance, and specific aims. More detailed information can be included when you are explaining program interventions. Some grant-writing specialists suggest that proposal writers begin each paragraph simply and then progress to more complex information or that writers alternate paragraphs that have less and more technical information (National Institutes of Health, National Institute of Diabetes and Digestive and Kidney Diseases, n.d.). Ultimately, as the grant writer, it is your decision as to how to include both broader, less technical descriptions and more technical information in a proposal. Keeping your audience in mind will help you decide which writing strategies to use.

If the staff of the health promotion program do not have the writing skills to create a structured, concise, and persuasive application with attention to specifications and a reasonable budget, consider asking for help from experienced grant writers. Some schools, hospitals, and community health organizations hire outside contractors as writers or editors. Whoever writes the application must first read the guidelines to learn the specifications, what information is required, and how it should be arranged. Standard proposal components are the narrative, budget, appendix of support material, and authorized signature. Sometimes proposal applications require abstracts or summaries, an explanation of budget items, and certifications. Table 9.2 is an overview of the potential components of a grant proposal, including the approximate number of pages for each component area.

First, the executive summary is a brief description of the proposed project. The executive summary should be a clear, concise statement of what problem is being addressed, why it needs to be addressed, how it will be addressed, and what will be changed as a result of the program.

TABLE 9.2    Overview of a Grant Proposal

| Component | Description | Number of Pages |
|---|---|---|
| Executive summary | Umbrella statement of your case and summary of the entire proposal | 1 page |
| Statement of need | Why the project is necessary | 2 pages |
| Project description | Nuts and bolts of how the project will be implemented and evaluated | 3 pages |
| Budget | Financial description of the project plus explanatory notes | 1 page |
| Information on organization | Organization history and governing structure; its primary activities, audiences, and services | 1 page |
| Conclusion | Summary of the proposal's main points | 2 paragraphs |

Second, the statement of need focuses on the project's purpose, goals, and measurable objectives, and it provides a compelling, logical reason why the proposal should be supported). The needs statement gives the project's background, providing a perspective on the conception of the project.

The project description needs to be concise and informative, and it needs to provide a hook for the reviewers in order to stir their interest and draw their attention to what makes your application unique. Make sure that the proposed program is aligned with the purpose and goals of the funding source. Describe your proposed interventions (methods and processes for accomplishing goals and objectives) and activities, the intended scope of work and expected outcomes, and required personnel functions, including the names of key staff members and consultants). Because the reviewers will probably read many similar proposals, a tailored and attention-getting description of the program will interest the funder. In addition, including a method of evaluation with intended outcomes and expectations will appeal to a funder's need for accountability. Prepare a logic model and a Gantt chart to illustrate the project flow, including start and end dates, a schedule of activities, and projected outcomes.

The budget portion of the application is a cost projection of how the project will be implemented and managed. Well-planned budgets reflect carefully thought-out projects. Be sure to include only the things the funder is willing to support. Many funders provide mandatory budget forms that must be submitted with the proposal. Don't forget to list in-kind and matching revenue, where appropriate. Overall, it is important to be flexible about a budget in case the funder chooses to negotiate costs.

Include information about your organization that validates its ability to successfully undertake the proposed effort. The organization information and supporting materials may sometimes include the same documents, and these are often arranged in an appendix. These materials may endorse the project and the applicant, provide certifications, add information about project personnel and consultants, provide additional detail in exhibit tables and charts, and so on. Names and addresses of board directors, insurance coverage, and current and past year organizational audits are items that funders commonly request from grant-seeking groups. Don't forget to prepare and gather any special documentation required—for example, signed releases for human subjects (National Institutes of Health, National Institute of Diabetes and Digestive and Kidney Diseases, n.d.). For projects that involve collaborations, cooperative agreements, or matching funds, cost sharing, and in-kind contributions from other organizations, supporting documents from these organizations frequently required. Most often theses documents are in the form of written letters from the organizations to the funder detailing their role and support. Typically these would be placed in a proposal appendix.

The conclusion is a succinct, crisp restatement of the program purpose, objective, interventions, and evaluation. Conclusions are read by grant reviewers and should always be written with these reviewers in mind. The program timeline and requested funding are not typically be included in the conclusion. The conclusion emphasizes the program's impact on the life quality of the target population. It is one final opportunity to clearly articulate your program and make a pitch for its funding.

In general, follow all instructions in order to minimize the risk of having a proposal returned because it exceeded the page limits or used too small a font. Look for the page and word limits in the grant proposal guide. Make it easy for the reviewers to find material by using strong headings, graphics, and tables. Graphical representations of timetables for experiments can effectively illustrate their flow and time frame. These basic techniques will help keep writing streamlined and well organized so that reviewers can readily glean the information that interests them. In addition, be sure to cite the appropriate references throughout the proposal.

## Technological Process

Submitting a grant proposal involves a potentially large number of technical requirements. At one time, the technical aspects of submitting a grant proposal involved the number of pages and number of copies to submit to the funder. However, with increased use of technology (particularly computers and the

Internet), submitting grant proposals has become more challenging. It is now common to submit proposals online through sites that require organizational or individual registration and passwords. The sites may require populating (completing) an online form and uploading files and materials in certain formats and with size restrictions. Although graphics, charts, and other visual elements break the monotony of text and can help reviewers grasp a lot of information quickly, they can be difficult to format with word processing software and they may not remain stable across different hardware and software platforms.

Help for technological problems encountered during the submission process may be limited. Typically, funders do not see technical problems as a reason for accepting proposals after the due date for grant submission.

Clearly, technology can make the grant-writing and submission process easier. However, technology can also add barriers to the already time-consuming endeavor of writing a grant, requiring a concentrated effort, commitment, and persistence on the part of grant seekers and grant writers. Thus the commitment of time and resources for writing a grant proposal might need to include some provision for technical training or outside support in order to compose and submit the application.

## Meeting the Funder's Needs

Once the first draft of a grant proposal is complete, sharpen the focus of the proposal. Reviewers will quickly pick up on how well the proposal matches the grant requirements. Remember that a proposal has two audiences: some reviewers who are not familiar with health promotion programs and interventions and some who have field experience of health promotion programs and thus have that sort of program knowledge.

Remember the following points:

- All reviewers are important because each reviewer typically gets one vote.
- Typically, there is a primary reviewer (or perhaps more than one) who is knowledgeable about health promotion programs; write to win over that reviewer.
- Write and organize your proposal so that the primary reviewer can readily grasp and explain what is being proposed.

Ultimately, a grant-making organization has the breadth and depth of knowledge, experience, and wisdom to understand and judge a large range of grant applications. Even if a funding organization is not familiar with all the techniques proposed in a grant, its reviewers can and will judge how well a proposal clearly communicates the desire for funding and the need for it. Finally, the following is a list of common reasons cited by reviewers of grant proposals for not approving them:

- Problem not important enough
- Program not likely to produce useful information or address health problem
- Program not based on health theory or evidence, and alternative not considered
- Health promotion interventions unsuited to the objective
- Proposal addresses a health problem other than the one asked for in the funding announcement.
- Technical problems (for example, exceeds page limitations, uses incorrect budget, lacks required information on organization, or lacks endorsement letters from partners)
- Problem more complex than program staff appear to realize
- Lack of focus in program's mission statement, intervention, and evaluation
- Lack of original or new ideas
- Proposed program not appropriate to address the proposed questions

## MAINTAINING RELATIONSHIPS WITH FUNDERS

All the elements of a personal relationship are present in the relationship between an organization that operates a health promotion program and an organization that funds the program. Expected as part of the relationship are trust, honesty, timeliness, and accountability, as well as transparency in the program's operation and delivery and provision of high-quality services and materials that achieve the program's goals and objectives.

Specific strategies for maintaining a good relationship with a funder include these:

- Schedule an initial meeting in order to gather information from the potential funder as well as to share information about your organization. Meeting preparation is critical. Prepare a concise, clear document that outlines your program's scope, responsibilities, timeline, and budget. In the meeting, work to establish mutually agreed-on measures of program success right from the beginning. Find out about current programs that are being funded and how program achievements are evaluated.) Find out about the stakeholders of the funding organization, including its board members.
- Engage in a frank discussion about funder attributions and recognitions for the health promotion program, and document decisions in writing. For

example, would the funder like to have its logo on every brochure, poster, checklist, and DVD related to the program? How will the funder's support be acknowledged in media interviews (for example, "Through our partnership with the Green Foundation, the health department has provided free bike helmets to children in our community."). Should reciprocal links be established between the Web sites of the funder and the health promotion program? Some funders seek constant and highly visible recognition, while others prefer to remain anonymous. To avoid missteps, it is important for health program staff to elicit these funder preferences prior to printing brochures, speaking with the media, or posting content and logos on the program's Web site.

- If the funder agrees, seek opportunities to leverage its contribution to attract additional funding and funders. Using this strategy can help you expand your health promotion program in several ways—by creating new materials, making additional presentations, achieving greater audience diversity, and penetrating different channels of communication. Some funders may wish to be listed as the founding funder, particularly if their initial contribution launched an organization or major program initiative. The founding funder may permit others to join the donor list, particularly if their brands do not compete. (For example, Coke and Pepsi would be competing brands and so would McDonald's and Burger King.) Others may want an exclusive partnership, which the longevity of the partnership and dollar amount contributed may warrant. Remember that loyalty is a two-way street, so it's important to discuss emerging funding opportunities with current funders to ensure that there are no actual or perceived conflicts of interest.

- Keep excellent financial records so that your organization can track income and expenses easily, quickly, and accurately. These records should be both computerized and on hard copy in case of technological glitches or natural disasters. Retain this documentation for at least three years in order to respond to auditors' requests. Work closely with the finance and administration staff responsible for monitoring the health promotion program's budget to ensure that all reporting requirements are being met. If there are anticipated cost overruns or unexpended funds, communicate these details immediately to the funder and the organization's finance and administration staff so that any necessary adjustments can be made prior to the end of the grant cycle.

- Find a champion within the foundation, corporation, or other funding source. Ideally, this individual's role should be to institutionalize your health promotion program within the funding organization in order to guarantee its continued support. Examples of helpful actions of a champion include ensuring that senior management is apprised of the health promotion program's achievements, influencing the public relations department to highlight the partnership in media interviews and its annual report, and establishing a cause-related marketing effort with the advertising department, if relevant. Health promotion program staff should strive to regularly equip this champion with the necessary tools (for example, the latest educational materials or evaluation reports) to help him or her manage internal relations pertaining to the partnership. In this way, if the champion leaves the funding organization, there will be others there who can adopt a leadership and advocacy role on the grantee's behalf.

- Be willing to admit it to the funder when a mistake is made or plans go awry, whether it be an unrealistic timeline, a budgetary miscalculation, a difficulty with program implementation, or neutral or negative results from a program evaluation. The funder might suggest solutions that the program staff have not considered and may be willing to invest more resources to rectify the shortcomings. After all, the funder has already made an investment in the health promotion program and is reluctant to see it fail. While no funder wants to throw good money after bad, few funders are willing to lose their entire investment. Honest and frequent communication is the key to winning partnerships.

Many other recommendations stem from common sense and simple courtesy. These include diversifying funding streams (for example, soliciting funds from foundations, corporations, federal agencies, trade associations, and individual giving), adding value to the partnership with fresh ideas and seized opportunities, setting realistic expectations (that is, underpromise and overdeliver), and thanking the funder frequently and sincerely for the support provided. After all, when it comes to health promotion programming, there is truth in the adage "no money, no mission!"

## FUNDRAISING

For health promotion programs operated by a small or large nonprofit organization, another resource that may be available to help with program funding is development staff (sometimes called *development officers*). These individuals have job titles such as fundraising coordinator, development director, or resource developer, and their job is to seek out and manage fundraising efforts for the organization. Development staff responsibilities can include but are not limited to writing grant proposals, researching foundation and corporation requests for proposals, and overseeing or implementing other fundraising strategies. They may work mostly behind the scenes, establishing a structure for effective fundraising.

Organizations use a variety of fundraising strategies:

- **Annual giving**. An annual giving program is any organization's yearly drive to raise financial support for its ongoing operating needs. Annual giving is about donor acquisition, repeating the gift, and upgrading the gift. Annual giving creates the habit of giving on a regular yearly basis.

- **Campaigns**. Fundraising campaigns have a specific set of defining points that include a specific goal, support of a particular project, and set starting and ending dates. The best way to run any campaign is to begin by defining its mission. After this definition, name the amount needed to achieve the mission, set a deadline, and then determine how donors will be recognized (for example with small gifts or listing in the annual report) (Pelletier, 2007).

- **Alumni and donor relations**. There are a number of key elements in cultivating a long-term and mutually rewarding relationship with a donor. Stewardship relates to resource management, and in the context of a donor's gift, that involves compliance with the donor's wishes with respect to application of the gift, effective management of the resources represented by the gift, and accountability. All donations should be acknowledged with a personalized letter of thanks with a charitable donation receipt attached.

- **Major gifts**. Many major gifts are given for a specific purpose, distinguishing them from an annual gift, which is usually unrestricted and available to fund current operations. Major gifts are likely to be given in a restricted manner in order to accomplish a specific purpose that is valued by the donor. Gifts can be solicited for specific purposes, to suit both the organization's needs and the donor's stated preferences.

- **Planned gifts**. When donors plan to give, they can donate a greater significant amount than they may have originally thought possible, and for some donors, planning ahead of time is the only way to make a substantial gift. Development officers who deal with planned gifts specialize in handling gifts with tax and estate implications for donors. These include gifts of outright cash and securities; gifts that provide a lifetime income to donors, such as pooled income fund gifts, charitable gift annuities, and charitable remainder trusts; and bequests, gifts of real estate, and gifts of tangible personal property, such as art, jewelry, antiques, and collectibles.

- **Special event fundraisers**. Often called *fundraising benefits*, special event fundraisers are social gatherings that generate publicity for an organization; raise money; charge a fee for attendance but offer some form of entertainment in exchange; and include extravaganzas (gala dinner-dances, concerts, cruises, or major sporting events), events for bargain hunters or gamblers (bingos, raffles, casino nights, garage sales, rummage sales, auctions, flea markets, or bake sales), or educational events (ranging from major speakers who fill large auditoriums to slide shows shown in community centers).

- **Mass fundraising**. Mass fundraising is generated from huge mailings that generate tens of thousands of donors and produce funds with the fewest strings attached. But mass fundraising via mailing and phoning, the pre-Internet techniques, has always suffered from the high cost of raising the money (Thompson, n.d). Recently the Internet has presented a major opportunity and strategy for mass fundraising with many organizations using a mix of Internet strategies including social networking sites, e-mails, and donations via organizational home pages.

The main goal of the development staff is to find individuals who are willing to donate funds to the organization. Congress provides tax incentives to entice individuals to donate (Texas Commission on the Arts, 2007). Regardless of tax breaks, individuals will donate if they have a motivating factor or if a major donation is planned by individuals connected with the organization. Development officers handle the annual giving program for an organization, and any annual development effort over time will offer planned giving prospects (Jordan & Quynn, 2000). The development office may also handle other donation campaigns such as direct mail solicitation; telefund or phone-a-thon programs that solicit pledges; special events, including annual fund donor dinners or lecture series; major gifts campaigns, for gifts ranging from $10,000 to $100,000 or more raised through the identification, cultivation, and solicitation of prospects and donors; foundation and corporation grants or charitable trusts; or a stewardship office that oversees an organization's endowed restricted funds (Walker, 2006, chap. 1). The development office may also encompass a prospects management office that tracks solicitation activity throughout an organization and that includes gift reporting and a processing department that keeps track of gifts and pledges. Regardless of which types of fundraising efforts are pursued, the members of the development office must understand the philosophies and goals of the organization in order to effectively solicit funds to assist the development of the organization.

Development offices are a benefit for health promotion programs. They can provide access to support and resources that might not otherwise be available to programs, due to programs' primary need to focus on implementation. Likewise, health promotion programs are often sought out by development offices, since the programs' focus on improving individuals' quality of life is attractive to funders. Furthermore development officers like to showcase the impact of an organization's programs on the target populations it serves. Health promotion programs are typically open to visitors and their work is easily understood by individuals who may not have technical health background or exposure to health programs.

## WORKING WITH BOARD MEMBERS

For health promotion programs operated by a small or large community health organization, another resource that is available to help with the funding programs is the organization's board of directors. By law, all nonprofit organizations (such as community health organizations) are required to have a board of directors to oversee the organization's mission, operation, and fiscal management. Most professional fundraisers will say that before boards get involved in fundraising, they must first be involved in the mission and governance of the organization. This involvement with the larger scope of the organization often leads to a more focused commitment to the fundraising program.

Like stakeholders in other aspects of a program, board members must be engaged in the planning process to determine with staff what the organization wants and what it will do. Involvement in planning builds ownership of the plans, which essentially become the organization's agenda for the future and the foundation for all subsequent fundraising. After goals, objectives, programs, and services have been determined, planning turns to translating these aspirations into real financial needs, which are often reflected in budgets. It is essential that board members participate in determining the financial needs if they are to be involved in serious fundraising in the future.

After this process has been completed, board and staff need to form a partnership in order to develop and implement a plan to secure the necessary funds to go forward with the plan. The actual fundraising task is immeasurably strengthened when a true partnership between board and staff is in place. Staff members manage the fundraising program, while board members get involved in the elements that suit their interests, skills, and capabilities. A good fundraising plan is explicit about both board and staff responsibilities. Exhibit 9.1 lists board and staff members' fundraising responsibilities.

Most people do not gravitate to fundraising naturally or easily. It can be helpful to involve board members in a process to explore their personal feelings about giving and asking. Most health promotion programs use a variety of methods to ask for money, such as direct mail appeals, special events, pledge programs, or products for sale. Perhaps the hardest way for an organization to raise money is for board, staff, and volunteers to ask people directly for donations (Vander, 2007). Experience has shown, however, that it is almost impossible to have a major gifts program without face-to-face solicitation of prospective donors.

---

## EXHIBIT 9.1
## Board and Staff Members' Fundraising Responsibilities

*Board Members*

- Provide input on the fundraising plan
- Organize and participate on fundraising committee
- Identify and cultivate new prospects and donors
- Ask peers for donations
- Always be an advocate for the agency
- Make introductions for staff to follow up
- Accompany staff on key visits to funders
- Help with expressions of thanks when appropriate

*Staff Members*

- Accompany board members on key visits to funders
- Help with expressions of thanks when appropriate
- Research new and existing donors
- Write stories about the impact of a program on program participants
- Write grant proposals
- Accompany board members on solicitation visits
- Take care of all logistics related to fundraising activities
- Develop a funding strategy incorporating all funding types and sources, keeping board members apprised of the status of all funded programs and grants

---

Asking a person for money face to face is an acquired taste. Few people love to do it initially. And being hesitant about asking for money is common. People hesitate to ask for money for a wide variety of reasons. For example, one can look at the role that money plays in American society to understand one source of the anxiety. Most people are taught that four topics are taboo in polite conversation: politics, money, religion, and sex. Many people were also raised to believe that asking people what their salary is or how much they paid for their house or their car is rude. In many families, the man takes care of all financial decisions. It is not unusual, even today, for wives or partners not to know how much their spouse or partner earns, for children not to know how much their parents earn, or for close friends not to know one another's income.

In working with board members and volunteers to ask directly (in person) for donations, frame the idea of asking in the context of support and urgency in addressing a health problem. Focus the process on how the organization is working to solve the health problem. Money is only one part of the process (but an important one). Be clear that the money is not being sought for personal gain or use but rather to address a human need larger than any one individual.

## SUMMARY

Health promotion programs need money in order to operate. Effective programs have staff members who understand the role of money in programs, the sources and types of funding, and the work involved in acquiring, managing, and reporting on program resources. Although talking about money may seem to be at odds with the goals of a health promotion program, in reality, it is a natural part of figuring out the value of health to a business, school, health care organization, or community. Furthermore, the clearer that program staff are about a program's goals and objectives and the effectiveness of the program in meeting those goals and objectives, the better positioned the staff will be to build funders' confidence that a program is effective and worth funding.

## FOR PRACTICE AND DISCUSSION

1. Locate a few health promotion programs that receive funding from at least three of the ten different funding sources listed in this chapter. Compare and contrast the programs. Discuss differences and similarities among the programs.
2. You are working with a community college to develop and implement a student health promotion program. As part of a planned meeting with a school staff member, you will be asked to discuss options that the college might consider in order to fund the health promotion program. Prepare a brief list of available options and examples of funding sources to pursue.
3. Contact the United Way in your area or region. How does this organization raise money, and whom does it fund? What organizations and programs get the most funding? What criteria must a program meet in order to receive funding? Who gets the least funding? Why are there differences in the funding amounts?
4. Staff members who participate in a lunchtime physical activity program sponsored by their employer, a small business, are asked to pay $2 a session. What are the pros and cons of charging fees for participation in a health promotion program? How can the fees be incentives and disincentives?

## KEY TERMS

Board members'
fundraising
responsibilities

Client fees

Collaborations and
cooperative agreements

Foundations

Fundraising

Fundraising field

Fundraising professionals

Grant-writing process

Grants

Health insurance

Infrastructure (operating,
core, or hard) funding

Matching funds, cost
sharing, and in-kind
contributions

Nonprofit sector

Private sector

Public funds

Public sector

Staff members' fundraising
responsibilities

Volunteers

## REFERENCES

Foundation Center. (2007). *Proposal writing short course*. Retrieved November 30, 2007, from http://foundationcenter.org/getstarted/tutorials/shortcourse/index.html.

Jordan, R. R., & Quynn, K. L. (2000). *Planned giving management, marketing and the law* (2nd ed.). Hoboken, NJ: Wiley.

National Institutes of Health. (2007, February). *Before you start writing*. Retrieved November 30, 2007, from http://www.niaid.nih.gov/ncn/grants/write/write_a1.htm.

National Institutes of Health, National Institute of Diabetes and Digestive and Kidney Diseases. (n.d.). *Writing a grant*. Retrieved November 30, 2007, from http://www.niddk.nih.gov/fund/grants_process/grantwriting.htm.

Pelletier, M. (2007). *The basics of managing a fundraising campaign*. Retrieved December 13, 2007, from http://www.helium.com/tm/309652/fundraising-campaigns-specific-defining.

Texas Commission on the Arts. (2007). *Fundraising and development*. Retrieved December 6, 2007, from http://www.arts.state.tx.us/toolkit/fundraising

Texas Education Agency. (1999, June). *A grantseeker's resource guide to obtaining federal, corporate and foundation grants*. Retrieved November 30, 2007, from http://www.tea.state.tx.us/opge/grantdev/seekers/document1.html.

Thompson, M. (n.d.). *Morris continued*. Retrieved December 13, 2007, from http://cagle.msnbc.com/news/DeanMorris/1.asp.

University of Toronto, Division of Business Affairs. (2007). *Fundraising and donations overview*. Retrieved December 13, 2007, from http://www.finance.utoronto.ca/gtfm/donations/overview.htm.

Vander, A. S. (2007). *Special event fundraising*. Retrieved December 13, 2007, from http://www.learningtogive.org/papers/index.asp?bpid=60.

Walker, J. I. (2006). *Nonprofit essentials: Major gifts*. Retrieved December 13, 2007, from http://media.wiley.com/product_data/excerpt/79/04717383/0471738379.pdf.

# PART FOUR

# EVALUATING AND SUSTAINING HEALTH PROMOTION PROGRAMS

# EVALUATING AND IMPROVING A HEALTH PROMOTION PROGRAM

DANIEL PERALES

ANDY FOURNEY

BARBARA MKNELLY

EDWARD MAMARY

## LEARNING OBJECTIVES

- Compare the scope and timing of formative, process, impact, and outcome evaluation

- Identify and discuss the elements to be considered in designing an evaluation framework

- Describe the role of evaluation is shaping program design, implementation, and sustainability

- Describe the shared components of the evaluation frameworks from the CDC, RE-AIM, and the Institute of Medicine's Obesity Project

- Explain the fundamental tasks in implementing program evaluation

- Discuss evaluation results in terms of dissemination, utility, and program improvement

H OW DO PROGRAM STAFF, stakeholders, and participants know whether a health promotion program has been implemented and is operating as planned? How do they know how and when it produces the results stated in the program's mission statement, goals, and objectives? Lots of time, energy, resources, and effort are spent by many people in implementing a health promotion program. At a certain point, it is only natural to ask, Is the program working and addressing the program participants' health concerns? This chapter discusses how to answer these questions through program evaluation. We describe the basic tools needed to design and implement a program evaluation as well as how to use and disseminate an evaluation's findings. The role of evaluation is discussed in the context of the overall design of a health promotion program and the ways in which evaluation can provide continual feedback to strengthen such programs. Finally, the nuts and bolts of implementing the tasks needed for evaluation are described.

Evaluation is not the last phase in the process of creating, operating, and sustaining a health promotion program. It is one of the phases, and in the most effective health promotion programs, runs parallel to the other phases, starting at the very beginning of the process when a program is being planned and continuing in tandem as the program is implemented and sustained in order to provide continual feedback to program staff, stakeholders, and participants.

## PROGRAM EVALUATION DEFINITION, TYPES, AND TERMS

*Program evaluation* is the systemic collection of information about a health promotion program in order to answer questions and make decisions about the program. The types of program evaluation are formative evaluation, process evaluation, impact evaluation, and outcome evaluation. While it is important to know what type of program evaluation needs to be conducted, first it is critical to know what questions are to be answered and what decisions are to be made with the collected information. Once this is known, it is possible to focus on accurately collecting information and on understanding that collected information.

Evaluation often seems like a heavy, complex activity to those who are not familiar with the real nature of evaluation. In essence, however, evaluation means answering some very basic questions and then reporting back to interested individuals and groups (that is, stakeholders) what was found. The questions evaluators might ask include

- What do the program participants, staff, and stakeholders want to know?
- Who are the primary audiences for the results?

- What decisions will be made based on the evaluation's findings and results?
- What kinds of information are needed?
- When is the information needed?
- Where can the information be acquired, and how?
- What resources are available for getting the information, analyzing it, and reporting it?
- What kind of report would be most useful to the program participants, staff, or other stakeholders?
- What might be some of the unintended consequences of program implementation?

The health theories and planning models (see Chapter Three, Tables 3.10 and 3.12) used in program planning and implementation will influence the evaluation questions as well as provide a framework for how they are answered. Furthermore, the theories and models might influence how the data are collected. Data collection methods are discussed later in this chapter.

Evaluation helps program staff, stakeholders, and participants think in a structured, systematic manner about the who, what, when, where, why, and how of a program. Evaluation is not a one-time report card but, ideally, an ongoing process that a health promotion program incorporates into its operation and management systems. Program evaluation is not the same as regular program monitoring. Program monitoring refers simply to keeping records on the nature of the participants, the services they receive, and their progress toward attaining program objectives. The purpose of monitoring is to provide systematically connected information on what was done, for whom, and where. These types of data are also called *tracking measures*. Program evaluation typically includes monitoring plus methods for determining more specifically and with more certainty that the program intervention and activities themselves produced the outcomes that are observed. In short, program evaluation addresses the question of what was done and whether the program itself was effective and why.

At one time, evaluation was viewed as something that is done to a program. An evaluator would come in and examine a program and its participants for the purpose of issuing a pass-or-fail report card for a funder or policymaker, presumably to contribute to a decision about whether to continue to fund the program or other similar ones. As a result, an antagonistic, "we-they" relationship frequently developed between evaluators and program staff. In addition, stakeholders often felt excluded from the process and the evaluation report did not provide recommendations on how to improve the program. In effect, the evaluation was often viewed as expensive and intrusive and adding little value to the program. These old images of evaluation still linger. However, today, evaluation is about systematic inquiry into the implementation, operation, and effectiveness of a health promotion program for the primary purpose of improving the program. It is a continual process that starts when the program is conceived and is best conducted as a collaboration among all stakeholders.

## Types of Evaluations

Different types of evaluations correspond to the type of information needed. An understanding of each type is important in order to select and carry out an evaluation that can answer stakeholders' questions and help make program decisions. In a comprehensive health promotion program with an outcome that can be measured within a program's funding period (generally one to three years), formative, process, impact, and outcome evaluation can all be conducted.

1. **Formative evaluation** involves gathering information and materials during program planning and development. It can be used to understand the needs assessment data gathered during the program planning process (Gilmore & Campbell, 2005). Indeed, Green and Kreuter (2005) view formative evaluation as an important part of the first four phases of the PRECEDE-PROCEED model, in which assessment helps to produce goals, objectives, and strategies for implementation.

   Fourney and Williams (2003) conducted a formative evaluation, grounded in the constructs of the health belief model and social cognitive theory, to develop a theory-based intervention to increase adherence to HIV therapies among low-literacy populations of African American women. The formative evaluation involved conducting focus groups to identify the determinants of adherence in order to develop an educational script, an illustrated cartoon book, and a ten-minute audiotape of the cartoon book. The focus groups were used to see whether the script resonated with the women, whether professors and upper-division students could identify the theoretical basis, and whether the women felt the illustrations were realistic and were like them. The formative evaluation provided confidence that the materials would be effective and would be used as intended by the women.

2. **Process evaluation** is about systematically gathering information during program implementation. It can be used to describe and assess to what extent the intended activities in health education interventions, organizational

policies, community action, and advocacy are being accomplished. A process evaluation is useful for formally monitoring implementation; for identifying necessary changes to the implementation; and, generally, for overall improvement of the health promotion program or any one of the individual strategies. A thorough process evaluation should include the following elements:

- Describing the environment of the health promotion program, including the individuals involved, the community, the broad socioeconomic environment, and the time frame
- Gathering and analyzing program-related documents such as meeting minutes, reports, memorandums, newsletters, and Web pages
- Describing the process used to design and implement the program intervention, including daily operation
- Tracking actual versus planned program activities (for example, services provided, participants reached, materials developed)
- Describing changes during the implementation from what was planned, including realities encountered in mobilizing the community, advocating for changes in legislation and policies, or implementing new policies
- Identifying and describing barriers to implementation, such as problems with language or access to services, that may have affected implementation and outcomes

Overall, a well-designed and well-monitored process evaluation can help a program director understand the elements that contributed to a health promotion program's success or the ways it could be improved in order to better achieve intended results. The results of a process evaluation may also help stakeholders describe external factors that limit achievement of the desired outcomes.

3. **Impact evaluation** measures the immediate effects of a health promotion program and the extent to which the program's goals were attained—that is, whether impacts were achieved that could lead to the program's ultimate desired outcome (for example, increased physical activity that could lead to a desired health status change). The primary question in an impact evaluation is, What has been the program's immediate effect on the participants? Early in program planning, the staff needs to determine the evaluation design that will be used for the impact evaluation. (Evaluation design is discussed in greater detail later in this chapter.) A key challenge in the design of an impact evaluation is developing a control group that is as similar as possible (in both observable dimensions, such as age, and unobservable dimensions, such as knowledge) to participants in the health promotion program, to allow comparison of a group that received the program with one that didn't. If the

evaluation design (for example, randomization of the two groups) permits, this comparison may result in conclusions about causality—that is, attributing observed changes to the program—as well as eliminate confounding factors. However, even when control groups are not possible, an impact evaluation must identify the measures consistent with the program goals and objectives.

Information generated by impact evaluations informs decisions on whether to expand, modify, or eliminate a particular aspect of a health promotion intervention (whether to enforce policies, change the focus of advocacy activities, or change educational methods, for example). In addition, impact evaluations can improve a program by addressing the following questions:

- Is the health promotion program achieving its intended goals?
- Can the impact be explained by the program's intervention, or is it the result of other factors that occurred simultaneously?
- Does the impact on knowledge, behavior, or policies vary across different groups of intended beneficiaries (for example, males, females, indigenous people), across regions, or over time?
- Are there any unintended effects of the health promotion program, either positive or negative?
- How effective is the health promotion program in comparison with alternative interventions?
- Given the intermediate effects on the target population, is the health promotion program worth the resources expended so far?

4. **Outcome evaluation** examines the changes in people during or after their participation in the health promotion program. Although the ultimate goal of health promotion programs is to improve a population's health status (for example, reduce rates of lung cancer), funding and time limitations often force program managers to choose outcomes that are proxy measures of long-term outcomes—for example, knowledge gains, attitude changes, skills acquired, or behavior changes. Furthermore, depending on its design, the outcome evaluation can examine changes in the short term (for example, hours or days after program participation), intermediate term (one to six months), and long term (six months to a few years). In effect, program outcomes are often observable and measurable milestones toward an ultimate goal that may take many years if not decades to accomplish. For example, although a smoking cessation program for teenagers may have a goal that 75 percent of the program participants will no longer be smoking after one year, the ultimate health status outcome (for example, presence or absence of lung cancer) in this group may not be known for many years. The outcome

objective of this particular program would not be a decrease in lung cancer mortality; rather, it would be the percentage of program participants who do not smoke after one year. Therefore, the outcome evaluation would focus on tracking and measuring the proportion of people who achieve the program's one-year cessation outcome.

## Evaluation Terms

A number of terms are used in discussing evaluation, regardless of the evaluation type. They reflect the common purpose of evaluation in general—to provide the best information to answer people's questions and help them make good decisions. Following is a list of some of the most common terms. Some of the same terms were mentioned in Chapter Four. In Chapter Four, the focus was on understanding the health needs of individuals in order to answer questions related to how best to design a program to meet those needs. In this chapter, the terms are used to help answer questions about whether the program met those needs.

- **Quantitative methods** involve the gathering and analysis of numerical data. Various techniques are then used to make sense of the numbers or scores in order to interpret the results of a program or intervention. Quantitative methods are more directive than qualitative methods; the evaluator determines the scope and direction of the evaluation questions. Numerical data might include a summary of demographic variables, pretest and posttest scores, attitude and self-efficacy ratings, and existing numerical data. Quantitative methods are commonly used in conducting evaluations of health promotion programs. Examples include tracking the number of participants in a weight management program, recording participants' scores on a survey of fruit and vegetable preferences, and comparing pretest and posttest scores on measures of knowledge before and after a pregnancy prevention program for adolescents.
- **Qualitative methods** involve the gathering of non-numerical data, including descriptions of the program, often from the perspectives and experiences of the program participants themselves. The data consist primarily of information gathered from interviews with key informants (for example, policymakers), observations of program intervention activities (for example, nutritious meal preparation), and focus groups with people who may share common values or experiences (for example, a gay and lesbian focus group discussing their experience and knowledge of tobacco use in the GLBT community). There are various methods for analyzing qualitative data, including a

constant comparison method that generates themes from data collected from interview transcripts, focus groups, or even visual representations such as videotapes and photos.

- **Mixed or integrated methods** involve a combination of qualitative or quantitative methods. The choice of which mix of methods to use is largely determined by the evaluation's question and purpose. Let's say, for example, that your evaluation question is, Did participants who attended a multiple-session stress reduction workshop reduce their self-perceived stress levels? To answer this question, you could use a pretest-posttest quantitative design in which you administer a short survey asking program participants to rate their levels of stress on a Likert scale, using a series of questions. Then, after the stress reduction program was completed, you would administer the same questionnaire. By comparing whether there was a statistically significant difference in median stress scores before and after the training, you could conduct a quantitative evaluation. However, if you wanted to determine how meaningful the training activities were in helping participants to reduce their stress, you would ask a different type of question altogether. A qualitative design would ask an open-ended question, allowing participants to express whatever way they wish to share with the evaluator. For example, the question could be, "Now that you have participated in a four-session stress reduction workshop, please tell us which activities were meaningful in helping you to reduce your stress and why you thought so?" This type of question allows participants an opportunity to provide the evaluator with very descriptive data about their experience within the context of the training workshop. It adds to the overall program evaluation by determining not just whether the program was effective but why it was effective and the meaning the workshop provided for the program participants—a much broader and more helpful evaluation.

- **Reliability** refers to the ability of evaluation instruments to provide consistent results each time they are used. Use of reliable instruments is integral to evidence-based practice. Evaluation instruments are used in data collection and are discussed later in the chapter.

- **Validity** refers to the ability of evaluation instruments to accurately measure what the evaluator wants to measure (for example, knowledge of how to prevent sexually transmitted diseases). Use of valid instruments is also integral to evidence-based programs.

- **Cultural relevance** means that evaluation instruments have been developed with consideration of how cultural differences (for example, in language or beliefs) can influence the manner in which qualitative and quantitative questions are perceived and answered.

# EVALUATION FRAMEWORKS

Evaluations, regardless of their type (for example, formative, process, outcome, or impact), are guided by a *framework*. Another word for framework is *process*: a consistent approach, structure, and format that helps program participants, staff, and other stakeholders understand the thinking that went into the evaluation, the type of questions asked, how the information was collected, and the type of report that might be expected. Three frameworks are discussed in this section.

Selecting a framework to use for an evaluation involves looking at evaluations of other health promotion programs to see what they have done. Look at the process (framework) that was used in the evaluation, including the evaluation type and methods. Consider the program goals and objectives and purpose of the evaluation. Likewise consider what process will lead to a program that is clearer and more logical, to stronger partnerships that allow collaborators to focus on achieving common goals, to integrated information systems that support more systematic measurement, and to lessons learned that can be used effectively to guide changes in the program and target population.

## CDC Evaluation Framework

The evaluation framework of the Centers for Disease Control and Prevention (1999) is widely used for evaluations of health promotion programs. The six steps are

1. **Engage stakeholders**, especially those involved in program operations (for example, collaborators, funding officials, and staff); those served or affected by the program (for example, clients, neighborhood organizations, academic institutions, elected officials, and opponents); and primary users of the evaluation results. They all have an investment in what will be learned and what will be done with the information.

2. **Describe the health promotion program**, including its mission and objectives; the need or problem addressed; the expected effects of the program on the need or problem; the intervention strategies and activities; the human, material, and time resources available; the program's stage of development; the program's social, political, and economic context; and a logic model that describes the projected sequence of events for bringing about change.

3. **Focus the evaluation design** in order to assess the issues of greatest concern to stakeholders while using time and resources efficiently, accurately, and ethically. Specifically, a focused evaluation design takes into consideration the evaluation's purpose, the users who will receive the results, and how

the evaluation will be used. Evaluation design should also focus on developing answerable evaluation questions, developing reasonable evaluation methods, and having agreements on the roles and responsibilities of those conducting the evaluation.

4. **Gather credible evidence** that will be perceived by stakeholders as believable and relevant for answering questions about the program and its implementation or effects. Stakeholders who were involved in planning the evaluation and gathering data are more likely to accept the evaluation's conclusions and to act on its recommendations.

5. **Justify conclusions**, including recommendations, by ensuring that they are linked to the evidence gathered and to explicit values or standards that were set with the stakeholders. Following this strategy will enable stakeholders to use the evaluation results with confidence.

6. **Ensure use of the results and share lessons learned** by having a strong and participatory evaluation design; preparing stakeholders to use the results by exploring the possible positive and negative implications of the findings; promoting stakeholder feedback by holding periodic discussions during the evaluation process and routinely sharing interim findings, provisional interpretations, and draft reports; following up with the stakeholders by advocating for use of the findings when decisions about the program are being made; and disseminating the findings through full disclosure and impartial reporting in a report that is tailored to the audience and that explains the evaluation's focus, its limitations, and its strengths and weaknesses.

## RE-AIM Evaluation Framework

The RE-AIM (reach, effectiveness, adoption, implementation, maintenance) evaluation framework recognizes the importance of both external validity (reach and adoption) and internal validity (effectiveness and implementation) in the evaluation of program interventions (Glasgow, Vogt, & Boles, 1999). It is useful in estimating public health impact, comparing different health policies, designing policies for increased likelihood of success, and identifying areas for integration of policies with other health promotion strategies. Questions that might be asked when using the RE-AIM framework to evaluate health promotion programs are shown in Table 10.1.

## Institute of Medicine Obesity Evaluation Framework

In 2007, the Institute of Medicine (IOM) of the National Academies published a report by the IOM Committee on Progress in Preventing Childhood Obesity,

TABLE 10.1    RE-AIM Dimensions and Template Questions for Evaluating
Health Promotion Programs

| RE-AIM Dimension | Evaluation Questions |
|---|---|
| Reach (individual level) | What percentage of potentially eligible participants (1) were excluded, (2) took part, and how representative were they? |
| Efficacy, effectiveness (individual level) | What impact did the intervention have on (1) all participants who began the program, (2) short-term and intermediate outcomes, and (3) both positive and negative (unintended) outcomes, including quality of life? |
| Adoption (population level) | What percentage of settings and intervention agents within these settings (for example, schools and educators, medical offices and physicians) (1) were excluded, (2) participated, and how representative were they? |
| Implementation (population level) | To what extent were the various intervention components delivered as intended in the protocol, especially when conducted by different staff members (for example, non-researchers) in applied settings? |
| Maintenance (both individual and population level) | *Individual level:* (1) What were the long-term effects (minimum six to twelve months following intervention)? (2) What was the attrition rate, were dropouts representative, and how did attrition affect conclusions about effectiveness? *Population level:* (1) To what extent were different intervention components continued or institutionalized? (2) How was the original program modified? |

comprising thirteen experts in diverse disciplines, including health-related disciplines, community development and mobilization, private sector initiatives, and program evaluation. Among the committee's findings was an evaluation framework that stakeholders can use to assess progress in a range of efforts to prevent childhood obesity across different sectors and settings, including schools, workplaces, health care organizations, and communities (Koplan, Liverman, Kraak, & Wisham, 2007).

The framework recognizes the impact of key contextual factors (for example, environmental, cultural, normative, and historical factors) that influence the potential impact of an intervention. The evaluation framework, shown in Figure 10.1, represents the resources and inputs, strategies and actions, and a range of

**FIGURE 10.1   Institute of Medicine's Obesity Evaluation Framework**

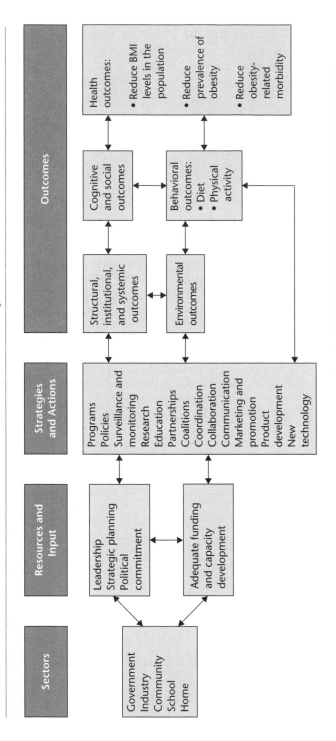

*Source:* Koplan, Liverman, Kraak, & Wisham, 2007, p. 43.

outcomes that are important in prevention of childhood obesity. The IOM obesity evaluation framework also categorizes outcomes based on the nature of the change: (1) structural, institutional, and systemic outcomes; (2) environmental outcomes; (3) population-level or individual-level cognitive and social outcomes; (4) behavioral outcomes (for example, dietary or physical activity behaviors); and (5) health outcomes (Koplan, Liverman, Kraak, & Wisham, 2007).

Whether process, impact, or outcome evaluation can be conducted depends on a program's intervention strategies and actions, the availability of evaluation resources and expertise (for example, for data collection and analysis), and the needs of stakeholders (Koplan, Liverman, Kraak, & Wisham, 2007). Although not part of the framework, the program's timeline is critical because it can affect the evaluation's depth. For example, short-term programs may result only in the measurement of increases in physical activity behaviors, whereas intermediate-term interventions might measure environmental changes in healthy food offerings in school lunches, and long-term interventions might actually measure biological changes such as decreases in the BMI of children involved in a program that promotes healthy foods and exercise.

This framework is focused on assessing policy and community interventions designed to influence food and physical activity environments. It is guided by a systems approach that explicitly takes into account the social contexts in which decisions are made and the multiple determinants of policy and community action (for example, projected health and economic impacts, feasibility, acceptability, and public demand). While focused on obesity prevention, this framework can guide more general evaluation efforts to assess and use scientific evidence in complex, multifactorial public health challenges (for example, violence, HIV/AIDS, and tobacco control).

## EVALUATION DESIGNS

Once the evaluator knows the type of evaluation and the framework that will be used, attention can be focused on the evaluation design. Selecting an evaluation design consists of two basic sets of tasks (Dignan & Carr, 1995).

The first task in selecting an evaluation design is to decide whether to use qualitative methods, quantitative methods, or a combination of the two. The program goals and objectives and the level of program development are reviewed to determine the important variables, resources, and constraints. This is followed by a review of the needs and expectations for the evaluation, including how the evaluation results will be used (for example, to help in the initial implementation or to contribute to the program's scientific validity). If the reviews point toward a need for descriptions and narratives about a program to provide understanding of participants' motivation, case studies, barriers, and other descriptive information from the participants, stakeholders, and staff, then qualitative methods would be selected. If the reviews point toward a need for numeric (hard) data, such as counts, ratings, scores, or classifications (for example, nutrition knowledge test scores, BMI measurements, or mortality rates related to lung disease), quantitative methods would be appropriate. It is also common and frequently advantageous to combine quantitative and qualitative methods (to use mixed methods) to take advantage of each method's strengths. Once there is a decision on the methods, decisions can be made about how to measure the variables (for example, with instruments, interviews, or observation) and how to analyze and report the data and findings.

The second task in selecting an evaluation design is to answer several key questions in order to match the needs of the evaluation with a design that ensures the evaluation can be completed (Centers for Disease Control and Prevention, 1999; Dignan & Carr, 1995). These questions include the following:

1. How much time do you have to conduct the evaluation?
2. When can you best collect the evaluation information—before the program begins, during implementation, or after the program ends?
3. How many individuals (program participants, stakeholders, staff) will be involved in the evaluation?
4. Do you have data analysis skills or access to statistical consultants?
5. Is it important to generalize your findings to other populations?
6. Are stakeholders concerned with validity and reliability?
7. Do you have the ability to randomize participants into experimental and control groups?
8. Do you have access to a comparison group?

Another aspect of selecting the evaluation design relates to the level of confidence needed for the evaluation findings. Questions 5, 6, 7, and 8 in the previous list address the scientific validity or level of confidence of an evaluation. In considering validity, we need to think about three primary approaches (Table 10.2) to designing an evaluation (Cook & Campbell, 1979). The *experimental design* is considered the gold standard; in this type of evaluation, participants are randomly assigned either to the experimental group (also known as the *treatment* or *intervention group*), which receives the intervention, or to the control group, which has the same demographic or other characteristics (for example, age, gender, race, alcohol consumption behavior) but does not receive the health promotion intervention. In both cases the participants are surveyed before the intervention (pretest) and

TABLE 10.2  Experimental Design Options

| Design Type | Design Considerations | Design Example |
|---|---|---|
| Experimental design: Random assignment Experimental group $O_{T1}$ I $O_{T2}$ Control group $O_{T1}$  $O_{T2}$ | May provide evidence of effectiveness May have predictive power Usually expensive Difficulty in finding enough participants Ethical considerations (who gets program benefit and who doesn't) | A school-based sex education intervention based on social cognitive theory and social network and social support theory is designed to prevent sexually transmitted diseases and unwanted pregnancies by increasing condom use among a sample of high school seniors of 2,411 randomly assigned high school students (Kvalem, Sundet, Rivø, Eilertsen, & Bakketeig, 1996). |
| Quasi-experimental: No random assignment with control group Experimental group $O_{T1}$ I $O_{T2}$ Comparison group $O_{T1}$  $O_{T2}$ | Experimental group may not have the same demographic variables as the control group Difficult to generalize results to other groups or situations | A program used the theory of planned behavior to increase risk perceptions and thereby reduce the use of alcohol and other drugs among university students. The program was evaluated through repeated anonymous random sample surveys of all students on the intervention campus and on a similar control campus that was not implementing prevention efforts during the same period. However, the campuses were not randomly assigned to intervention versus control conditions (Miller, Toscova, Miller, & Sanchez, 2000). |
| Pre-experimental: No random assignment and no control group: Experimental group $O_{T1}$ I $O_{T2}$ No comparison group | No predictive power Can be strengthened by doing multiple measures over time | A statewide program in California to prevent the illegal sale of tobacco to minors uses baseline observations of underage fifteen- and sixteen-year-old youth volunteers who seek to purchase tobacco from store clerks and calculates the percentage of merchants who sold to the underage youths. An educational intervention occurs after the baseline observation, which in turn is followed by a follow-up observation (a sting) approximately nine months later (California Department of Public Health, 2007). |

*Note:* O = measurement (for example, questionnaire, survey); I = intervention (for example, education, medication); T1 = pretest time; T2 = posttest time.

after the intervention (posttest) in order to see whether the desired change has occurred. The *quasi-experimental design* has the same structure as the experimental design, but the participants are not randomly selected. The *pre-experimental design* has neither randomization nor a comparison group. These different evaluation designs provide different levels of confidence in the findings about a program's effectiveness and success.

## DATA COLLECTION AND ANALYSIS

After the decisions about evaluation type, framework, and evaluation design have been made, the evaluator's focus turns to collecting the desired information (data). The data collected during an evaluation are used to answer questions about the program's processes, its immediate impact, and its final outcomes. Data collection involves the process of collecting, managing, organizing, analyzing, synthesizing, and summarizing the data in order to make sense of them and answer the evaluation's overall questions. Evaluation methods such as instruments, observations, interviews, and focus groups are used to collect data. The most effective evaluations of health promotion programs use methods that are validated and reliable. The programs listed in the National Registry of Evidence-Based Programs and Practices (http://www.nrepp.samhsa.gov) and the National Cancer Institute's Research-Tested Intervention Programs (http://rtips.cancer.gov/rtips/index. do) all use such methods (see Chapter Five, Figures 5.1 and 5.2). However, as indicated in Table 10.3, the decision about which data collection method to use depends on what is being measured. And what is being measured is based on the questions posed by the evaluation. Once these are known, then a specific instrument or set of focus group questions can be selected.

## EVALUATION REPORTS

An evaluation report is commonly used to report the outcome of an evaluation. While reports can have different styles, it is important that they provide user-friendly information to stakeholders in a timely fashion. The timing of formative or process evaluations is important; quick feedback is typically needed in order to provide useful information to stakeholders as the staff work to implement the program. Typically, summative or outcome evaluations are written and presented at the end of a program year. In some cases, a program status report at midyear or for another time period is required. In all cases, evaluators and program managers

TABLE 10.3    Changes to Be Measured and Nutrition-Related
Examples of Data Collection Methods

| What Is Being Measured | Quantitative Data | Qualitative Data |
|---|---|---|
| Awareness | Written instrument (yes-no items) to measure awareness of public service announcements on healthy eating | Interviews (intercept surveys) at local supermarkets to measure awareness of a healthy eating campaign |
| | Telephone survey to measure awareness of a healthy nutrition social marketing campaign | Focus groups to measure awareness of a nutrition-related social marketing campaign |
| Knowledge | Written or oral knowledge questionnaire (pretest and posttest on Likert scale items or multiple-choice items) to measure knowledge gained from a nutrition education seminar | Interviews to measure knowledge about the nutritional value of fruits and vegetables |
| | | Focus groups with children to gather information on their knowledge of the nutritional value of certain fruits and vegetables |
| Attitudes | Written instrument (pretest and posttest on Likert scale items or value scale items) to measure attitudes and preferences of children about certain fruits and vegetables | Interviews with mothers of small children to identify their attitudes toward feeding their children fresh fruits and vegetables |
| | | Focus groups with children to gather information on their attitudes toward certain fruits and vegetables |
| Behavior | Self-reports, using an instrument with scaled responses to measure the frequency and types of healthy eating behaviors | Interviews with individuals to gather information on their eating behaviors |
| | Observations of children in a cafeteria setting to count different types of foods consumed | Focus groups with teenagers to discuss the unusual eating behaviors of teens |
| | | Observations of children in a cafeteria setting to gather information on their eating behaviors |
| Skills | Scaled measurement of the degree to which students in the nutrition education program can skillfully prepare or cook fruits and vegetables | Comments based on observations of people in a nutrition education program as they prepare recipes using fruits and vegetables |

*(Continued)*

TABLE 10.3   Changes to Be Measured and Nutrition-Related
Examples of Data Collection Methods (Continued)

| What Is Being Measured | Quantitative Data | Qualitative Data |
|---|---|---|
| Policy changes | Measurement of the number of children who consume vegetables before and after a school district implements a policy that requires salad bars in school cafeterias | Interviews with children in a school that has salad bars, to gather their opinions on what they like or don't like in the salad bars since a policy that mandates salad bars was implemented |
| Organizational changes | Records documenting the number and demographic profile of people who go to a food bank for food but now also receive information on how to prepare nutritious food and how to access the food stamp program | Interviews with food bank staff to gather their opinions on whether the food bank's new nutrition education and food stamp outreach activities are having a positive effect on their clients |
| Environmental changes | Survey of the farmers' markets in the county to document the size of the markets, types of produce provided, and the cost of the produce | Observations of and interviews with people attending a new farmers' market, to identify their satisfaction with the market |
| Health status | Medical tests and screenings to measure heart disease status<br><br>Health risk appraisals to measure risk of heart disease | Interviews with patients to gather opinions and identify factors that contribute to their overall health status |
| Quality of life | Proxy measures (clean food, clean water, and availability of organic produce) | Interviews to gather people's opinions on the overall quality of nutrition in their community |

participating in the evaluation must keep the reporting needs of the stakeholders in mind. The following are basic sections of an evaluation report:

- **Cover page**. At minimum, a cover page will include a *title* for the evaluation, the *date* the report was completed, and the *author* (or authors). Ideally, a reader will know the evaluation's focus and recognize its timeliness after just a quick glance at the cover page. Evaluation photos or organizational logos are often used on the cover page to help convey the evaluation's topic and to spark interest. Contact information or funder information might also be included on the cover.

- **Executive summary**. As the name implies, this section summarizes the evaluation report for the "executive," which today really means readers with little time who need to quickly know the main points. Given that this describes the vast majority of people, a well-written executive summary can greatly increase the size of the audience that learns, at least, the major evaluation findings. An executive summary must concisely address the evaluation's purpose, approach, and key findings or recommendations.

- **Introduction and evaluation questions**. This section provides important background information and frames the overall report. The introduction should explain why the evaluation was undertaken, by whom, and for whom. In addition, the specific questions the evaluation was designed to address must be clearly stated. The method or approach of an effective evaluation always follows from the question (or questions) that it is trying to answer. Well-defined and compelling questions are essential to a good evaluation report. The introduction also typically provides a description of the program or intervention that is being evaluated.

- **Methods and results**. The methods section describes how the evaluation was carried out. Typically, the greatest detail pertains to the evaluation design, the sources of information used, and how this information was collected and analyzed. For example, this section will describe how data collection tools like surveys or in-depth interview guides were constructed, how respondents were selected or sampled, and the analysis techniques that were used. Evaluation results consist of a summary and presentation of the analyzed information.

- **Findings and recommendations**. This section describes what was learned through the evaluation. In the section the answers to the original evaluation questions are given. This section also typically includes acknowledgment of limitations that may have influenced the evaluation's results and findings. Recommendations are the future actions suggested by the findings; this section is tailored to the evaluation's intended principal audience. In the traditional program evaluation paradigm, recommendations were often generated by the external evaluator as his or her "expert" suggestions to the program implementers. However, in more participatory evaluation approaches, diverse program stakeholders and direct participants in the program are involved in the development of recommendations based on the findings.

Evaluation reports take different shapes and forms based on the audience for the report and how the report will be used. Aim for a publication that is short enough to be read in one sitting at the time it is received or viewed and attractive enough that the reader will want to take time to look through it. If the report goes on the "to read" pile, the opportunity for it to be seriously considered may have been missed. Often it is helpful to prepare one or two pages of *evaluation highlights* that provide an overview of the evaluation and the significant findings. (See Exhibit 10.1 for an example of evaluation highlights.) Always consider how the evaluation findings will be used. Ask what questions the evaluation is answering.

## Exhibit 10.1
## Evaluation Highlights for Community Trials Intervention to Reduce High-Risk Drinking

The Community Trials Intervention to Reduce High-Risk Drinking (RHRD) is a multi-component, community-based program developed to alter alcohol use patterns of people of all ages—for example, drinking and driving, underage drinking, acute (binge) drinking, and related problems. The program's aim is to help communities reduce various types of alcohol-related accidents, violence, and resulting injuries.

The program uses a set of environmental interventions, including

- Community awareness
- Responsible beverage service (RBS)
- Prevention of underage alcohol access
- Enforcement
- Community mobilization

### Target Population

Each of the six intervention and comparison communities located in northern and southern California and South Carolina had approximately 100,000 residents. The communities were racially and ethnically diverse and included a mix of urban, suburban, and rural settings.

### Benefits

The program brings about

- Reductions in intentional and unintentional alcohol-related injuries (for example, car and household accidents, assaults)
- Mobilization of community members and key policymakers
- Increased enforcement of drinking and driving laws
- Decreased formal and informal youth access to alcohol
- Responsible alcoholic beverage service and sales policies

### How It Works

For the RHRD program to be successful, the implementing organization must first determine which program components will best produce the desired results for its community. The RHRD program uses five prevention and health promotion components:

- **Alcohol access:** Assists communities in using zoning and municipal regulations to restrict alcohol access by controlling the density of alcohol outlets (for example, bars, liquor stores)
- **Responsible beverage service:** Assists servers and retailers of alcoholic beverages in developing policies and procedures to reduce intoxication and driving after drinking

- **Risk of drinking and driving:** Increases actual and perceived risk of arrest for driving after drinking through increased law enforcement and sobriety checkpoints
- **Underage alcohol access:** Reduces youth access to alcohol through increased enforcement of laws that prohibit alcohol sales to minors and by training alcohol retailers to avoid selling to minors and those who provide alcohol to minors
- **Community mobilization:** Provides communities with the tools to form the coalitions needed to implement and support the interventions of the preceding four prevention components

## Evaluation Design

The project evaluation used a longitudinal, multiple-time series design across three intervention communities. The matched comparison communities served as no-treatment controls. Within this design, the effects of project interventions can be determined by comparing outcomes to those from matched comparison communities.

Data sources included

- A community telephone survey including self-reported measures of drinking as well as drinking and driving
- Traffic crash records
- Emergency room surveys
- Local news coverage of alcohol-related topics
- Roadside surveys conducted on weekend evenings

## Outcomes

- 51 percent decline in self-reported driving with blood alcohol "over the legal limit" in the intervention communities compared with the comparison communities
- 6 percent decline in self-reported amounts consumed per drinking occasion
- 49 percent decline in self-reported "having had too much to drink"
- 10 percent reduction in nighttime injury crashes
- 6 percent reduction in crashes in which the driver had been drinking
- 43 percent reduction in assault injuries observed in emergency rooms
- 2 percent reduction in hospitalized assault injuries

## Proven Results

- Decreased alcohol sales to youths
- Increased enforcement of laws prohibiting drunk driving
- Implementation and enforcement of RBS policies
- Adoption of policies that limit the dense placement of alcohol-selling establishments
- Increased coverage of alcohol-related issues in local news media

Make sure these answers are clearly stated in both the brief evaluation highlights and the full evaluation report.

The evaluation report is best used to bring program staff, participants, and stakeholders together to help address the health concerns of the target population. Think strategically about the groups of individuals whose questions are answered by the evaluation. As the report is being prepared, include these individuals and groups in the report-writing process. For example, small details about the format of the data presentation (for example, graphs, pie charts, or tables) form one area where it can be helpful to solicit input on how people perceive that the evaluation findings will be shared and with whom. Prepare tailored reports in different formats (for example, one or two pages of highlights, a single-page executive summary, the full report, a podcast) to match the interests of the groups receiving the evaluation report.

Evaluators may want to consider using Web sites or other media outlets (for example, radio, television, podcasts, or YouTube videos) to disseminate an evaluation report. Web sites have the advantage of wide distribution and easy access; however, computer access (and, possibly, technical support) would be required in order for all interested individuals and groups to access the report. Finally, think about how the report fits with the overall program communication plan (see Chapter Eight). Consider how the process of developing and pretesting the message of the evaluation report can enhance the evaluation findings and recommendations to be used to improve the program. View the report as part of the overall communication plan to provide program staff, stakeholders, and participants with health communications that are both consistent and effective.

## EVALUATION AND PROGRAM DESIGN

As we mentioned earlier in the chapter, in the planning and development of a health promotion program, evaluation is frequently viewed as the last phase of program development, something conducted only after a program is complete. Sometimes this is referred to as a *linear evaluation model*. However, it is a mistake to think that evaluation happens only after a program ends. In fact, evaluation should be part of program planning, and planning should be part of evaluation. Ideally, evaluations start at the beginning of a health promotion program, occurring in parallel with planning and implementation in order to provide a continual information feedback loop that will help the program staff to improve and shape a health promotion program. This feedback cycle characterizes the *circular evaluation model*. The evaluation feedback loop (Figure 10.2) provides information that, through dialogue and reflection, contributes to decision making and planning, which in turn leads to action. The action then prompts a new cycle of information and feedback. The similarities in terminology and processes between a

FIGURE 10.2   Program Evaluation Feedback Loop in the
Circular Evaluation Model

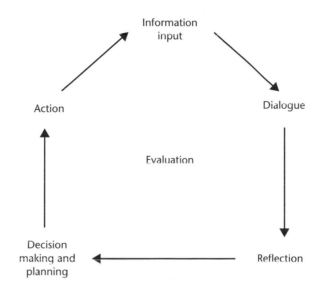

needs assessment (discussed in Chapter Four) and a program evaluation (discussed in this chapter) are consistent with a circular evaluation model. Furthermore it highlights the connection between the needs assessment and evaluation—what is evaluated in a program is the product of the priorities determined by the needs assessment, and the evaluation assesses how effectively these priorities have been implemented and addressed. In other words a program evaluation assesses which needs of the participants have been met by a program and which still need to be addressed. Thus program evaluation is a form of needs assessment.

The importance of the circular evaluation model has grown as health promotion programs work to eliminate health disparities. For example, a process evaluation using mixed methods (attendance data and brief telephone calls to check participants' program satisfaction and get feedback on program logistics) can provide program staff, stakeholders, and participants with quick feedback on how well matched a program is to the participants. The process evaluation would help staff to make adjustments to ensure a program's cultural competence. At the same time, this would require that the program evaluation itself be culturally competent (see Chapter Two), in order to adequately reflect the issues of the program participants.

One way to understand how evaluation is used throughout the life cycle of a program is to examine the role of evaluation in the PRECEDE-PROCEED model (Green & Kreuter, 2005), which was discussed in Chapter Three (Figure 3.2). As displayed in Table 10.4, the model begins with formative evaluation in the

**TABLE 10.4** The Evaluation Phases of the PRECEDE-PROCEED Model

| Conditions to Be Evaluated | Phases 1–5: Formative Evaluation | Phases 6, 7, and 8: Process, Impact, and Outcome Evaluation |
|---|---|---|
| Quality of life | Phase 1: Social assessment<br><br>Review the literature or assess and document the feelings, needs, concerns, assets, and community capacity that describe quality of life. | Phase 8: Outcome evaluation<br><br>Measure the factors that describe overall changes in the quality of life. |
| Health conditions | Phase 2: Epidemiological assessment<br><br>Review the literature or assess and document health conditions, including morbidity, mortality, disability, and risk factors. | Phase 8: Outcome evaluation<br><br>Measure and describe the epidemiological indicators that represent changes in health conditions. |
| Genetics<br>Behavior<br>Environment | Phase 2: Epidemiological assessment<br><br>Review the literature or assess and document indicators of health, including genetic, behavioral, and environmental factors that affect quality of life. | Phase 7: Impact evaluation<br><br>Measure and describe the epidemiological and social indicators that represent changes in behavior and environments that affect health status. |
| Predisposing factors<br>Enabling factors<br>Reinforcing factors | Phase 3: Educational and ecological assessment<br><br>Review the literature or assess and document the cognitive and social antecedents that influence behaviors that in turn affect health. | Phase 7: Impact evaluation<br><br>Measure changes in the impact objectives that reflect the predisposing, enabling, and reinforcing factors that promote healthy behaviors and environments. |
| Health program<br>Educational strategies<br>Policy<br>Regulation<br>Organization | Phase 4a: Intervention alignment<br><br>Phase 4b: Administrative and policy assessment<br><br>Review the literature or assess and document administrative resources, regulations, and policies that can affect educational and environmental factors and shape program implementation. | Phase 6: Process evaluation<br><br>Document and measure process objectives that address program capacity, the activities and strategies that constitute the intervention, and the response of practitioners and participants to the intervention's processes. |
| Program operation | Phase 5: Implementation<br><br>Implement activities that deploy program resources, implement policy and organizational changes, and coordinate the program's interventions. | Phase 6: Process evaluation<br><br>Document and measure program capacity, the activities that constitute the intervention, and the response of practitioners and participants to the intervention's processes. |

first five PRECEDE phases and uses process, impact, and outcome evaluation in the PROCEED phases (Phases 6–8) to measure and document change in people and their environments.

## IMPLEMENTING AN EVALUATION

The nuts and bolts of doing an evaluation may include finding and working with an evaluator and dealing with costs, time frame, and participant rights.

### Finding and Working with an Evaluator

Most program directors do not have the time, personnel resources, or desire to carry out a formal evaluation; therefore, it is not uncommon for funding agencies (for example, federal and state agencies and foundations) to require that program directors hire an external evaluator. An external evaluator may be requested if a funding agency feels that an external (and thus objective) evaluator will conduct a stronger evaluation. Selecting a program evaluator is an important management task. A good evaluator provides timely program information to refine and keep a program on track. In addition, a good evaluator accurately documents the program's experiences and effectiveness. This information is useful to a program's stakeholders and for seeking future funding.

Ideally, the program director and stakeholders of a health promotion program decide what the evaluation goals should be. Then, a program evaluator can help the program staff determine what the evaluation methods should be and how the resulting data will be analyzed and reported back to the program and its stakeholders. The degree of evaluator involvement may vary, depending on financial resources, but at a minimum, an evaluator should be hired to identify the appropriate evaluation design and methods and how the data can be collected. The program might find a less expensive resource to apply the methods (for example, to conduct interviews or send out and analyze results of questionnaires).

If no outside help can be obtained, the staff and stakeholders of the program can still learn a great deal by applying the data collection methods and analyzing the results themselves. However, there is a risk that data about the strengths and weaknesses of a program will not be interpreted objectively if the data are analyzed by the people who are responsible for ensuring the program is a good one—that is, if program directors are policing themselves. This caution is not meant to fault program directors but to recognize the strong biases inherent in trying to objectively look at and publicly (at least within the organization) report about programs. Therefore, if at all possible, have someone other than the program managers determine and examine the results of an evaluation.

If an external evaluator is sought, the first step in the process is to develop a clear description of evaluation needs that can be distributed to potential evaluators. This description should include an overview of the program's location, its purpose, the population served, a brief description of the program's objectives and elements (intervention, policies, community action, or advocacy), and the funder's requirements for evaluation.

Evaluators can be found at universities and colleges and through the American Evaluation Association and its network of state and regional affiliates. In addition, some foundations and agencies—such as the W. K. Kellogg Foundation, the Robert Wood Johnson Foundation, and federal and state departments of health and human services—maintain directories of evaluators. Another way to find evaluators is through word of mouth from colleagues who work in similar programs.

Although an evaluator is usually not considered a member of the program staff, he or she should be considered an important member of the program team. The evaluator's level of involvement will depend on the evaluation budget and contracted time to work on the evaluation. For example, the following list shows a number of activities that an evaluator would complete. As part of the budget and contracting process, the amount of time the evaluator will need for each activity would be projected.

- Attend program meetings or conference calls.
- Help program staff and relevant program stakeholders design the evaluation.
- Design the data collection instruments in collaboration with program staff and key stakeholders.
- Help design the data collection methods and monitor their implementation.
- Provide oversight of the database, even though staff may enter the data.
- Analyze the data or subcontract and provide oversight of the analysis.
- Write the evaluation report.
- Present findings to stakeholders.

## Evaluation Costs

An evaluation's cost is related to the complexity of the program being evaluated and the program's internal resources and expertise. Small programs with a single health education intervention may require an outside evaluator only to design the evaluation and develop and pretest the data-gathering instruments that the project staff will administer and analyze themselves. This work may cost a few thousand dollars. A common variation of this approach is a program that uses

staff for the activities that require legwork (for example, administering instruments, conducting observations and interviews, and doing data entry), while the
evaluator conducts the evaluation design, instrument development, data analysis, and report writing. These types of evaluations can range from $10,000 to
$25,000, depending on the program's size, timeline, and intervention methods.
For example, a program evaluation that requires traveling to multiple sites and
interviewing many key informants will be more expensive than one in which
program participants complete pretest and posttest instruments in a classroom
setting. The Council on Foundations (2003) notes that several factors can increase
evaluation costs, including

- A desire to attribute causal impact to the program, which means using an
  experimental design with a control group (and hence more data collection
  and analysis)
- Programs that focus on whole communities rather than specific groups of
  individuals
- Multi-site rather than single-site programs
- Programs that try to make relatively small reductions in problems, so that
  evidence of impact is hard to discern
- A need to collect primary data, when suitable records or published statistics
  are not available
- Designs that require data collection in person
- Designs that require collecting data at multiple points in time
- A need for data that must be collected through highly technical procedures

## Time Frame for Evaluation

If the purpose of evaluation is program improvement, then the evaluation needs
to continue as long as the program stakeholders seek to improve the program.
*Continuous program improvement* is often the stated purpose of evaluation, and if it is,
then evaluation in some form should continue as long as the program operates.

However, program evaluations are rarely funded for the life of a program.
Sometimes the evaluation is funded for only the first two or three years of a
program, and often this time frame is not long enough. It may be unrealistic to
expect a new program to attain even some of its short-term outcomes or, certainly,
its long-term outcomes in as little as two or three years. Given this reality, most
programs build evaluation into the program infrastructure in order to ensure a
continual flow of information back to the stakeholders. Identification and reporting of selected program indicators is a common strategy used by most health

promotion programs; annual values of key indicators over a period of years are shown for comparison purposes.

## Ethical Considerations

Data from program participants is gathered and analyzed in the course of program evaluation. Program participants have rights that need to be protected. In university research settings and increasingly in non-academic settings, many research and evaluation projects involving human participants must undergo a review by an independent institutional review board (IRB). The IRB must be composed of members who have enough experience, expertise, and diversity to make an informed decision on whether research is ethical, whether informed consent is sufficient, and whether appropriate safeguards have been put in place. *Informed consent* means advising clients about the nature of the data collection or research and obtaining their approval to participate (San José State University, 2007). Individuals being asked to participate in research and evaluations have the following rights (San José State University, 2007):

- To be asked to participate as a subject in a study involving human subjects in an open, honest, and non-coercive manner
- To be told the project is research on evaluation
- To be told what the study is investigating
- To be told exactly what will be required, including where and when the study will occur and what materials or devices will be employed
- To be clearly informed of any possible risks or inconveniences, including psychological stress, physical stress, or harm
- To be told about any possible benefits that might reasonably be expected from participation in the study
- To be told about any appropriate alternative procedures
- To be encouraged to ask questions concerning the study before and during the course of the study
- To be informed of any changes during the course of the study that might affect a person's willingness to continue to participate in the study
- To be told of any psychological or medical help available in the event of harm
- To be assured that no service to which a person is otherwise entitled will be lost or jeopardized if a person chooses not to participate in the study
- To be informed that a person has the right to choose not to participate in the study or in any part of the study

- To withdraw from the study at any time without affecting their relationship with any participating organization
- To receive a copy of their signed and dated consent form, or if a consent form is not used, to be given a list of appropriate contact numbers that can be used in the event of harm or complaints

Providing confidentiality or anonymity is necessary when gathering information on sensitive issues, especially those related to sexual behaviors or substance use. Care should be taken to protect the confidentiality or anonymity of participants. Identifying information such as names and addresses should not be collected unless it is necessary. Furthermore, collected data should be safely stored (for example, in a locked cabinet) and identifying information should be destroyed as soon as it is no longer needed. Data collectors should be trained in confidentiality issues.

Finally, the cultural and social competence of an evaluation is characterized by respect and acceptance of the differences found in diverse communities, whether the differences are related to race, ethnicity, socioeconomic status, sexual orientation, disability, age, gender, or other attributes. Sensitivity to diversity is evidenced by the active involvement of staff who are drawn from the program participants (Chapter Two) and by continual self-assessment of staff attitudes toward cultural and social differences, in order to eliminate bias.

## SUMMARY

Program evaluation is a method of assessing whether a health promotion program is achieving the desired results. Program evaluation involves systematically collecting information in order to answer evaluation questions and make program decisions. Evaluation that is integrated into the overall program design from its inception provides a continual information feedback loop for ongoing program modification and decision making in order to strengthen the program. Finally, as part of implementing a program evaluation, program staff and stakeholders must know how to select an evaluator, determine the evaluation's time frame and costs, and take steps to ensure that participant rights are protected.

## FOR PRACTICE AND DISCUSSION

1. What are the relationships between an evaluation's framework, design, and methods? What are the advantages and disadvantages of quantitative and qualitative methods? What is the role in an evaluation of the health theories discussed in Chapter Three (see Table 3.10)?

2. Select one program from the National Registry of Evidence-Based Programs and Practices (http://www.nrepp.samhsa.gov) and one from the National Cancer Institute's Research-Tested Intervention Programs (http://rtips.cancer .gov/rtips/index.do). What are these programs' evaluation designs and methods (for example, instruments, focus groups, or observations)? What evidence of the methods' validity and reliability is stated? How are the evaluation findings reported?

3. Discuss the differences between viewing evaluation as the last phase of a program (linear model) and viewing evaluation as a source of continual feedback and input (circular model).

4. You are evaluating a workplace-based nutrition and physical activity program with 300 employee participants. As part of the initial program phase, each employee participates in a confidential health review that includes a physical examination by a physician, blood cholesterol screening, body mass index (BMI) measurement, and health risk appraisal. This information is also available, with employee names removed, for the evaluation.

   a. What are the ethical considerations in conducting the evaluation?

   b. How will you ensure that the evaluation is culturally competent?

   c. What types of quantitative and qualitative evaluation measurements will you use (see Table 10.3) and why?

5. Using the evaluation highlights in Exhibit 10.1, identify what the evaluation resource and implementation considerations were likely to have been. How would the findings from the evaluation report most likely have been used, and by whom?

## KEY TERMS

CDC evaluation framework

Circular evaluation model

Cultural competence

Evaluation costs

Evaluation design

Evaluation ethics

Evaluation highlights

Evaluation report

Formative evaluation

Impact evaluation

Institute of Medicine obesity evaluation framework

Linear evaluation model

Mixed or integrated methods

National Registry of Evidence-Based Programs and Practices (NREPP)

Outcome evaluation

PRECEDE-PROCEED model

Process evaluation

Program evaluation

Qualitative methods

Quantitative methods

RE-AIM evaluation framework

Reliability

Research-Tested Intervention Programs (RTIPs)

Validity

# REFERENCES

California Department of Public Health. (2007). *Results from the 2007 Youth Tobacco Purchase Survey.* Retrieved November 8, 2009, from http://www.cdph.ca.gov/HEALTHINFO/NEWS/Pages/Update-01.aspx.

Centers for Disease Control and Prevention. (1999, September). Framework for program evaluation in public health. *Morbidity and Mortality Weekly Report, 48*(RR11), 1–40.

Cook, T. D., & Campbell, D. T. (1979). *Quasi-experimentation: Design and analysis issues for field settings.* Boston: Houghton Mifflin.

Council on Foundations. (2003). *Evaluation approaches and methods.* Retrieved November 8, 2009, from http://classic.cof.org/Learn/content.cfm?ItemNumber=1379.

Dignan, M. B., & Carr, P. A. (1995). *Program planning for health education and promotion* (2nd ed.). Philadelphia: Lea & Febiger.

Fourney, A. M., & Williams, M. L. (2003). Formative evaluation of an intervention to increase compliance to HIV therapies: The ALP project. *Health Promotion Practice, 4*(2), 165–170.

Gilmore, G. D., & Campbell, M. D. (2005). *Needs and capacity assessment strategies for health education and health promotion* (3rd ed.). Sudbury, MA: Jones & Bartlett.

Glasgow, R. E., Vogt, T. M., & Boles, S. M. (1999). Evaluating the public and community health impact of health promotion interventions: The RE-AIM framework. *American Journal of Public Health, 89*(9), 1322–1327.

Green, L. W., & Kreuter, M. W. (2005) *Health program planning: An educational and ecological approach* (4th ed.). New York: McGraw-Hill.

Koplan, J. P., Liverman, C. T., Kraak, V. I., & Wisham, S. L. (Eds.). (2007). *Progress in preventing childhood obesity: How do we measure up?* Washington, DC: Institute of Medicine & National Academies Press.

Kvalem, I. L., Sundet, J. M., Rivø, K. I., Eilertsen, D. E., & Bakketeig, L. S. (1996). The effect of sex education on adolescents' use of condoms: Applying the Solomon four-group design. *Health Education & Behavior, 6*(1), 34–47.

Miller, W. R., Toscova, R. T., Miller, J. H., & Sanchez, V. (2000). A theory-based motivational approach for reducing alcohol/drug problems in college. *Health Education & Behavior, 27*(6), 744–759.

San José State University. (2007). *Human subjects—Institutional review board.* Retrieved November 8, 2009, from http://www.sjsu.edu/gradstudies/Research/irb.html.

# CHAPTER ELEVEN

# LEADERSHIP FOR CHANGE AND SUSTAINABILITY

DAVID A. SLEET

SARA L. COLE

## LEARNING OBJECTIVES

- Explain catalyzing and mastering change to build resources and capacity, including effective leadership

- Discuss the benefits and process of engaging participants and building support

- Discuss professional preparation and practice of health education and health promotion professionals through continuing education and credentialing

- Describe how to enhance the impact and sustainability of health promotion programs

I N THE MOST EFFECTIVE health promotion programs, all staff, stakeholders, and program participants share leadership responsibilities. Consistent with the view of program evaluation as a continual loop of information and feedback that is not limited to the end of a program, program staff, stakeholders, and participants are constant sources of information (evaluation) that are critical as a program faces change and seeks sustainability. Leaders attend to the details of running the program while keeping in mind the big picture of what the program is striving to achieve. Four areas of leadership in which staff, stakeholders, and participants can exercise leadership are (1) catalyzing and mastering change, (2) building support for a program at a site, (3) promoting professionalism in health promotion, and (4) enhancing the impact and sustainability of health promotion programs. Leadership is often associated with formal structures and titles (for example, president, director, or supervisor), each with specific tasks, responsibilities, and authority. Leadership can also be informal and personal. Everyone has leadership ability. Recognizing the leadership ability of people is important in effective health promotion programs.

## CATALYZING AND MASTERING CHANGE

Health promotion programs promote change; it is the nature of their mission, purpose, and structure. Health promotion programs must use a variety of strategies to accommodate changes among the various influences on health that affect a program's participants. People's health is influenced on multiple levels, including the intrapersonal, interpersonal, and population levels, creating the potential for employment of many interventions simultaneously (Chapter One, Table 1.1). The intrapersonal level focuses on individual behaviors, knowledge, attitudes, beliefs, and personality traits. The interpersonal level deals with interactions between and among people—for example, families, friends, and peers. The population level includes institutional factors, social capital factors, and public policy. Institutional factors may be rules, regulations, policies, or informal structures that constrain or promote behaviors. Social capital includes social networks and norms among individuals, groups, and organizations. Public policy includes local, state, and federal policies and laws that regulate or support disease prevention practices, including early detection, disease control, and disease management (McLeroy, Bibeau, Steckler, & Glanz, 1988).

Leading a health promotion program requires awareness of the ecological context of the health issue, which presents intervention opportunities that range from promoting changes in individuals' behavior to advocating for changes in social policy and the environment. At the same time, programs need to change enough or change quickly enough to keep up with individual or social needs or they may not remain viable or survive for long. For health promotion programs, mastering change is a process of supporting and engaging people and resources in the context of an evolving and dynamic environment in order to enhance program staff members' and participants' health status, develop networks of people committed to health promotion, and improve health promotion program outcomes and impacts (Senge, 1999). McKenzie, Neiger, and Thackeray (2009) have identified six realities that complicate the ability of health promotion programs to be flexible and agile in their response to change:

1. **Health status can be changed, but it requires hard work and patience**. Health promotion programs can contribute to the health of environments, individuals, families, communities, workplaces, and organizations, but it takes time; change is hard work. Addressing health problems is more like a marathon than a short-distance sprint. One example is that it took over 200 years to eradicate smallpox from the earth, and that was after the vaccine had been discovered. While health promotion programs may focus on individual change, important changes in policies, laws, social norms, consumer products, and environments will be necessary to keep everyone safe and healthy.

2. **Building consensus that shapes health promotion programs takes time**. One person does not determine the success of a health promotion program; rather, health promotion programs are the result of input from different groups and individuals—for example, stakeholders, practitioners, and the target population. The name for this process is *consensus building*: the process of achieving general agreement among program participants and stakeholders about a particular problem, goal, or issue of mutual interest. It is best when it can occur in an environment of frank and honest discussion aimed at hearing and addressing people's concerns. Collaboration with and support of all stakeholders maximizes the process. Engaging stakeholders can facilitate desired environmental changes; however, reaching consensus among these groups often requires compromises—for example, other needs of the target population may need to be met before program goals can be accomplished.

3. **Stakeholder engagement is critical**. Throughout this book the importance of stakeholder engagement has been emphasized. Program participants and staff are key stakeholders but so are family members of participants, funders, colleagues, other individuals at a program site, government officials, labor unions, health care groups, or schools, to name a few. They have a vested interest in improving health and safety for everyone at a site. Identifying and

engaging all the stakeholders can be difficult, but it is critical. It requires dedicated resources—time, money, and people—to find stakeholders and to keep them engaged in the program in a way that supports mutual goals.

4. **The power of various partners to effect change may not be equal, but their contributions are equally important**. For example, a hypertension control program might engage partners from low-income minority communities, community health organizations, faith-based groups, businesses (for instance, barber shops and beauty shops) as part of a coalition to screen and refer high-risk individuals. While there would be major differences in the size of each group and the resources each could offer, each would contribute in ways that would add value to the program.

5. **Translation of research to practice is necessary, but it is not automatic**. As part of planning, implementing, and evaluating health promotion programs, a cycle of continual feedback between researchers and practitioners is necessary. Just because an intervention has worked in a research study does not mean it will work in a school, workplace, health care organization, or community. Effective health promotion program staff stay current on what research says about effective interventions and, more important, will know how to effectively translate this research into action. This role, which health promotion staff can assume, is sometimes described as being a *knowledge broker* for the setting.

6. **Resistance and reluctance on the part of individuals and organizations is to be expected**. A key focus in health promotion is voluntary action that people take to improve their own health. The needs and past experiences of individuals and organizations will affect their participation in a program. Resistance should be expected because change is difficult and maintaining old habits is comfortable. Likewise, often people know they should change but they are reluctant due to perceived barriers. Frequently, using the transtheoretical model stages of change can help program staff to tailor their strategies to overcome resistance and reluctance, thereby improving the health of a target population at a site.

Peter Senge's book *The Fifth Discipline* codifies many of the experiences of organizations in successfully dealing with change and learning how to change into a set of five practices for building learning capabilities in organizations (Senge, 1990). It is recommended that program staff, stakeholders, and participants be aware of and incorporate the five learning practices (which Senge calls *learning disciplines*) into their daily work.

- **Personal mastery**. This discipline of aspiration involves formulating a coherent picture of the results that people most desire to gain as individuals (their personal vision) alongside a realistic assessment of the current state of their life today (their current reality). Learning to cultivate the tension between vision and reality can expand people's capacity to make better choices and to achieve more of the results that they have chosen.

- **Mental models**. This discipline of reflection and inquiry focuses on developing awareness of the attitudes and perceptions that influence thought and interaction. By continually reflecting on, talking about, and reconsidering these internal pictures of the world, people gain more capability in governing their actions and decisions.
- **Shared vision**. This collective discipline establishes a focus on mutual purpose. People learn to nourish a sense of commitment in a program by developing shared images of the future they seek to create and the principles and guiding practices by which they hope to get there.
- **Team learning**. This discipline involves group interaction. Attending to group dynamics and processes, staff members can transform their collective thinking, learning to mobilize their energies and actions to achieve common goals and create synergy for creative and thoughtful problem solving.
- **Systems thinking**. In this discipline, people learn to better understand interdependency and change and thereby learn to deal more effectively with the forces that shape the consequences of their actions. Appreciation of feedback and complexity are important in leading and growing a program.

## ENGAGING PARTICIPANTS AND BUILDING SUPPORT

Leadership of a health promotion program requires the use of strategies to engage program participants, staff, and stakeholders. Regardless of the program setting (for example, school, workplace, health care organization, or community), effective programs engage people and build support for health promotion. This section discusses five widely used strategies to engage people in health promotion programs: partnerships; coalitions; networking, outreach, and referrals; online communities; and community empowerment and organizing. The strategies all have roots in the community mobilization concept of individuals taking action that is organized around specific community issues, particularly health issues (see Chapter Three). The strategies are proactive and focus on building honest, trusting, and respectful relationships in order to maximize individuals' program participation and benefits. The strategies have some commonalities with the advocacy strategies discussed in Chapter Seven. Advocacy strategies focus on the broad environment (that is, public policy) but can also be used in local settings to influence organizations. Similarly, the strategies discussed in this chapter, while primarily used to build support within a setting, can also be used when trying to influence the broader environment. Thus, the five strategies discussed here and the advocacy strategies in Chapter Seven complement one another.

## Partnerships

*Partnerships* involve organizations that develop mutually beneficial relationships built on trust and commitment (Exhibit 11.1). Partnerships can extend the reach and effectiveness of a program. In partnerships the member organizations are generally equal in their relationships and there is mutual agreement on their goals and objectives. For example, the Chicago Neighborhood Housing Services has

---

**EXHIBIT 11.1**
**Benefits of Partnerships**

Partnerships achieve goals that individual organizations cannot achieve alone by

- Combining the full force of their members to change local laws, policies, and norms
- Integrating and coordinating prevention services to improve quality and responsiveness
- Minimizing duplication of services
- Fostering diverse ideas and talents
- Mobilizing resources

Partnerships inspire communities to try new approaches by

- Encouraging the participation of organizations that have never worked together
- Creating unique collaborations among diverse partnership organizations
- Bringing together new talents and approaches to health promotion

Partnerships make it easier for organizations to work together by

- Helping communities to acknowledge and take responsibility for their health problems
- Motivating organizations outside the health care system to work within it
- Improving communication and trust among groups that might ordinarily compete with each other

---

*Source*: Adapted from the Center for Substance Abuse Prevention, n.d.

partnerships with banks, other housing organizations, and the city government to develop and support high-quality, safe, and affordable housing for young families and the elderly in Chicago. Sometimes the housing service works alone and sometimes it works with partners. Frequently, Chicago Neighborhood Housing Services and one or more partners will conduct joint projects (that is, partnerships), share resources, and make referrals to each other. Creating partnerships supports and extends partners' own influence at a site. More work can be accomplished when health promotion programs partner with organizations and agencies to reach a common goal. Forming and maintaining strong partnerships has been shown to increase the efficiency and effectiveness of health promotion programs. For example, partnerships with organizations, agencies, or programs that have a vested interest in the well-being of a community, such as county agencies, senior citizens' centers, unions, Chambers of Commerce, businesses, Head Start, law enforcement, or schools may help establish or maintain a community-based health promotion program (Harden, 1995).

Partnerships also require nurturing, support, and information sharing. Partnering creates an opportunity for program participants and organizations to share their views on health and to learn from one another (Butterfoss, 2007). Above all, partnerships must be mutually beneficial. Developing partnerships with business, industry, public organizations, or nonprofits might provide fertile ground for a program to piggyback a new intervention within an established intervention framework. For example, the Centers for Disease Control and Prevention partnered with Meals on Wheels to provide safety education to homebound older adults when delivering nutritious meals to their homes (Sleet, 2007).

## Coalitions

A *coalition* is a formal, long-term alliance among organizations (and individuals too) that are working together toward a common goal (Butterfoss & Whitt, 2003). Coalition building is important in health promotion. Governance and oversight of the coalition and its work must reflect the collaboration through representatives from many settings, organizations, and individuals (Harden, 1995). In contrast to the partnerships discussed earlier, where partners are generally equal in their relationships and there is mutual agreement on their goals and objectives, a coalition is generally organized by a particular group and that group generally runs the coalition. In addition, coalitions are generally organized for a particular purpose. Coalition members may not necessarily view themselves as active workers toward the goals of the coalition but may want to add their voice and support to a group fighting to address a health issue. Coalition members frequently do not share resources, staff, or materials but may simply write letters, send e-mails, and make telephone calls to key decision makers. For example, the Steel Valley Coalition

Against Drunk Driving was formed to increase the numbers of organizations in support of addressing drunk driving among young people in the old small steel towns of southwest Pennsylvania.

The development of coalitions is a key ingredient for successful implementation of health promotion programs. The members of a coalition might help decide in which neighborhood to conduct the program, which department at a work site gets to pilot a program, how to address barriers to implementing a program in a particular setting, or what resources the program can gather to improve the chances of success in meeting program goals. Coalitions not only can be an important political force for change but can increase the efficiency of program implementation, improve participant and organization buy-in, and increase capacity. A strong coalition can also increase sustainability by continuing to implement a program long after the original implementers have left.

Coalition building and collaboration are not easy. There are many opinions about how to successfully employ coalitions to promote health, including a formal community coalition action theory that consists of fourteen constructs and twenty-three testable propositions to increase local support and capacity (Butterfoss, 2007). Ultimately, the program (and its potential health outcomes) must be seen as valuable to each member of the coalition (Harden, 1995). Following are some guidelines from the Gay-Straight Alliance Network (n.d.) to help ensure coalition success:

- **Choose unifying issues**. The most effective coalitions unite around a common issue. Make sure the creation of group goals involves all members, rather than just one or two members who decide the goals and then invite others to join.
- **Understand and respect each group's self-interest**. There must be a balance between the goals and needs of the coalition and those of the individual organizations.
- **Respect each group's internal process**. It is important to understand and respect the differences among groups. These differences are often visible in processes or chains of command for decision making, so structure the decision-making process carefully. Sometimes it is advisable to agree to disagree. Commit to learning about the unique values, history, interests, structure, and agendas of the other groups and organizations.
- **Distribute credit fairly**. Recognize that contributions will inevitably vary, and appreciate all contributions. Each organization will have something different to offer. Each contribution is important, so be sure to acknowledge them all, whether they consist of volunteers, meeting space, funding, copying, publicity, leafleting, passing resolutions, or other resources.

- **Give and take**. It is important to build on existing relationships and connections with other organizations. Do not just ask for or expect support; be prepared to give it.
- **Develop a common strategy**. The strength of a coalition is in its unity. Work together with other organizations to develop a strategy that makes sense for everyone. The tactics you choose should be ones that all members can endorse. When tactics are not endorsed by all members, they should be applied by individual organizations, independent of the coalition.
- **Be strategic**. Building coalitions in and of itself requires a good strategy. Which organizations to ask, who asks them, and in which order to ask them are all questions to figure out.
- **Ensure consistency**. To ensure consistency, organizations should send the same representatives to each coalition meeting. This practice helps meetings run more smoothly. These individuals should also be authorized to make decisions for the organizations they represent.
- **Formalize the coalition**. It is best to make explicit agreements. Make sure everyone understands members' rights and responsibilities. Be clear in order to help prevent conflicts.

## Networking, Outreach, and Referrals

Networking, outreach, and referrals have their roots in social network and social support theory (discussed in Chapter Three). It is known from research that social networks and social support can influence health (positively or negatively). At least five primary pathways have been identified through which they influence health: (1) provision of social support, (2) social influence, (3) social engagement, (4) person-to-person contact, and (5) access to resources and material goods (Ayres, 2008; Csorba et al., 2007; Twoy, Connolly, & Novak, 2007).

Networking in health promotion is the action of building alliances to address a health problem or concern. It is not about waiting until a problem appears but rather, deliberate action to know people, resources, and organizations. However, it does not have to be a carefully choreographed process of meeting and greeting people. It's much better done on a more informal basis, but remember that networking is always a two-way street. It must benefit both parties (whether individuals, programs, or organizations) and help them to be most effective, so as you ask your network for help when you need it, be prepared to return the favor when asked. Networking has the power to bring together stakeholders whose particular focuses have given them different ways of thinking, methods, and strategies for building a smarter and more knowledgeable health care constituency (Berkowitz, 2002).

Program outreach is the intentional sharing of information about a program with specific individuals and groups for the purpose of educating them about the program and for developing support for program participants. Standard materials that might be used for outreach are program brochures, program staff business cards, and flyers. All outreach materials need to contain clear and concise contact information, including names of people to contact, telephone numbers, e-mail addresses, Web sites, and street addresses (with directions). Typically, these materials will be part of the program communication plan discussed in Chapter Eight. Furthermore, these materials are developed following the processes discussed in Chapter Eight.

Referral is the process of connecting a person to a program. Program staff identify where potential program participants are and who can direct these individuals to the program. For example, in a school, teachers, nurses, counselors, and parents refer students to health programs. Students might also sign up independently of an adult (a process called *self-referral*). In work settings it is common for a supervisor to refer employees to health programs; in addition, many individuals in work settings self-refer as a result of workplace health screenings. Like networking, referrals are a two-way process. Frequently individuals are attracted to a program but then find that this program does not address their needs. In these situations, program staff can help the individual by making a referral through a network formed by staff of other programs and resources, helping the individual to contact and potentially enroll in a health program designed to address his or her health concern.

Networking, outreach, and referrals are effective means of improving implementation. Today most people are aware of the impact of technology through sites such as Facebook and LinkedIn, which encourage and support networking, outreach, and referrals at a personal level as well as at a growing program level. However, going beyond current technology to promote health means that health promotion program stakeholders (including staff and participants) are working across the ecological model of health at all levels to improve their grasp of health problems, pool their knowledge and expertise with others, and jointly develop ways to solve individual health problems across a range of settings. Telephone conversations, meetings, and social gatherings offer opportunities to build a program staff network to bring together organizations, agencies, and people who have the experiences, resources, and talents to create a multidisciplinary team to solve problems.

## Online Communities

Using the Internet to form online health promotion communities is one of the most recent innovations in creating communities. Social networking technologies offer opportunities for information sharing and support. An online community can be a powerful tool for bringing constituents together to share their concern about an issue. The term *online community* represents the concept of convening people in virtual space and describes a range of online activities, including electronic collaboration, networking, Web-based discussions, and participation in electronic mailing lists.

As part of a health promotion program, an online community can be used in a variety of ways in order to

- Increase the visibility of an issue of concern.
- Mobilize concerned citizens to advocate for a political agenda.
- Facilitate shared learning between constituents, staff, and other like-minded individuals and organizations.
- Support fundraising efforts by connecting with donors or members.
- Announce current events to the public.
- Recruit volunteers for an organization.
- Discuss challenges with colleagues and peers.

## Community Empowerment and Organizing

*Community empowerment* begins with the feeling among individuals at a site that they have the power to make a difference in their situation. Friedman (1992) identified three levels of power that an individual must possess in order to feel empowered: social, political, and psychological. *Social power* is achieved when an individual has access to information, knowledge, and skills. Social power also includes financial resources and participation in social organizations. Once social power is achieved, political power is possible (Friedman, 1992).

*Political power* is the power of voice and collective action. This collective voice helps to create change within a community. *Psychological power* is established when an individual feels a sense of personal power or the ability to create change (Friedman, 1992). When all three levels of empowerment are achieved, community mobilization can occur.

*Community organizing* refers to efforts to involve individuals at a site in activities ranging from defining needs for prevention of health problems to obtaining support for prevention programs. All of the strategies discussed in this section (partnerships, coalitions, and so forth) may be used when organizing people at a site. The process involves working with and through constituents to achieve common goals. Organizing emphasizes changing the social and economic structures that influence health. Organizing can include elements of bottom-up (grassroots or citizen-initiated) strategies and top-down (outside-in or leader-initiated) strategies. In bottom-up strategies, the people at the site define the problems and decide on the solutions, while in top-down strategies, an outside expert (an external or self-appointed leader) facilitates change. Because leaders from the site (for example, school, workplace, health care organization, or community) understand their local culture, politics, and traditions better than outsiders, their participation is essential in tailoring prevention programs to local needs (McKenzie, Pinger, & Kotecki, 2008).

Program staff take a number of steps to empower and organize a group of people at a site. First, the problem or issue must be identified, either by people at the site (grassroots) or by a planner or consultant from outside the site. Grassroots efforts tend to be more successful, so it is best to let people at the site identify and prioritize their own issues. If the issue is to be identified by an outsider, he or she must gain entry into the setting, often by approaching a formal or informal leader. The outsider must meet the local leader on his or her own terms (McKenzie, Pinger, & Kotecki, 2008).

Once access is granted, the people must be organized. Organizing is often initiated by a core group of volunteers who get others involved in the work of the group. Coalitions of groups might be formed to address specific interests. Assets, resources, strengths, and weaknesses are assessed in order to determine the capacity of the organization or community to tackle the problem. Determining priorities and goals helps to move the process along, so that an intervention can be created. Partnerships can be formed to work on joint proposals and projects (McKenzie, Pinger, & Kotecki, 2008).

An example of organizing in a community setting is described by Gielen, Sleet, and Green (2006) in summarizing a successful effort to reduce alcohol-related trauma. A partnership between community organizations and university researchers was formed in order to focus on changes in the social and structural contexts of alcohol use that would facilitate changes in individual behavior. Researchers asked communities to customize and prioritize their initiatives based on local concerns and interests and worked to implement evidence-based prevention policies and activities. Specific components of the mobilization effort were directed toward responsible beverage service and toward preventing drinking and driving, underage drinking, and alcohol access. Coalitions, task forces, and media advocacy were used to raise awareness and support for effective policies among members of the public and decision makers. An evaluation of the impact of the efforts demonstrated significant reductions in alcohol consumed, drinking and driving, nighttime injury crashes, alcohol-related crashes, and alcohol-related assaults (Holder et al., 2000).

# ENSURING COMPETENCE THROUGH CREDENTIALING

Having program staff with the requisite competencies is an important key to sustaining a high-quality health promotion program. The Institute of Medicine notes, "As weaknesses in the public health infrastructure have become more obvious, the need to certify and credential the public workforce has grown" (Institute of Medicine, 2003, p. 206). Developing and nurturing professionalism in health promotion is a responsibility of program staff, stakeholders, and participants, who need to expect and demand that all staff members hold professional credentials. All health and medical professions have similar credentialing processes. This section details as a model the credentialing process for health educators.

Health education as a profession has moved to credential practitioners in health promotion and health education competencies. *Health education* and *health promotion* (while not synonymous terms) refer to "efforts that enable and support people to exert control over the determinants of health and to create environments that support health" (Allegrante et al., 2009). Credentialing health educators is a vehicle for creating a competent workforce to plan, implement, and evaluate health promotion programs.

The United States has a dual system of quality assurance: individuals can become credentialed as health education specialists, and programs in institutions of higher education can be accredited by specific accrediting bodies (Figure 11.1). Health education teachers in public schools are required to have a teaching license from the state in which they are teaching. Health educators working in jobs outside the public school system can obtain a voluntary credential by passing an examination administered by the National Commission for Health Education Credentialing, Inc. (NCHEC). Many health education teachers also obtain this credential.

A *certified health education specialist* (CHES) is a health educator who has successfully completed the competency-based exam given by NCHEC. NCHEC contributes to health promotion by certifying health education specialists, promoting professional development, and strengthening professional preparation and practice. These objectives are accomplished by creating standards for university programs that train health educators, developing and administering a national exam, and creating continuing education opportunities for health educators (National Commission for Health Education Credentialing, n.d.).

The CHES areas of responsibility on which the competencies and subcompetencies are based describe, in general terms, the skill set that is necessary for

FIGURE 11.1   Credentialing of Individual Health Educators and
Professional Preparation Programs in the United States

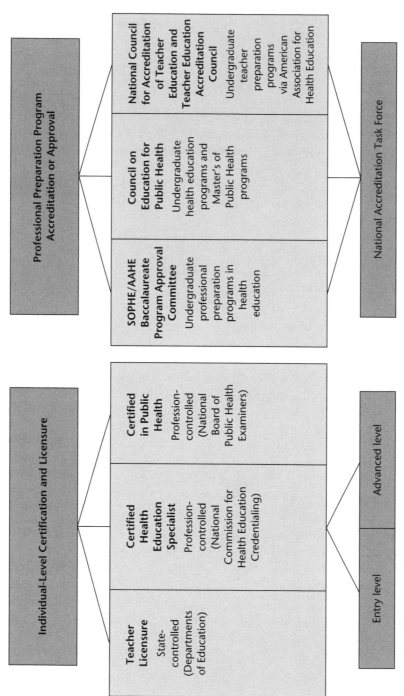

Source: Adapted from Cottrell et al., 2009.

a certified health educator and useful for just about anyone who is conducting a health promotion program. The CHES areas of responsibility are

- Assessing individual and community needs for health education
- Planning effective health education strategies, interventions, and programs
- Implementing health education strategies, interventions, and programs
- Conducting evaluation research related to the impact of health education programs
- Administering and budgeting for health education programs
- Serving as a health education resource person
- Communicating and advocating for health and health education

The basic CHES competencies are to be met by those graduating from baccalaureate and master's degree programs with less than five years of experience in the field. A written examination is taken, and those passing the examination are known as certified health education specialists. A candidate who wants to take the CHES examination must (1) possess a bachelor's, master's, or doctoral degree from a regionally accredited institution of higher education; (2) have an official transcript demonstrating course titles in health education; and (3) have completed a minimum of twenty-five semester hours or thirty-seven quarter hours of course work in health education (Cottrell et al., 2009).

Individuals having received CHES status must earn seventy-five hours of continuing education credits every five years in order to maintain their certification. Though credentialing is not mandatory for health educators, certification is highly recommended and is often specified as a requirement or a highly desirable qualification on job postings. Credentialing informs potential employers of the skills and competencies they can expect from prospective health education workers.

The NCHEC is now also implementing an advanced level of certification, in response to growing awareness in the field that the entry-level certification was not reflective of the scope of practice of many health educators. The *master certified health education specialist* (MCHES) process, to be implemented in 2011, includes a review of experience documentation and an exam.

Another credentialing source became available in 2008 to all public health professionals (including health educators) with a master's or doctoral degree from a public health program. This new credential, *certified in public health* (CPH), is accredited by the Council on Education for Public Health (CEPH). The National Board of Public Health Examiners (NBPHE) was created in 2005 to ensure that graduates of CEPH-accredited institutions have the knowledge and skills to be successful in public health. Like NCHEC, NBPHE does this by creating and administering a voluntary exam. To sit for the exam, one must have earned a graduate degree from a CEPH-accredited program or school.

The CPH exam focuses on the five core competencies of public health: biostatistics, environmental health sciences, epidemiology, health policy and management, and social and behavioral sciences (Gebbie et al., 2007). Each of these competencies is important for successful public health (and health promotion) practice, regardless of the individual's specialization or discipline. How the CHES and CPH certifications will articulate with each other has not been fully worked out at this time (Taub, Allegrante, Barry, & Sakagami, 2009).

## ENHANCING PROGRAM IMPACT AND SUSTAINABILITY

In a time of limited resources, *program sustainability* is important. While clearly an ineffective program should not be continued, there are still many effective programs that are not yet sustainable. In a perfect world, a program must be both effective and sustainable to receive continued support and resources. Although there have been examples of programs that were sustained despite evidence that they were not effective, health promotion program leadership requires skill in maintaining and sustaining effective programs.

Swerissen and Crisp (2004) suggest that one approach to understanding what it will take to sustain a health promotion program is to consider sustainability in the context of the level of the intervention and the strategies employed. Swerissen and Crisp's levels and corresponding strategies are shown in Table 5.1 in Chapter Five. Table 11.1 adds a new column to Table 5.1 in order to show the four health promotion intervention levels, corresponding strategies, and sustainability factors. For example, programs focused on individual behaviors such as smoking, nutrition, and physical activity have relatively short implementation time frames but require ongoing resources and support. And while health promotion programs dedicated to institutional change through advocacy take a lot of time and resources, once the desired change is in place, it continues to support the desired health behavior after the program has ended. Examples of such programs are those focused on policy, such as legislation that created smoke-free workplaces or policies that enforce lower blood alcohol levels for drivers.

Dutton (2000) has suggested some questions that program staff, stakeholders, and participants might ask in order to help sustain an effective program:

- **Does the health promotion program have a clear and honest understanding of its current reality?** Program staff should actively seek information and evaluations and not wait for the government, funders,

TABLE 11.1    Health Promotion Program Interventions and
Sustainability Factors

| Intervention Level | Intervention Strategies | Program Sustainability |
|---|---|---|
| Health promotion interventions for individuals | Focus on information, education, and training in order to promote change in knowledge, attitudes, beliefs, and behavior in regard to health risks such as smoking, eating, physical activity, and injury prevention | Requires a relatively short time frame for initial implementation but ongoing resources if program is to be maintained |
| Policy and practices of organizations | Focus on organizational change and consultancy in order to change organizational policies (rules, roles, sanctions, and incentives) and practices in order to produce changes in individuals' risky behavior and greater access to social, educational, and health-promoting resources | Requires few ongoing resources once organizational change has been implemented, but a longer-term time frame for establishing the program and a systematic process for withdrawal of resources |
| Environmental actions and social change at sites | Focus on social action and social planning at existing sites and on creating new sites (for example, organizations, networks, or partnerships) in order to produce change in organizations and redistribute resources that affect health | Often requires significant resources over an extended time frame, but resources may be systematically withdrawn once new sites have been created and resource redistribution occurs |
| Public advocacy | Focus on social advocacy in order to change legislative, budgetary, and institutional settings that affect community, organizational, and individual levels | Often requires significant resources over an extended time frame, but resources may be withdrawn once institutional change has been achieved |

*Source*: Adapted from Swerissen & Crisp, 2004.

or stakeholders to request them. Staff should seek feedback by talking with participants, asking them how they feel, what they think, and what improvements can be made. Program staff should always challenge the program's underlying assumptions and revise them if necessary.

- **Is the understanding of current reality shared throughout the health promotion program and used to sustain and improve the program?** The program staff should share knowledge, build on current knowledge, and support learning by participants, staff, and stakeholders.

Programs should improve over time, using feedback to make relevant modifications.

- **Is knowledge translated into effective action toward a desired future?** Staff, stakeholders, and program participants should make use of new knowledge to improve their health. Knowledge that is passed on to participants should be relevant. Programs need benchmarks or indicators to measure progress toward goals. Program staff need to develop program priorities, and staff and participants should share these priorities.

## SUMMARY

Leadership is the responsibility of health promotion program staff, stakeholders, and participants. Leading a health program requires people to view change as part of sustaining that program. Program stakeholders have many options available for developing, maintaining, and sustaining health promotion programs. Some keys to maximizing success are creating a supportive and engaged setting for a program; employing professional, credentialed, and qualified staff; and developing a clear, honest, and shared understanding by staff, stakeholders, and program participants of the program's goals, objectives, and strategies.

## FOR PRACTICE AND DISCUSSION

1. How do health promotion programs in your community cope with change? What are the effects of the six realities of health promotion programs identified by McKenzie, Neiger, and Thackeray (2009) on your local health promotion programs?

2. How might the strategies for engaging participants that are discussed in this chapter be used differently in different health promotion program settings? Compare and contrast how schools, work sites, health care organizations, and community health programs might approach program change and sustainability.

3. Building culturally competent health promotion programs requires individuals (staff, stakeholders, and participants) to take leadership in sharing their views and thoughts (evaluations) of a program. How can staff and other stakeholders invite and develop a climate of shared leadership to sustain programs that are culturally competent and that eliminate health disparities?

4. Investigate credentialing for other health professions (for example, physicians, nurses, diabetes educators, or physical therapists). What organizations are

involved in individual-level certification and licensure? What organizations are involved in accreditation of professional preparation programs? How are these organizations similar to and different from the organizations involved in credentialing and accreditation in health education?

5.  How can the staff, stakeholders, and participants of a health promotion program close the gap between the program's current reality and its desired future? How can they identify benchmarks of progress?

## KEY TERMS

Certified Health Education Specialist (CHES)

Certified in Public Health (CPH)

Change

Coalition

Collaboration

Community empowerment

Community organizing

Consensus building

Individual-level certification and licensure

Mastering change

Networking

Outreach

Partnerships

Professional preparation program accreditation

Program sustainability

Referral

## REFERENCES

Allegrante, J. P., Barry, M. M., Airhihenbuwa, C. O., Auld, M. E., Collins, J. L., Lamarre, M. C., et al. (2009). Domains of core competency, standards and quality assurance for building global capacity in health promotion: The Galway Consensus Conference Statement. *Health Education & Behavior, 36*(3), 476–482.

Ayres, C. G. (2008). Mediators of the relationship between social support and positive health practice in middle adolescents. *Journal of Pediatric Health Care, 22*(2), 94–102.

Berkowitz, B. (2002). The importance of partnership in the public health system. In B. DeBuono & H. Tilson (Eds.), *Advancing healthy populations: The Pfizer guide to careers in public health.* New York: Pfizer Pharmaceuticals.

Butterfoss, F. D. (2007). *Coalitions and partnerships in community health.* San Francisco: Jossey-Bass.

Butterfoss, F. D., & Whitt, M. D. (2003). Building and sustaining coalitions. In R. J. Bensley & J. Brookins-Fisher (Eds.), *Community health education methods* (2nd ed.) (pp. 325–356). Sudbury, MA: Jones & Bartlett.

Center for Substance Abuse Prevention. (n.d.). *What works in prevention* [Pamphlet]. Rockville, MD: U.S. Department of Health and Human Services, Substance Abuse and Mental Health Services Administration.

Cottrell, R. R., Lysoby, L., King, L. R., Airhihenbuwa, C. O., Roe, K. M., & Allegrante, J. P. (2009). Current developments in accreditation and certification for health promotion and health education: A perspective on systems of quality assurance in the United States. *Health Education & Behavior, 36*(3), 451–463.

Csorba, J., Sörfozo, Z., Steiner, P., Ficsor, B., Harkány, E., Babrik, Z., et al. (2007). Maladaptive strategies, dysfunctional attitudes and negative life events among adolescents treated for the diagnosis of "suicidal behaviour." *Psychiatria Hungarica, 22*(3), 200–211.

Dutton, J. (2000). How do you know your organization is learning? In P. Senge, N. Cambron-McCabe, T. Lucas, B. Smith, J. Dutton, & A. Kleiner, *Schools That Learn.* New York: Doubleday.

Friedman, J. (1992). *Empowerment: The politics of alternative development.* Cambridge, MA: Blackwell.

Gay-Straight Alliance Network. (n.d.). *Justice for all: Coalition building.* Retrieved January 12, 2008, from http://www.gsanetwork.org/justiceforall/coalition.htm.

Gebbie, K., Goldstein, B., Gregorio, D., Tsou, W., Buffler, P., Petersen, D., et al. (2007). The National Board of Public Health Examiners: Credentialing public health graduates. *Public Health Reports, 122*(4), 435–440.

Gielen, A. C., Sleet, D. A., & Green, L. W. (2006). Community models and approaches for interventions. In A. C. Gielen, D. A. Sleet, & R. J. DiClemente (Eds.), *Injury and violence prevention: Behavioral science theories, methods, and applications* (pp. 65–82). San Francisco: Jossey-Bass.

Harden, C. M. (1995). Community partnerships: Principles for success. *AHA News, 31*(13), 6.

Holder, H., Gruenewald, P., Ponicki, W., Treno, A., Grube, J., Saltz, R., et al. (2000). Effects of community-based interventions on high-risk driving and alcohol-related injuries. *Journal of the American Medical Association, 284*(18), 2341–2347.

Institute of Medicine. (2003). *Who will keep the public healthy?* Washington, DC: National Academies Press.

McKenzie, J. F., Neiger, B. L., & Thackeray, R. (2009). *Planning, implementing, and evaluating health promotion programs: A primer* (5th ed.). San Francisco: Pearson Benjamin Cummings.

McKenzie, J. F., Pinger, R. R., & Kotecki, J. E. (2008). *An introduction to community health* (6th ed.). Sudbury, MA: Jones & Bartlett.

McLeroy, K. R., Bibeau, D., Steckler, A., & Glanz, K. (1988). An ecological perspective on health promotion programs. *Health Education Quarterly, 15*, 351–377.

National Commission for Health Education Credentialing. (n.d.). *Mission and purpose.* Retrieved December 12, 2007, from http://www.nchec.org/aboutnchec/about.htm.

Senge, P. M. (1990). *The fifth discipline: The art and practice of the learning organization.* New York: Random House.

Senge, P. M. (1999). The challenges of profound change. In P. Senge, A. Kleiner, C. Roberts, R. Ross, G. Roth, & B. Smith, *The dance of change: The challenges of sustaining momentum in learning organizations.* New York: Doubleday.

Sleet, D. A. (2007, April). *Unintentional injury prevention: Healthy People 2010 progress review for the Assistant Secretary for Health.* Washington, DC: Centers for Disease Control and Prevention, National Center for Injury Prevention and Control.

Swerissen, H., & Crisp, B. (2004). The sustainability of health promotion interventions for different levels of social organization. *Health Promotion International, 19*(1), 123–130.

Taub, A., Allegrante, J. P., Barry, M. M., & Sakagami, K. (2009). Perspectives on terminology and conceptual and professional issues in health education and health promotion credentialing. *Health Education & Behavior, 36*(3), 439–450.

Twoy, R., Connolly, P. M., & Novak, J. M. (2007). Coping strategies used by parents of children with autism. *Journal of American Academic Nurse Practitioners, 19*(5), 251–260.

# PART FIVE

# HEALTH PROMOTION PROGRAMS IN DIVERSE SETTINGS

# CHAPTER TWELVE

# PROMOTING HEALTH IN SCHOOLS AND UNIVERSITIES

MARLENE K. TAPPE

DIANE D. ALLENSWORTH

JIM GRIZZELL

## LEARNING OBJECTIVES

- Discuss the health and other benefits to faculty, staff, and students of offering health promotion programs in schools and universities

- Discuss the challenges and opportunities of offering health promotion programs and services in schools and universities

- Describe the history of school and university health promotion programs and services

- Describe current approaches to the design, implementation, and delivery of school and university health promotion programs

- Describe administrative, clinical, and academic careers in school and university health promotion, including paid and volunteer opportunities for students

**T**HERE ARE 55.5 MILLION STUDENTS in elementary, middle, and high school and 18 million college students in the United States (National Center for Education Statistics, 2007). Schools and universities, therefore, are ideal sites for health promotion because they are efficient places for reaching almost all K–12 children and adolescents and many young adults. Students, however, are not the only audience for health promotion activities in schools and universities. Schools and universities also serve as efficient sites for health promotion initiatives for adults. Schools are a work site for 9.8 million faculty and staff (National Center for Education Statistics, 2007) and have been promoted as ideal sites for workplace health promotion because, beyond the immediate health benefits that accrue to school and university staff, these staff members can then serve as healthy role models for students. Creating healthy schools and healthy universities has been a quest for many years and will continue to be so because of the opportunities for health promotion programs to reach so many people.

## RATIONALE FOR PROMOTING HEALTH IN SCHOOLS AND UNIVERSITIES

The rationale for heath promotion in schools and universities extends beyond the fact that schools and universities are very efficient sites for conducting health promotion programs. Health promotion programs are needed in schools and universities not only because large numbers of young people congregate in these settings but also because these children, adolescents, and young adults face a number of serious health threats (Centers for Disease Control and Prevention, 2009a). These threats include asthma, overweight and obesity, diabetes, injury and violence, unintended pregnancy, and sexually transmitted diseases, including HIV infection. Health promotion in schools and universities is also important because children, adolescents, and young adults consolidate their health-related behaviors and attitudes as they make the transition from childhood to adulthood. Further, health promotion in schools and universities is important because young people make choices that influence both their current and their future health (Centers for Disease Control and Prevention, 2009a). The Centers for Disease Control and Prevention (2009a) has identified six risk behaviors related to the leading causes of morbidity and mortality in the United States for adolescents and adults: alcohol and other drug use; sexual behaviors leading to HIV, other sexually transmitted diseases, and unintended pregnancy; behaviors that lead to intentional and unintentional injuries; tobacco use; physical inactivity; and imprudent dietary behaviors. Further, conducting health promotion programs in schools is valuable because there is a link between quality school health programs and academic achievement (Centers for Disease Control and Prevention, 2009b).

Health and academic achievement are inextricably intertwined. Academic achievement is related to both a reduction in health disparities and a reduction in health risk behaviors (see Chapter Two). The Centers for Disease Control and Prevention (2009b) notes that one of the major indicators for the overall well-being of youth and a primary predictor and determinant of adult health outcomes is academic success. Conversely, health problems such as chronic illness, physical and emotional abuse, or hunger can lead to absenteeism, inability to pay attention in class, poor test scores, and academic failure (Centers for Disease Control and Prevention, 2009b). Further, there is a perfect correlation between engaging in high-risk behaviors and receiving poor grades. Students who receive D's and F's are more likely to engage in high-risk behaviors than are students who have mostly A's and B's (Figure 12.1). Given the link between health and academic achievement, national education organizations have identified the need to embed health programs and policies in the education environment of all students (American Association of School Administrators, 2009; Council of Chief State School Officers, 2004; National Association of State Boards of Education, 2009; National School Boards Association, 2009).

**FIGURE 12.1    Relationship Between Grades and Risk Behaviors**

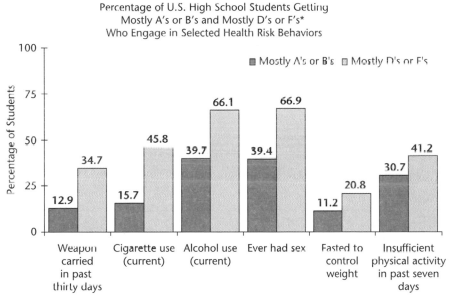

Percentage of U.S. High School Students Getting
Mostly A's or B's and Mostly D's or F's*
Who Engage in Selected Health Risk Behaviors

* As reported by students.
*Source*: www.cdc.gov/HealthyYouth/health_and_academics/index.htm

## EVOLVING ROLE OF PROMOTING HEALTH IN SCHOOLS AND UNIVERSITIES

The use of schools and universities for health promotion can be traced to political leaders as well as health and education leaders. In the colonial period, Benjamin Franklin (1749) outlined a plan for education that included recommendations for instruction related to healthy eating, physical activity, and temperance. In 1836, Mount Holyoke was the first college to have a course in hygiene (Lockhart & Spears, 1972). At about the same time, the father of American education, Horace Mann (1838), suggested that students need to understand concepts related to diet and exercise essential for the maintenance of health. A few years later, the landmark public health document known as the *Shattuck Report* recommended that children receive health instruction in schools. Shattuck, Banks, and Abbott (1850) also recommended assessing sickness among students enrolled in schools and universities, seeking proof of vaccination as a requirement for school enrollment, using guidelines for the construction of healthy and safe schools, and hiring sanitary (health) professors in colleges and medical schools.

By the beginning of the twentieth century, a variety of other strategies to promote the health of students were found in schools and universities. These included the use of hygiene textbooks for students of all ages (for example, Johonnot & Bouton, 1889), as well as textbooks for future teachers about the health of children and adolescents and how to teach hygiene (for example, Terman 1914). Additional health promotion strategies included the appointment of doctors as school sanitarians (Lincoln, 1886), development of a system for the medical inspection of schools (Burks & Burks, 1913), screening of students for health problems (Gulick & Ayres, 1917), use of nurses to supplement the work of doctors in schools (Brainard, 1922), establishment of a school lunch program (Gunderson, 1971), and implementation and practice of the profession of school psychology (Wallin, 1914). Over time, these initiatives evolved into local, state, national, and international initiatives to promote the health and learning of students in schools and universities.

## CURRENT ROLE OF PROMOTING HEALTH IN SCHOOLS AND UNIVERSITIES

Present-day approaches to health promotion in schools and universities clearly reflect the propositions made many years earlier in regard to the role of responsibility of schools and universities. Today, health promotion in schools is based on an eight-component model. Programs following this model were originally labeled comprehensive school health programs (Allensworth & Kolbe, 1987; Allensworth, Lawson, Nicholson, & Wyche, 1997; Kolbe, 1986) but are now referred to as coordinated school health programs.

## Coordinated School Health Programs

The eight components of *coordinated school health programs* (Centers for Disease Control and Prevention, 2008b; also see Figure 12.2) are disciplines and services that most schools have but that are not necessarily organized to work together. Following is a brief description of each component:

1. **Health education**: classroom instruction that addresses the physical, mental, emotional, and social dimensions of health; promotes knowledge, attitudes, and skills; and is tailored to each age or developmental level—designed to motivate and assist students in maintaining and improving their health and to reduce their risk behaviors.
2. **Physical education**: planned, sequential instruction that promotes lifelong physical activity—designed to develop basic movement skills, sports skills, and physical fitness as well as to enhance mental, social, and emotional abilities.

## FIGURE 12.2    Coordinated School Health Programs

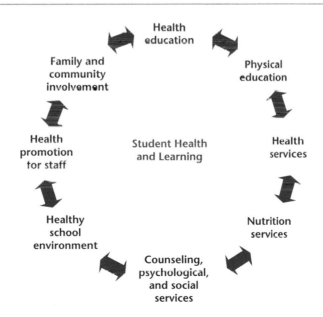

3. **Health services**: services that promote the health of students; identify and prevent health problems and injuries; and ensure appropriate preventive services, emergency care, referral, or management of acute or chronic health conditions.

4. **Nutrition services**: integration of nutritious, affordable, and appealing meals and nutrition education in an environment that promotes healthy eating habits.

5. **Counseling, psychological, and social services**: services that prevent and address problems, facilitate positive learning and healthy behavior, and enhance healthy development by providing assistance that focuses on cognitive, emotional, behavioral, and social needs of students.

6. **Healthy school environment**: a setting designed to provide both a safe physical plant and a healthy and supportive environment that fosters learning and addresses the physical, emotional, and social climate of the school.

7. **Health promotion for staff**: assessment, education, and fitness activities for school faculty and staff—designed to maintain and improve the health and well-being of school staff members, who serve as role models for students.

8. **Family and community involvement**: partnerships among schools, families, community groups, and individuals—designed to maximize resources and expertise in addressing the healthy development of children, youths, and their family members.

The word *coordinated* is used to emphasize the interaction that is needed between these eight components in order to maximize the contributions of each component to the health and learning of students. A coordinated school health program is defined as "an integrated set of planned, sequential, school-affiliated strategies, activities, and services designed to promote the optimal physical, emotional, social, and educational development of students. The program involves and is supportive of families and is determined by the local community needs, standards, and requirements. It is coordinated by a multidisciplinary team and accountable to the community for program quality and effectiveness" (Allensworth, Wyche, Lawson, & Nicholson, 1995).

Coordinated school health programs link the goals of public health and education to promote both students' health and their learning. The goals of coordinated school health programs, according to Kolbe (2002), include improving students' health knowledge, attitudes, and skills (for example, decision making); improving students' health behaviors (for example, use of safety equipment such as seat belts); improving students' health outcomes (for example, reduced motor vehicle fatalities); improving students' educational outcomes (for example, high school or college completion); and improving their social outcomes (for example, employment).

Exhibit 12.1 illustrates the broad variety of coordinated health programs in K–12 schools. The listed components are offered in addition to schools' health education, physical education, and counseling and guidance curricula. The illustration is for a K–12 program, but many of the same topics are addressed by universities with age-appropriate programs that are matched to college students' needs.

A variety of processes are critical to coordinating a school health program at the local level, including

- Securing administrators' support and commitment
- Establishing a school health council at the district level and school health teams at the school level
- Identifying a school health leader at the school level and a school health coordinator at the district level who coordinate the school activities
- Developing an annual action plan for continual improvement of the coordinated school health program
- Implementing multiple strategies (universal interventions and targeted interventions for high-risk students)
- Addressing both health risk and protective factors among students
- Engaging students in health promotion initiatives
- Engaging all school staff in health promotion initiatives

At the state level, the Centers for Disease Control and Prevention (CDC) suggests that state education agencies and state health departments work collaboratively to support local educational and health agencies in implementing the processes critical to coordinating school health programs. In addition to cross-agency collaboration, the CDC encourages state health and education agencies to engage other state agencies, state voluntary health organizations, and other professional associations in a state coordinating council in order to promote the health and learning of children and youths. In addition, the CDC funds a variety of states and large cities in order to implement activities that support school health programming at the local level. In most states, the CDC also supports activities related to HIV prevention and administration of the Youth Risk Behavior Survey.

## Health-Promoting Universities

The basic components and principles of coordinated school health programs also apply to the promotion of student health on the campuses of colleges and universities. The World Health Organization has promoted the concept of

## EXHIBIT 12.1
## Coordinated School Health Program Showing K–12 Components Additional to School Curricula

*Health Education*

- Obesity prevention programs
- Student health advocate programs
- Diabetes prevention program
- Professor Peace (conflict resolution program)
- Programs for special focus weeks: nutrition, asthma, dental

*Physical Education*

- SPARK (Sports, Play and Active Recreation for Kids)
- Girls on the Run (after-school physical activities for girls)
- Wii fitness bundles
- Walking and running clubs
- Heart rate monitors

*Health Services*

- Mobile dental clinic
- Immunizations
- School and sports physicals
- Asthma education
- School health clinic plus service partnerships with local hospitals

*Nutrition Services*

- School breakfast and lunch program
- Implementation of Healthier Options for Public Schoolchildren's suggested changes in the placement or offering of foods and beverages to increase the sale of healthy foods (for example, fruits) and beverages (for example, water) and decrease the sale of less healthy foods (for example, cookies) and beverages (for example, soda)
- Removal of deep fryers from school kitchens
- Individualized student and family nutritional coaching
- Multicultural food appreciation and selections

## Counseling, Psychological, and Social Services

- Student Assistance Program
- Partnerships with local community mental health and drug and alcohol programs
- Social, emotional, and behavioral support
- Promoting positive behavior in the classroom

## Healthy School Environment

- Continuous improvements in wellness policies
- Juvenile justice liaison officers
- Building security
- Anonymous tip line
- CPR training
- First Aid training
- School climate improvement action plan

## Health Promotion for Staff

- Health screenings at local medical centers
- Assessments of health risks
- Health newsletter
- Workplace wellness health promotion program, as part of the district's health benefit package for faculty and staff, including an on-site program (such as smoking cessation)

## Family and Community Involvement

- Family fitness night
- Community walking program
- Summer fitness and games program
- Family health fairs
- Clothing bank
- Back to School Blitz (getting ready for school program)
- After-school and extended school day programs
- Service agreements with community health organizations (for example, physical health exams, mental health care)

both *health-promoting schools* (World Health Organization, Expert Committee on Comprehensive School Health Education and Promotion, 1997) and *health-promoting universities* (Tsouros, Dowding, Thompson, & Dooris, 1998). The outcomes or goals of a health-promoting university are similar to those for coordinated school health programs. These goals include improving the health of students, university personnel, and the wider community as well as integrating health into the university's culture, structure, and processes (Tsouros, Dowding, & Dooris, 1998). The key objectives in achieving these goals include the following: promoting healthy and sustainable planning and policy decision making throughout the university; ensuring healthy work environments; providing healthy and supportive social environments for students, staff, and the local community; establishing and enhancing primary health care; facilitating personal and social development among students and staff; ensuring a healthy and sustainable (that is, *green*) physical environment; encouraging wider academic interest in health promotion (for example, health education classes) and research; and creating community partnerships for health (Tsouros, Dowding, & Dooris, 1998). Elements that have been found to be important in starting and sustaining a health-promoting university initiative include the following: a senior-level advocate who will argue for the initiative and make funding available for start-up; funding for a coordinator to facilitate the formation and implementation of the initiative; early successes and securing long-term funding for the initiative; formation of a steering committee and continued networking by the coordinator and the committee in order to establish broad-based legitimacy, ownership, and accountability for the initiative; and an initiative that responds dynamically to the context in which it is developed and implemented (Dooris & Martin, 2002).

## Health Promotion Initiatives in Schools and Universities

Health promotion initiatives in schools and universities protect and promote student health in a variety of ways. Course work in health education and physical education provides students with the health-related knowledge, skills, and motivation for engaging in a healthy lifestyle. Unfortunately, only 56.6 percent of all K–12 schools require students to receive health instruction as part of a specific course or class and just 78.3 percent of schools require students to receive some physical education (Kann, Brener, & Wechsler, 2007). In order to build support for health education and physical education, the American Cancer Society, the American Diabetes Association, and the American Heart Association (2008a, 2008b, 2008c, 2008d) collaborated to release joint statements and fact sheets emphasizing the benefits of health education and physical education in schools. Although quality health and physical education programs across the curriculum can help the majority of students choose health-enhancing behaviors, some students who have already begun to engage in risky health behaviors may need additional and more intensive health promotion strategies to address those high-risk behaviors (see the Institute of Medicine's model of preventive intervention in Chapter Five).

The university setting is an opportunity for reaching a large number of young people and providing them with the knowledge, skills, and attitudes to enhance not only their personal health but also that of the families they will establish and the communities in which they will live (Kupchella, 2009). Some universities require all students to take health education and physical education courses as part of their core curriculum, whereas other universities provide students with opportunities to take these courses as a way to fulfill their general education requirements.

Initiatives to promote physical activity are integrated into the physical education component of the school health programs and are also an important aspect of health promotion in universities. In school settings, opportunities for physical activity include not only physical education but also recess, intramural activities, physical activity clubs, and interscholastic sports. In addition, in some schools, students have access to facilities (for example, fitness centers), spaces (for example, tennis courts), and equipment (for example, treadmills) for engaging in exercise. Universities often provide students with a wide range of opportunities for physical activity and exercise. In addition to fitness centers, these opportunities include interscholastic, club, and intramural sports as well as noncredit exercise classes and clubs (for example, swing dance) that enable students to participate in a wide range of physical activities.

Health services in schools and universities offer health education, including peer education programs to provide students with the knowledge, skills, and attitudes to engage in health-enhancing behaviors and avoid health risks. Health services in schools and universities also provide screenings to identify health problems (for example, vision problems) that interfere with learning as well as traditional health care services for treating immediate health problems and injuries.

School and university nutrition services include more than traditional school lunch programs and residence hall meal plans. Many schools now offer school breakfast programs and are working to provide healthier food choices throughout the school day in classroom snacks, school lunches, vending machines, and school stores. Many universities are providing a wider array of dining choices (for example, vegetarian), and some campuses are involved in initiatives to use campus-grown or locally grown and produced foods. Unfortunately, beverages and foods sold on school and university campuses commonly include sports drinks, soda pop, fruit drinks that are not 100 percent juice, and snacks that are high in fat, salt, and sugar.

The remaining components of coordinated school and university health programs are also important to student health and learning. Counseling, psychological, and social services in schools and universities provide students with personal and academic guidance, services to prevent and reduce mental health problems, and services to address social circumstances that may interfere with health (for example, providing low-cost options for health care) and learning (for example, financial support for purchasing textbooks or other education supplies). Healthy school and university environments include services to provide a healthy and safe physical and social learning and working environment as well as policies that support and enable healthy behaviors (for example, alcohol-free, tobacco-free, and drug-free school and university campuses). Health promotion services on school and university campuses not only enable staff to engage in and model healthy behaviors but also increase their productivity and reduce staff absenteeism and health insurance costs. Family and community involvement in schools includes enlisting family members in support of classroom learning (for example, homework to practice skills in refusing alcohol, cigarettes, or drugs), inviting family and community members on school health councils, and engaging community services and resources to support health and learning among students (for example, service-learning opportunities). Family involvement on university campuses includes not only activities designed to engage family members in university events (for example, family weekends) but also, on some campuses, programs to help families and students adjust to life on campus. Community involvement includes the formation of coalitions to promote health and prevent health problems associated with high-risk behavior by university students.

## RESOURCES AND TOOLS

A number of unique resources are available to help in planning, implementing, and evaluating health promotion programs in school and university settings. Most of these resources were developed in the last twenty-five years to help schools and universities deal with the range of health issues and problems that they are asked to address.

### Youth Risk Behavior Survey

The Centers for Disease Control and Prevention conducts the biannual Youth Risk Behavior Survey (YRBS) in odd-numbered years (for example, 2009) (Brener et al., 2004). This survey identifies, by state and by some large cities, the extent of high school students' participation in the six CDC risk behaviors. The YRBS can be used by local planners to identify local problems and compare their students with other students in their state or in the nation. When local students are engaged in higher levels of one or more risk behaviors (for example, tobacco use) than their state or national cohorts, planners can motivate stakeholders in the local community to take actions to address the risk behaviors. Although the entire survey can be used by any local school, there is often reluctance to administer a health survey to students because of time constraints or concerns related to the sensitive nature of some of the questions on the survey (for example, those pertaining to students' sexual risk behaviors). Alternative ways to obtain similar data are by polling students in health classes or using a limited number of questions from the survey. For example, teachers have used the portion of the survey most relevant to a particular health lesson or have solicited students' anonymous responses via an audience response system. Students find the immediate results available through an audience response system useful and thought-provoking. Tabulating the results by class and by grade level over a semester can provide a school health team with the necessary data to plan needed and targeted health promotion initiatives within a school.

## School Health Profiles

Complementing the YRBS is the School Health Profiles survey (Balaji et al., 2008). This biannual survey is conducted by the CDC in the even-numbered years (for example, 2010), between administrations of the YRBS. The School Health Profiles survey currently assesses secondary school programs, services, and policies related to health education; physical education and physical activity; health services; healthy and safe school environments; and family and community involvement in secondary schools. The survey is used to describe initiatives and identify long-term and short-term trends related to health programs and policies in secondary schools (Balaji et al., 2008). Local school professionals—for example, the members of a school health council—can use the survey to identify how the programming, services, and resources provided to their students compare with what other schools within their state provide to students in order to enhance student health and learning.

## School Health Policies and Programs Study

Approximately every six years, the CDC conducts the School Health Policies and Programs Study (SHPPS), an in-depth examination of school health programs and policies in schools, districts, and states (Kann, Brener, & Wechsler, 2007). SHPPS assesses all eight components of coordinated school health programs by surveying fifty state departments of education and a national, representative sample of districts and elementary, middle, and high schools. The results provide school and public health practitioners as well as all those who care about the health and safety of youths with an analysis of current school health programming. The survey gathers data pertaining to *Healthy People* objectives, and it helps states and districts determine their needs and priorities in regard to technical assistance and professional development related to coordinated school health programs. SHPPS helps school administrators, teachers, and other community members determine how their own school health policies and programs compare with those that have been implemented nationwide. SHPPS also helps local school and community personnel determine the extent to which their district is implementing policies and practices that evidence has shown to be effective. Because SHPPS has been administered since 1995, it is possible to assess how school health policies and programs have changed over time (Kann, Brener, & Wechsler, 2007).

## School Health Index

The CDC's School Health Index is a self-assessment and planning tool that schools can use to improve local initiatives related to coordinated school health programs (Centers for Disease Control and Prevention, 2005a, 2005b). The School Health Index includes modules linked to each of the eight components of coordinated school health programs. Each module contains questions to assess school strengths and weaknesses related to the component (for example, health education) in general as well as five specific health topics: safety, physical activity, nutrition, tobacco use, and asthma. Each module also includes a planning activity for school personnel to complete once they have conducted the self-assessment process. Local school personnel can use the School Health Index to assess and plan improvements in any or all of the components of coordinated school health programs.

The School Health Index has two paper versions—one for elementary schools (Centers for Disease Control and Prevention, 2005a) and the other for middle and high schools (Centers for Disease Control and Prevention, 2005b). In addition to the paper versions, there is an online version of the tool.

## Characteristics of an Effective Health Education Curriculum

Both public health and education emphasize the use of evidence-based programs and curricula. In order to facilitate the use of evidence-based health education, the Centers for Disease Control and Prevention (2008a) conducted a review of effective programs and solicited input from experts in school health education to identify the characteristics of effective health education curricula. The fourteen CDC characteristics reflect evidence that effective health education curricula emphasize the teaching of functional knowledge (that is, essential health concepts), shape personal values and group norms for healthy behavior, and develop essential skills that students need in order to adopt and maintain healthy behaviors. The CDC characteristics guided the revision of the National Health Education Standards and the performance indicators that accompany them (Joint Committee on National Health Education Standards, 2007) and provide important guidance for the development and evaluation of effective health education curricula.

## The National Health Education Standards

The National Health Education Standards (Joint Committee on National Health Education Standards, 1995, 2007) provide a framework for state and local initiatives related to school health education curriculum, instruction, and assessment. Performance indicators are provided that identify the key concepts, skills, or elements of skills that students need to know or be able to do as well as the beliefs, values, and norms that students need to espouse in order to demonstrate achievement of each standard. The original National Health Education Standards (Joint Committee on National Health Education Standards, 1995) reflected the paradigm shift in school health education from a focus on the facts and concepts students should know to a focus on the health-related skills that students should be able to demonstrate as a result of health instruction. The revised National Health Education Standards (Joint Committee on National Health Education Standards, 2007) reflect a shift in focus from health literacy to students' ability to engage in health-enhancing behaviors as a result of health instruction (Tappe, Wilbur, Telljohann, & Jensen, 2009). The eight national standards and the performance indicators aligned with each standard identify the important concepts, skills, and attitudes that students need in order to engage in health-enhancing behaviors and avoid health risks. The eight standards are shown in Exhibit 12.2.

National Health Education Standard 1 and the performance indicators aligned with it emphasize the functional knowledge that students need in order to engage in healthy behaviors. Standards 2, 3, 4, 5, and 6 and the performance indicators aligned with them emphasize the skills or elements of skills that students need in order to engage in health-enhancing behaviors as delineated in Standard 7. Standard 8 and the performance indicators aligned with it emphasize the elements of advocacy that students need in order to advocate for personal, family, and community health (Tappe, Wilbur, Telljohann, & Jensen, 2009).

---

**EXHIBIT 12.2**
## National Health Education Standards

1. Students will comprehend concepts related to health promotion and disease prevention to enhance health.
2. Students will analyze the influence of family, peers, culture, media, technology, and other factors on health behaviors.
3. Students will demonstrate the ability to access valid information, products, and services to enhance health.
4. Students will demonstrate the ability to use interpersonal communication skills to enhance health and avoid or reduce health risks.
5. Students will demonstrate the ability to use decision-making skills to enhance health.
6. Students will demonstrate the ability to use goal-setting skills to enhance health.
7. Students will demonstrate the ability to practice health-enhancing behaviors and avoid or reduce health risks.
8. Students will demonstrate the ability to advocate for personal, family, and community health.

---

*Source*: Joint Committee on National Health Education Standards, 2007.

---

Many states have adopted or adapted the original or revised National Health Education Standards as state standards for health education. In addition, most states and districts have adopted policies that require districts and schools to use national, state, or local health education standards (Kann, Telljohann, & Wooley, 2007).

### Health Education Curriculum Analysis Tool

The Health Education Curriculum Analysis Tool (HECAT) (Centers for Disease Control and Prevention, 2007) is a tool to help school districts, schools, and others analyze health education curricula on the basis of the National Health Education Standards (Joint Committee on National Health Education Standards, 2007) and the CDC's characteristics of an effective health education curriculum (Centers for Disease Control and Prevention, 2008a). The HECAT includes questions to help in the analysis of the overall characteristics of a curriculum as well as the specific health-related behaviors, functional knowledge, skills, and subskills addressed in the curriculum. Results from the HECAT can be used in selecting or developing health education curricula and in improving health education in local schools.

## ACHA-National College Health Assessment

In 1998, the American College Health Association (ACHA) created a work group to develop the ACHA-National College Health Assessment (ACHA-NCHA), an instrument to collect information on a broad range of student health behaviors and perceptions (American College Health Association, 2008). Since the spring of 2000, the ACHA-NCHA has annually collected data from over 450,000 college students at almost 400 institutions of higher education (American College Health Association, 2008). The ACHA-NCHA collects data about smoking, contraception, mental health, relationship difficulties, sexual behaviors, exercise, preventive health practices, perceptions of drug and alcohol use, and health links to academic performance. ACHA-NCHA data were used in formulating the Healthy Campus 2010 objectives (American College Health Association, 2002). The major impediments to academic success in course work that were reported by students include stress; colds, flu, or sore throats; sleep difficulties; concern for a troubled friend or family member; relationship difficulty; depression, anxiety, or seasonal affective disorder; Internet use or computer games; death of a friend or family member; sinus infection, ear infection, bronchitis, or strep throat; and alcohol use (American College Health Association, 2008).

## Standards and Guidelines for Higher Education

CAS Professional Standards for Higher Education is a tool that can be used by health promotion program staff at the college level to compare their campus with the ideal campus (Council for the Advancement of Standards in Higher Education, 2009) and to support the development of health promotion programs on their campus. The Council for the Advancement of Standards in Higher Education (2008) promotes standards for student affairs, student services, and student development programs. The standards are meant to foster student learning, development, and achievement. In 2005, health promotion services became one of over thirty functional areas within the standards (Allen et al., 2007). The standards cover criteria related to a higher education institution's mission, programs, leadership, organization and management, human resources, financial resources, legal responsibilities, equity and access, campus relations, external relations, diversity, ethics, and assessment and evaluation (Allen et al., 2007).

## Standards of Practice for Health Promotion in Higher Education

The Standards of Practice for Health Promotion in Higher Education (American College Health Association, 2005a) provide guidelines for health promotion in the university setting. The first edition of the standards, published in 2001, was the culmination of work by the ACHA-appointed Task Force on Health Promotion in Higher Education (American College Health Association, 2005a; Zimmer, Hill, & Sonnad, 2003). Three years later, ACHA published a revised edition of the standards (Allen et al., 2007; American College Health Association, 2005a). The standards address the following topics:

1. Integration with the learning mission of higher education
2. Collaborative practice
3. Cultural competence
4. Theory-based practice
5. Evidence-based practice
6. Professional development and service (American College Health Association, 2005a)

### Vision into Action: Putting the Standards into Action

ACHA published *Vision into Action: Tools for Professional and Program Development Based on Standards of Practice for Health Promotion in Higher Education*, in spring 2005 (American College Health Association, 2005b), as a companion piece to the standards (American College Health Association, 2005a). It contains the first comprehensive health promotion assessment tool. It includes professional and program self-assessment and development worksheets and a CD.

### Data Sources

Table 12.1 is a summary of online sources of health data and health policies that may be useful to those who are planning and running programs in school and university settings. At each Web site listed, you will find reports of current projects, conference announcements, and funding opportunities.

## CHALLENGES

Although economy of scale is a good reason to implement health promotion programs at both schools and universities, such initiatives present challenges—for example, understanding the culture and goals of schools and universities, gaining access to students, and communicating with teachers and faculty in order to gain their support. First and foremost, those from public health or community agencies who wish to provide health promotion programming to students must understand

**TABLE 12.1  External Sources of Data on Health and Health Promotion**

| Source | What the Source Describes | Content | Examples of Findings |
|---|---|---|---|
| School Health Profiles survey http://www.cdc.gov/ healthyyouth/profiles/index .htm | Health policies and activities in secondary schools | School health education requirements and content | Percentage of high schools with a physical education requirement |
| | | Physical education requirements | Percentage of schools with a written policy that protects the rights of students or staff with HIV infection or AIDS |
| | | Asthma management activities | |
| | | Comprehensive food practices and policies | |
| | | Family and community involvement | Percentage of schools with healthy foods in vending machines |
| | | School health policies | |
| Youth Risk Behavior Survey http://www.cdc.gov/yrbs | Health risk behaviors of high school students | Unintentional injuries and violence | Prevalence of high school students who participated in recommended level of physical activity during the past seven days |
| | | Tobacco use | |
| | | Alcohol and other drug use | |
| | | Sexual behaviors that contribute to unintended pregnancy and sexually transmitted diseases, including HIV infection | Prevalence of students in grades 9–12 who used tobacco products during the past thirty days |
| | | Unhealthy dietary behaviors | |
| | | Physical inactivity | |
| National Association of State Boards of Education, State School Health Policy Database http://www.nasbe.org/healthy_ schools/hs/index.php | Searchable database of state-level school health policies | Legal codes, rules, standards | State health education mandates |
| | | Administrative orders, mandates, resolutions | State education mandates on prevention of HIV, sexually transmitted diseases, and pregnancy |
| | | Other means of exercising authority | |

(*Continued*)

TABLE 12.1 External Sources of Data on Health and Health Promotion (Continued)

| Source | What the Source Describes | Content | Examples of Findings |
|---|---|---|---|
| State and local level health surveys (for example, Youth Tobacco Survey, Communities That Care Youth Survey) http://www.cdc.gov/tobacco/data_statistics/surveys/nyts/index.htm http://ncadi.samhsa.gov/features/ctc/resources.aspx | State- and local-level health-related knowledge, attitudes, skills, and behaviors of students, other groups of youths, parents, and community groups | Various attitudes and behaviors of students and parents pertaining to health and health risks Depends on survey focus | Percentage of middle school students who report current use of any tobacco product Percentage of students who report that their family has clear rules about alcohol and drug use Percentage of students who report using drugs in the last thirty days Percentage of students who feel safe at school Percentage of parents who approve of HIV prevention education in schools |
| ACHA-National College Health Assessment http://www.acha-ncha.org | Health risk behaviors of college students | Alcohol, tobacco, and other drug use Sexual health Weight, nutrition, and exercise Mental health Personal safety and violence | Prevalence of students who engage in vigorous aerobic exercise Prevalence of students who used tobacco products during the past thirty days Prevalence of impediments to academic performance |

that the chief goal and mission of educational institutions is education and learning—not health. Furthermore in recent years schools have had added pressure to focus on academics, with the emphasis on accountability for students passing high-stakes state and national tests established by the No Child Left Behind Act; therefore, there is little time left in the curriculum for new programs, particularly those that might be viewed as not central to the role of schools. So the health promotion program staff who work outside the school or university and want to secure instructional time for health promotion must focus on the educational impact of the intervention and frame the arguments for partnerships in terms of educational outcomes as well as health outcomes (for example, by emphasizing the ways in which addressing students' health problems and concerns eliminates barriers to learning that interfere with students' being fully engaged in their studies).

It is also important for health promotion program staff to understand that the process for gaining access to K–12 students is more formal than it is for working with university students. Health promotion program staff from nonschool settings must respect the hierarchy in schools. To work with students and teachers, one must seek approval of the principal. To work in a district, one must seek the approval of the superintendent. At the district level, one should also approach the coordinator for health and physical education (or the district coordinator for school nursing or the district coordinator for counseling) to secure support for the school's or the district's participation in a health promotion initiative. Gaining access to students in institutions of higher education often depends on gaining approval at the department level. If access to students in a particular course is required, the department chairperson or individual faculty member is the person to approach for approval. Health promotion program staff who want to work with students directly might need to contact the director of residence halls or the dean of student life for permission.

Communication with education staff should be succinct and free of health promotion jargon. Language used by public health officials occasionally differs somewhat from that used by education staff. For example, for health workers, *surveillance* means assessment of morbidity and mortality, whereas for K–12 educators, it means using a camera to monitor student behavior. Beyond awareness of the occasional definition that differs, health promotion program staff who are approaching education staff from outside should be prepared to talk about links between the curriculum or lessons they would like to provide and state or national education standards and performance indicators. Further, the health promotion program staff should be able to identify research-based best practices that will be used and the proposed initiative's characteristics that bode well for successful outcomes.

Even health promotion initiatives that are organized by college or university personnel face a number of barriers. Health promotion on campus is usually conducted with limited resources. Further, the strategies that are used to promote health on campus are often limited to awareness activities, written information, and didactic presentations (Zimmer, Hill, & Sonnad, 2003). More research on best practices and a greater understanding of effective strategies for promoting individual and community change is needed in order to improve health promotion on college and university campuses. In addition, health promotion on college and university campuses should be led by professionals who have the skills to assess health needs and to plan, implement, and evaluate interventions, not by clinical health professionals who staff university clinics.

## CAREER OPPORTUNITIES

Over time a variety of professional organizations have emerged to support health professionals who work in schools—for example, health educators, school nurses, physicians, physical educators, counselors, psychologists, social workers, dieticians, and others who are interested in promoting the health and learning of children and adolescents. Given their strong links with community organizations, many of these same professionals could be working in health departments or other community agencies, but instead they are targeting the majority of their professional practice to improving the health and well-being of students in schools or colleges.

Professional health education organizations with an interest in promoting the health of K–12 students include the American Public Health Association, the Society for Public Health Education, the Society of State Directors of Health, Physical Education, and Recreation, the American Association for Health Education (an organization within the American Association for Health, Physical Education, Recreation, and Dance), and the American School Health Association. Health educators working in K–12 schools are most likely to be members of the American Association for Health Education or the American School Health Association. The American College Health Association is the primary professional organization for health educators working in college and university health services. Health educators working in state departments of education are best represented by the Society of State Directors of Health, Physical Education, and Recreation. It is not unusual, however, for health educators to belong to more than one national health education organization as well as state affiliates of these organizations.

A variety of other national organizations represent school and university personnel as well as others involved in health promotion activities. Organizations that serve those interested in initiatives in K–12 schools include, among others, the following: National Association for Sport and Physical Education (an organization within the American Association for Health, Physical Education, Recreation, and Dance), National Association of School Nurses, National Athletic Training Association, American School Food Service Association, National Association for School Psychologists, American School Counselor Association, School Social Work Association of America, National Association of Social Workers, National School Transportation Association, National Education Association, American Federation of Teachers, Association for Supervision and Curriculum Development, American Association of School Administrators, Council of Chief State School Officers, National Association of State Boards of Education, National School Boards Association, and National Parent Teacher Association. Organizations that serve those interested in initiatives in colleges and universities include the National Association of Student Affairs Professionals and NASPA: Student Affairs Administrators in Higher Education.

A wide variety of professional opportunities are available for individuals who are interested in a career in promoting the health and learning of students in school and university settings. Individuals who are interested in teaching students in K–12 settings must pursue degrees that will allow them to meet state standards for teacher certification by completing degrees or programs in elementary education, health education, or physical education. Other school-based or school-linked professionals who directly influence the health and learning of students in K–12 settings include school principals, superintendents, curriculum directors, school nurses, school physicians, athletic trainers, school food service directors, dieticians, school counselors, school psychologists, school social workers, and health educators involved in on-site health promotion for school staff. Community health educators who work in health organizations (for example, local affiliates of the American Cancer Society) or agencies (for example, local public health departments) can partner with schools by collaborating individually with school professionals or collectively as members of school health councils or by offering school-based or community-based programs designed to influence the health and learning of youths. School and community health educators can also influence the health and learning of students by working in health education centers (for example, the Robert Crown Center for Health Education; see www.robertcrown .org). In addition, school and community health educators can work in state agencies (for example, state departments of education or health) and organizations (for example, state or regional affiliates of the American Heart Association) as well as national agencies (for example, the Centers for Disease Control and Prevention) and organizations (for example, the American Diabetes Association) to influence the health and learning of youth.

Individuals interested in health promotion careers in university settings often need advanced degrees (a master's or doctoral degree) that will allow them to meet the employment requirements of colleges and universities. Individuals who are interested in teaching health education courses are usually employed by academic departments, whereas other health educators are employed by units of the university that are organized to serve students (for example, student services) and staff (for example, human resources). For instance, health educators may work in student health services, campus recreation departments, or faculty health promotion services. In addition, university settings provide a wide variety of other career opportunities that are directly linked to promoting students' health and learning.

## SUMMARY

Schools and universities offer tremendous opportunities for health promotion. The role of schools and universities in promoting and protecting the health of children, adolescents, and young adults has been recognized throughout history. In recent years, however, many initiatives have been put in place to support health promotion activities in school and university settings. Future professionals can take part in a wide variety of partnerships to promote the health of children, adolescents, and young adults. Students who are interested in pursuing careers in health promotion are encouraged to join professional organizations that will support their professional preparation and development as health promotion specialists in school and university settings.

## FOR PRACTICE AND DISCUSSION

1. Use the rationale for health promotion in school and university settings to create a brief (three-minute) presentation to justify the provision of health promotion programs in school or university settings.
2. Think about a specific elementary school, middle school, high school, or university. Identify and describe the programs, services, and policies that are designed to promote or protect student health in this school or university.
3. Use the Internet to explore the results of one of these surveys: Youth Risk Behavior Survey, School Health Profiles, School Health Policies and Programs Study, or ACHA-National College Health Assessment. Select a specific risk behavior assessed in the Youth Risk Behavior Survey or the ACHA-National College Health Assessment or a specific component of coordinated school

health programs assessed in the School Health Profiles or the School Health Policies and Programs Study, and describe the results related to a specific risk behavior or component of coordinated school health programs.

4. Use the Internet to explore three of the organizations that serve professionals who work in school or university settings to promote the health of students. For each organization, identify its mission, the professionals that it serves, and its important initiatives.

5. Using the resources and tools described in this chapter, design a four-hour training session on promoting student health for new community college staff members.

6. A school district is advertising a new job for an individual to plan, implement, and evaluate health promotion programs for its elementary school students. Prepare a list of interview questions that the school district's human resource director can use to evaluate the job candidates.

## KEY TERMS

ACHA-National College Health Assessment

Characteristics of an effective health education curriculum

Coordinated school health program

Counseling, psychological, and social services

Family and community involvement

Health education

Health Education Curriculum Analysis Tool

Health promotion for staff

Health services

Health-promoting universities

Healthy school environment

National Health Education Standards

Nutrition services

Physical education

School Health Index

School Health Policies and Programs Study

School Health Profiles

Standards of Practice for Health Promotion in Higher Education

Youth Risk Behavior Survey

## REFERENCES

Allen, N., Fabiano, P., Hong, L., Kennedy, S., Kenzig, M., Kodama, C, et al. (2007). Introduction to the American College Health Association's "Standards of practice for health promotion in higher education." *Journal of American College Health Association*, *55*, 374–375.

Allensworth, D. D., & Kolbe, L. J. (1987). The comprehensive school health program: Exploring an expanded concept. *Journal of School Health*, *57*, 409–412.

Allensworth, D., Lawson, E., Nicholson, L., & Wyche, J. (Eds.). (1997). *Schools and health: Our nation's investment.* Washington, DC: National Academies Press.

Allensworth, D., Wyche, J., Lawson, E., & Nicholson, L. (Eds.). (1995). *Defining a comprehensive school health program: An interim statement.* Washington, DC: National Academies Press.

American Association of School Administrators. (2009, February). *American Association of School Administrators' position statements. Position statement 18: Providing safe and nurturing environment.* Retrieved May 23, 2009, from http://www.aasa.org.

American Cancer Society, American Diabetes Association, & American Heart Association. (2008a). *Facts. Learning for life: Health education in schools.* Retrieved May 23, 2009, from http://www.everydaychoices.org/082008/Health%20Ed%20Fact%20Sheet%20ACS%20ADA%20AHA%205.27.08%20_final_.pdf.

American Cancer Society, American Diabetes Association, & American Heart Association. (2008b). *Facts. Learning for life: Physical education in schools.* Retrieved May 23, 2009, from http://www.everydaychoices.org/082008/PE%20Fact%20Sheet%20AHA%20ACS%20ADA%205.27.08%20[Final].pdf.

American Cancer Society, American Diabetes Association, & American Heart Association. (2008c). *Health education in schools: The importance of establishing healthy behaviors in our nation's youth.* Retrieved May 23, 2009, from http://www.everydaychoices.org/082008/Health%20Ed%20Statement%20ACS%20ADA%20AHA%205.27.08%20_final_.pdf.

American Cancer Society, American Diabetes Association, & American Heart Association. (2008d). *Physical education in schools: Both quality and quantity are important.* Retrieved May 23, 2009, from http://www.everydaychoices.org/082008/PE%20in%20Schools%20Statement%20ACS%20ADA%20AHA%205.27.08%20_final_.pdf.

American College Health Association. (2002). *Healthy campus 2010: Making it happen.* Baltimore, MD: Author.

American College Health Association. (2005a). *Standards of practice for health promotion in higher education.* Retrieved May 23, 2009, from http://www.acha.org/info_resources/SPHPHE_statement.pdf.

American College Health Association. (2005b). *Vision into action: Tools for professional and program development based on Standards of Practice for Health Promotion in Higher Education.* Retrieved May 23, 2009, from http://www.acha.org/info_resources/SPHPHE.cfm.

American College Health Association. (2008). American College Health Association–National College Health Assessment spring 2007 reference group data report (abridged). *Journal of American College Health, 56,* 469–479.

Balaji, A. B., Brener, N. D., McManus, T., Hawkins, J., Kann, L., & Speicher, N. (2008). *School Health Profiles: Surveillance of health programs among secondary schools.* Retrieved August 16, 2008, from http://www.cdc.gov/healthyyouth/profiles/pdf/Profiles_2006.pdf.

Brainard, A. M. (1922). *The evolution of public health nursing.* Philadelphia: Saunders.

Brener, N. D., Kann, L., Kinchen, S. A., Grunbaum, J. A., Whalen, L., Eaton, D., et al. (2004). Methodology of the Youth Risk Behavior Surveillance System. *Morbidity and Mortality Weekly Report, 53*(RR-12), 1–12.

Burks, F. W., & Burks, J. D. (1913). *Health and the school: A round table.* New York: Appleton.

Centers for Disease Control and Prevention. (2005a). *School Health Index: A self-assessment and planning guide. Elementary school version.* Retrieved May 23, 2009, from http://www.cdc.gov/HealthyYouth/SHI/pdf/Elementary.pdf.

Centers for Disease Control and Prevention. (2005b). *School Health Index: A self-assessment and planning guide. Middle school/high school version.* Retrieved May 23, 2009, from http://www.cdc.gov/HealthyYouth/SHI/pdf/MiddleHigh.pdf.

Centers for Disease Control and Prevention. (2007). *Health Education Curriculum Analysis Tool.* Retrieved May 23, 2009, from http://www.cdc.gov/healthyyouth/hecat/index.htm.

Centers for Disease Control and Prevention. (2008a, November). *Healthy youth! CDC's school health education resources (SHER): Characteristics of an effective health education curriculum.* Retrieved May 23, 2009, from http://www.cdc.gov/healthyyouth/SHER/characteristics/index.htm.

Centers for Disease Control and Prevention. (2008b, September). *Healthy youth! Coordinated school health program.* Retrieved May 23, 2009, from http://www.cdc.gov/healthyyouth/CSHP.

Centers for Disease Control and Prevention. (2009a, March). *Healthy youth! Adolescent health.* Retrieved May 23, 2009, from http://www.cdc.gov/healthyyouth/AdolescentHealth/index.htm.

Centers for Disease Control and Prevention. (2009b, March). *Healthy youth! Student health and academic achievement.* Retrieved May 23, 2009, from http://www.cdc.gov/HealthyYouth/health_and_academics/index.htm.

Council for the Advancement of Standards in Higher Education. (2008). *CAS mission statement.* Retrieved May 23, 2009, from http://www.cas.edu/index.html.

Council for the Advancement of Standards in Higher Education. (2009). *CAS professional standards for higher education* (7th ed.). Washington, DC: Author.

Council of Chief State School Officers. (2004). *Policy statement on school health.* Retrieved May 23, 2009, from http://www.ccsso.org/content/pdfs/SchoolHealthPolicyStatement.pdf.

Dooris, M., & Martin, E. (2002). The health promoting university—From idea to implementation. *Promotion and Education, 9*(Suppl. 1), 16–19.

Franklin, B. (1749). *Proposals relating to the education of youth in Pensilvania.* Retrieved May 23, 2009, from http://www.archives.upenn.edu/primdocs/1749proposals.html.

Gulick, L. H., & Ayres, L. P. (1917). *Medical inspection of schools.* New York: Russell Sage Foundation.

Gunderson, G. W. (1971). *The National School Lunch Program background and development.* Retrieved March 16, 2008, from http://www.fns.usda.gov/cnd/lunch/AboutLunch/ProgramHistory.htm.

Hoag, E. B., & Terman, L. M. (1914). *Health work in the schools.* New York: Houghton Mifflin.

Johonnot, J., & Bouton, E. (1889). *Lessons in hygiene, or the human body and how to take care of it.* New York: American Book Company.

Joint Committee on National Health Education Standards. (1995). *National Health Education Standards: Achieving health literacy.* Atlanta, GA: American Cancer Society.

Joint Committee on National Health Education Standards. (2007). *National Health Education Standards: Achieving excellence* (2nd ed.). Atlanta, GA: American Cancer Society.

Kann, L., Brener, N. D., & Wechsler, H. (2007). Overview and summary: School Health Policies and Programs Study, 2006. *Journal of School Health, 77,* 385–397.

Kann, L., Telljohann, S. K., & Wooley, S. F. (2007). Health education: Results from School Health Policies and Programs Study 2006. *Journal of School Health, 77,* 408–434.

Kolbe, L. J. (1986). Increasing the impact of school health promotion programs: Emerging research perspectives. *Health Education, 17*(5), 47–52.

Kolbe, L. J. (2002). Education reform and the goals of modern school health programs. *State Education Standard, 3*(4), 4–11.

Kupchella, C. E. (2009). Colleges and universities should give more broad-based attention to health and wellness—at all levels. *Journal of American College Health, 58*, 185–186.

Lincoln, D. F. (1886). The sanitary conditions and necessities of school-houses and school-life. In *Public health: The Lomb prize essays* (pp. 65–98). Retrieved May 23, 2009, from http://books.google .com/books?id=5ZUVxH09nV8C&printsec=frontcover&dq=The+Lomb+Prize&lr= &as_brr=0&ei=E9pwSLz-MpPgiQHoifiUBA.

Lockhart, A. S., & Spears, B. M. (1972). *Chronicle of American physical education: Selected readings, 1855–1930.* Dubuque, IA: W. C. Brown.

Mann, H. (1838). Physical education. *Common School Journal, 1*(1), 10–11.

National Association of State Boards of Education. (2009). *Public education positions of the National Association of State Boards of Education.* Retrieved May 23, 2009, from http://www.nasbe.org/ index.php/file-repository?func=startdown&id=789.

National Center for Education Statistics. (2007, August). *Table 1: Projected number of participants in educational institutions, by level and control of institution, Fall 2007.* Retrieved May 23, 2009, from http://nces.ed.gov/programs/digest/d07_001.asp?referrer=report.

National School Boards Association. (2009, April). *Beliefs and policies of the National School Boards Association.* Retrieved May 23, 2009, from http://www.nsba.org/FunctionNav/AboutNSBA/ NSBAGovernance/BeliefsandPolicies.aspx.

Shattuck, L., Banks, N. P., & Abbott, J. (1850). *Report of a general plan for the promotion of general and public health, devised, prepared and recommended by the commissioners appointed under a resolve of the legislature of Massachusetts, relating to a sanitary survey of the state.* Retrieved May 23, 2009, from http://biotech .law.lsu.edu/cphl/history/books/sr/index.htm.

Tappe, M. K., Wilbur, K. M., Telljohann, S. K., & Jensen, M. (2009). Articulation of the National Health Education Standards to support learning and healthy behaviors among students. *American Journal of Health Education, 40*, 245–253.

Terman, L. M. (1914). *The hygiene of the school child.* New York: Houghton Mifflin.

Tsouros, A., Dowding, G., & Dooris, M. (1998). Strategic framework for the Health Promoting Universities project. In A. Tsouros, G. Dowding, J. Thompson, & M. Dooris (Eds.), *Health promoting universities: Concept, experience and framework for action* (pp. 121–137). Copenhagen: World Health Organization.

Tsouros, A., Dowding, G., Thompson, J., & Dooris, M. (Eds.). (1998). *Health promoting universities: Concept, experience and framework for action.* Copenhagen: World Health Organization.

Wallin, J.E.W. (1914). *The mental health of the school child.* New Haven, CT: Yale University Press.

World Health Organization, Expert Committee on Comprehensive School Health Education and Promotion. (1997). *Promoting health through schools* (World Health Organization Technical Report Series 870). Geneva: World Health Organization. Retrieved August 14, 2008, from http://www.who.int/wormcontrol/documents/en/trs_870.pdf.

Zimmer, C. G., Hill, M. H., & Sonnad, S. R. (2003). A scope-of-practice survey leading to the development of Standards of Practice for Health Promotion in Higher Education. *Journal of American College Health, 51*, 247–254.

# CHAPTER THIRTEEN

# PATIENT-FOCUSED HEALTH PROMOTION PROGRAMS IN HEALTH CARE ORGANIZATIONS

LOUISE VILLEJO

CEZANNE GARCIA

KATHERINE CROSSON

## LEARNING OBJECTIVES

- Discuss the evolving role of patient-focused health promotion programs in the health care organizations

- Identify core components of effective patient-focused health promotion programs

- Identify and discuss resources and tools for patient-focused health promotion programs

- Explore the opportunities and challenges of patient-focused health promotion programs

- Describe administrative, clinical, and programming careers in patient-focused health care organizations

HEALTH CARE ORGANIZATIONS include for-profit, nonprofit, public, community, and academic hospitals and medical care clinics that provide both routine and emergency services; home health agencies that provide in-home care designed to replace or reduce the need for more expensive hospitalization; and physician organizations such as health maintenance organizations and preferred provider organizations (Breckon, Harvey, & Lancaster, 1998). Traditionally, health care organizations have directed their efforts toward the provision of medical care, including acute care, long-term care, rehabilitation, and psychiatric care, and hospitals have been viewed as the center of the medical care delivery system (Johnson, 2000). However, in recent years, given significant changes in the health care system, health care organizations have devoted more attention to health promotion programs. These health promotion programs reflect collaboration between practitioners in medicine and public health. And while practitioners in medicine and public health have worked together on health problems in the past and have continued to have ample opportunities to do so, only recently have need, incentives, and supportive organizational structures come together to promote the design, implementation, and evaluation of a wide range of health promotion programs in health care organizations (Lasker, 1997).

## EVOLVING ROLE OF PROGRAMS IN HEALTH CARE ORGANIZATIONS

Traditionally, health care institutions and organizations have focused on their long-established role as centers for the care of the sick and injured, relegating the responsibility for health promotion to the public health system, educational institutions (schools), and other community agencies. However, during the 1980s and 1990s, as the health care system became more complex and health care costs rapidly increased, the where, how, and what of medical services changed. Hospitals, once seen as the center for most medical services and programs, decentralized many of their functions and began to provide many programs and services in free-standing ambulatory settings in the community and in homes. Concerns about health care finances led to the implementation of managed health care, which focused on cost containment and efficient service delivery. Many benefits and consequences related to these late twentieth-century changes are still being felt and debated in the twenty-first century, and one outcome that has remained is the continuing need to provide education, skills training, and information for patients and their family members, staff members of health care organizations, and community members.

For patients and families in the 1980s and 1990s, individuals known as *patient advocates* began to exert their influence on the health care system. They were fervent about the need for change in the health care system and wanted health care providers to listen to patients' concerns; respect their lifestyles; and communicate with rather than dictate to patients, their families, and significant others. In many cases, they had had a personal experience of being patients or were family members or friends of a patient. The advocates worked closely with advocacy groups, relying on their close identification with the patient population to assess informational and educational needs, as well as lobby on behalf of the patient population for patient-centered services within the health care environment (Davenport-Ennis, Cover, Ades, & Stovall, 2002).

One of the most visible advocacy groups brought forward the voices of breast cancer patients and their families. The National Breast Cancer Coalition, a private organization, mobilized women's groups nationwide and demanded that the president and Congress allocate more funds for breast cancer research. Their successful efforts resulted in the establishment of the National Action Plan on Breast Cancer, a public-private partnership that resulted in a significant rise in awareness of breast cancer issues nationwide and the funding and implementation of research, dissemination of information, and outreach aimed at breast cancer prevention and treatment. In addition to setting agendas for action, these advocates also worked to increase patient and family awareness of the disease. They were so skillful and successful at raising funds and increasing public awareness that they were often able to claim spots on hospital boards or federal scientific review committees. Many other patient advocacy groups modeled their activities on the successful work of the breast cancer advocates. Patient advocates continue to have a major influence on the delivery of health care in the United States, in addition to ensuring that the needs of patients and their families are met (National Action Plan on Breast Cancer, 2000).

During this same time period, the U.S. Department of Veterans Affairs took steps to integrate health promotion programs into its system by appointing patient education coordinators within its nationwide hospital system and assigning an individual to supervise their work (Rose Mary Pries, personal communication, 2008). In northern and southern California, Kaiser Permanente installed health education coordinators in each of its hospital facilities who were responsible for planning, promoting, implementing, and evaluating education and health promotion activities for patients and their families. These educators were accountable to their facilities management team and to a regional health education coordinator (Squyres, 1982). In 1989, the National Cancer Institute (NCI) created the Cancer Patient Education Network (CPEN). Individuals responsible for patient education at NCI-designated comprehensive cancer centers constituted the CPEN's initial membership. Almost twenty years later, this group is a private organization working in partnership with the NCI and includes membership from Canada as well as non-NCI-designated cancer facilities.

In the 1980s and 1990s, hospital operations were scrutinized and focused on efficient service delivery and on staffing. Discussion of patient safety and outcomes was spurred by revelations of inefficient and even dangerous conditions in hospitals that led to negative health consequences and even death for some patients. In addition to the compelling need to improve safety and quality in health care, improving working conditions in health care organizations became a priority as competition increased for health care staff and future shortages in medical and health care staffing were predicted. Health care organizations became sites for workplace health promotion programs that took into consideration the unique characteristics of the medical setting (for example, the provision of services twenty-four hours a day, seven days a week; patient lifting as a cause of back injuries; and the threat of contracting blood-borne diseases).

Outreach into the community by health care organizations also grew during this period. Public health initiatives, blended with scientific advances and technological advances in particular, introduced new health interventions to prevent and in some cases eliminate health problems by addressing them early. The greatest growth for these interventions occurred in primary care sites in hospital-based health care systems and independent clinics.

Today, a range of health promotion programs operate within health care organizations. For example, Exhibit 13.1 shows selected components of the health promotion program at the M. D. Anderson Cancer Center in Houston, Texas. The programs at the Anderson Center, as well as programs in other health care organizations, are focused on but not limited to

- Education, information needs, decision making, rights, and privacy of patients and family
- Patient safety (for example, medical error reduction) and positive health outcomes
- Health needs of staff members, including medical, administrative, support, and maintenance staff (for example, food service and nutrition, physical activity, stress management)
- Workplace safety (for example, disposal of hazardous waste and blood, reduction of needle sticks, measures to protect against infectious disease)
- Community outreach through health promotion and health education programs, particularly on public health matters

The health professionals involved with such programs range from physicians, health educators, and nurses to medical social workers and allied health professionals (for example, physical therapists and occupational therapists), safety coordinators, and health coordinators. The programs are viewed as integral to the organizations' mission and help to create a supportive, caring, health-promoting environment. Exhibit 13.1 demonstrates this integral role by highlighting a program's specific attention to creating a supportive social and physical environment and integrating programs into the overall operation of the organization.

## EFFECTIVE PROGRAMS IN HEALTH CARE ORGANIZATIONS

Some of the components of health promotion programs in health care organizations are similar, if not identical, to programs that are implemented at work sites for employees (Chapter Fourteen) and in community settings for members of the public (Chapter Fifteen). For example, in Exhibit 13.1, both staff and community health promotion programs are mentioned. Unique to health care organizations, however, are health promotion programs that historically have been patient-focused and associated with patient education to help people to make informed medical and health decisions and develop skills needed to participate in their health care. In today's world, individuals are more involved in their own health care decisions. The increased involvement reflects an increase in health promotion programs and managed care that has created shorter hospital stays in response to the need for cost containment and increasing demand for outpatient and in-home services. In Exhibit 13.1, patient-focused programs include patient and family health education, behavioral health promotion, and cancer prevention that focuses on minority and underserved populations.

Patient-focused health promotion programs, with their roots in patient and family education, have been an integral component of health care for decades but have been transformed through the years as significant changes have been made through strengthening of the evidence base and changes in how health care is delivered and financed in an increasingly multicultural society in which individuals are living longer and patients and their families are managing their health with the aid of new resources and evolving technologies. For years, patients and their families relied on physicians and nurses as their main sources of health education; these professionals shared information about a disease, discussed proposed treatments and potential side effects of treatment, and prepared the patient and family for a return to their home environment or another health care setting. In the mid-1970s, health education specialists joined health care teams in hospitals and clinics nationwide. They possessed a unique set of skills that enabled them to assess patients' educational needs and design and implement interventions that strengthened and reinforced the health care team's messages. Professionally

## EXHIBIT 13.1
## Selected Components of the Health Promotion Program at the M. D. Anderson Cancer Center

*Program Areas*

- **Patient and family health education**. Provide programs for each medical specialty area, including
  - Twenty-five specific disease programs with educational resources to help manage the cancer experience (database of 2,500 items of printed materials in multiple languages)
  - Classes (for example, management of cancer-related fatigue, pain management, bowel management, and caregiver support)
  - Computer-based education
  - Health campaigns (for example, diabetes awareness, Fatigue Week, patient safety)
  - Nutrition and cancer programs (for example, guest chef program, organic foods, nutrition for those touched by cancer)
  - Weekly PIKNIC (Partners in Knowledge News in Cancer) educational sessions (for example, Chemobrain: Is It Real?; Finding Reliable Information—We're Here for You; Important Psychosocial Services for Patients, Survivors, and Caregivers; Caregivers: "I've Got Feelings Too!")
- **Community health promotion and public health education**. Provide education, outreach, and communications programs that increase awareness and understanding of cancer and the programs and services of the M. D. Anderson Cancer Center. These programs serve as the institutional gateway to community organizations. Serving over 90,000 people, community education programs include a speakers bureau, exhibits, publications, institutional tours, puppet shows, and community partnerships.
- **Behavioral health promotion**. Provide research-driven clinical care to promote a healthy lifestyle and encourage changes in order to reduce cancer risk, improve adherence to cancer treatment, enhance survivors' coping with long-term consequences of cancer treatment, and provide a model of optimal care for cancer-related psychosocial and behavioral issues.
- **Cancer prevention**. Advance the science and application of cancer prevention and population sciences and eliminate the unequal burden of cancer in minority and underserved populations through multidisciplinary programs in research, clinical service, and education. Programs seek to identify lifestyle factors, genetic predispositions, and molecular events that contribute to the development of cancer; develop, implement, and evaluate interventions that reduce carcinogenic risk and progression or the adverse psychological and physical impact of cancer; explore new approaches to the assessment and management of cancer risk through early detection, genetic counseling, and clinical interventions; develop, implement, and evaluate community programs to reduce cancer risk; train health care professionals

in the delivery and application of prevention services; and create educational and behavioral support systems.

- **Staff work-life balance and wellness promotion**. Provide employee benefit programs to promote work-life integration and wellness. M. D. Anderson is the first National Cancer Institute–designated comprehensive cancer center and the first health care system to receive the CEO Cancer Gold Standard accreditation. The Gold Standard focuses on risk reduction, early detection, and quality cancer care. To be accredited, organizations must offer a series of benefits and programs that lower the risk of cancer through lifestyle changes, including eliminating the use of tobacco, exercising regularly, and maintaining a healthful diet. Providing preventive screenings and access to the best available treatment, including clinical trials, for employees and their family members is also a key criterion for accreditation.

### Supportive Social and Physical Environment

- Four learning centers on campus provide the latest information on cancer care, support, and prevention as well as general health and wellness issues. Staff members are available to provide skilled, personalized service.
- Place of Wellness Center is an environment in which all persons touched by cancer can enhance their quality of life through programs that complement medical care and focus on the mind, body, and spirit. Most programs are offered free of charge, except acupuncture and full body massage, which are provided for a nominal fee.
- Exercise rooms and stretching equipment are placed through the institution, which also has an outdoor track.
- An institutional art program promotes an environment of optimism and hope.

### Integration with Operations

- Health promotion efforts are included in new employee orientation, customer service training, and job orientation in all clinical disciplines.
- All health promotion programs are promoted on an institutional intranet site.
- Patient Education Online is a Web-based database that allows staff members to access about 2,500 patient education information sheets from their computers.
- Training in patient teaching is available to enhance the clinical staff's patient teaching skills.
- Over 200 patient education videos are available twenty-four hours a day, seven days a week, through Video on Demand, the in-house cable system.
- Channel 21, the patient information system, is a closed-circuit cable channel dedicated to communicating news and information to patients and caregivers. Channel 21 is broadcast on flat-screen televisions in outpatient and supportive care waiting areas throughout M. D. Anderson's main campus.
- *myMDAnderson*, a secure, personalized Web site, includes patient education print materials, class schedules, and videos and other resources to help patients take an active role in their cancer care.

prepared in the behavioral sciences, group dynamics, counseling, education theory, community organization, and the diffusion of innovations and practices, health educators were ideally suited for roles on health care teams.

At the same time, the consumer health care movement was evolving and there was a growing awareness that to achieve the best possible health care outcomes, patients and their families needed to be actively engaged in decision making about their own health care. Health education specialists were able to assist patients and their families in building collaborative relationships with the members of their health care team, advising and counseling them about how to access health information and use the knowledge and advice they received from the members of the health care team in order to make patient-centered and family-centered best choices about health. Many patients embraced this shared ownership of the health care decision-making process and now view it as a personal responsibility.

In the planning, implementation, and evaluation of effective patient-focused health promotion programs in health care organizations, four qualities are important:

- Focus on the needs of patients and families and on their partnership role
- Incorporation of evidence into practice
- Interdisciplinary, collaborative approach
- Commitment to quality performance, improvement, and continual evaluation

## Focus on Patients' and Families' Needs

*Patient- and family-centered care* is "an approach to the planning, delivery, and evaluation of health care that is grounded in mutually beneficial partnerships among health care patients, families, and providers" and built on the four core concepts of dignity and respect, information sharing, participation, and collaboration (Institute for Family-Centered Care, 2008b) (see Exhibit 13.2). In less than a decade, patient- and family-centered care has emerged from relative obscurity to an approach that holds promise for transformational change in health care. By creating capacity for patients and families as allies for quality in the health care system, the driving forces of change in our health care system can become more patient- and family-centered rather than predominantly system- or clinician-centered. This approach strives to maintain a balance between technically competent care and emotionally supportive care, and it requires patient and family education programs in order to integrate self-care, safe care at home, psychosocial support, and complementary and alternative medicine practices. In addition, there is a

## EXHIBIT 13.2
## Four Core Concepts of Patient- and Family-Centered Health Promotion Programs

- **Dignity and respect.** Health care practitioners listen to and honor the perspectives and choices of patients and family members. The knowledge, values, beliefs, and cultural backgrounds of patients and family members are incorporated into the planning and delivery of care.
- **Information sharing.** Health care practitioners communicate and share complete and unbiased information with patients and families in ways that are affirming and useful. Patients and families receive timely, complete, and accurate information in order to effectively participate in care and decision making.
- **Participation.** Patients and families are encouraged and supported in participating in care and decision making at the level they choose.
- **Collaboration.** Patients, families, health care practitioners, and hospital leaders collaborate in policy and program development, implementation, and evaluation; in health care facility design; and in professional education, as well as in the delivery of care.

*Source*: Adapted from Institute for Family-Centered Care, 2008b.

need to strengthen the integration of health promotion resources and interventions as integral components of clinical decision-aid and treatment education for patients and their families in order to foster healthy eating, physical activity, and mental health care and discourage tobacco use and alcohol abuse.

## Incorporation of Evidence into Practice

Patient focused health promotion programs in health care organizations have been strengthened by a wide variety of patient and family education standards developed by panels of experts. The experts translate research and best practice evidence into practice standards, resulting in high-quality, outcome-oriented patient and family education programs. Furthermore, the ever-evolving research base has strengthened evidence-based practices in patient and family health promotion and improved understanding of the links between patient and family behavior and health outcomes. Examples of these informative and useful standards include

- Accreditation standards for health care settings developed by the Joint Commission (2009)

- Clinical practice standards developed by panels of experts to identify what should be done in clinical decision making and predominantly identified with the U.S. Preventive Services Task Force of the Agency for Healthcare Research and Quality
- Institution-specific or system-specific practice guidelines that are defined as part of policy and procedure guidelines within most health care organizations or within specific patient and family education practice domains within a health care system, such as the Indian Health Service's procedural blue book on patient and family caregiver education (Indian Health Service, 2008)
- Disease-specific or practitioner-specific guidelines that customize practice standards and tailor the design of patient and family education programs to disease-specific or practitioner-specific domains, such as the American Diabetes Association's (2009) clinical practice recommendations and standards of care; the guidelines for establishing comprehensive cancer patient education services from the Cancer Patient Education Network (2002); the publication *Partnering with Patients and Families to Design a Patient and Family-Centered Health Care System: Recommendations and Promising Practices*, from the Institute for Family-Centered Care (2008b); and information on providing a patient-centered medical home from the American Academy of Family Practice (2009).

Decision-aid tools have demonstrated the value of integrating evidence-based practices with patient's personal values. Patient decision aids typically are multimedia tools or booklets designed to communicate the best available evidence on treatment or screening options to patients and their families in ways that encourage them to engage in meaningful dialogue with their health care provider in order to choose an intervention that is consistent with the evidence and with the patient's personal values. Part of a widespread movement to create mechanisms for clinician and patient collaboration in treatment and screening decision making, these tools are designed to translate the research evidence and help patients apply this information to everyday care experiences (O'Connor et al., 1999). Decision aids are used most often in contexts of preference-sensitive health decisions (Barry, Mulley, Fowler, & Wennberg, 1988) or decisions for which the benefit-harm ratio is uncertain. Thus the strategy of using decision aids depends on the patient's valuation of the potential benefits and harms. Promising work to measure the efficacy of decision aids and the prospects for their widespread adoption and implementation is currently being conducted (Holmes-Rovner et al., 2007).

## Interdisciplinary, Collaborative Approach

An interdisciplinary, collaborative approach is vital to patient-focused health promotion programs. Such programs work in partnership with clinically trained

professional teams (of physicians, nurses, social workers, dietitians, physical therapists, and pharmacists, for example) and patients and their families to guide the
development of interventions that will enable patients to manage and live with
their disease, adapt new health behaviors, and learn new skills. Interdisciplinary
clinical teams help guide health promotion practice at the institutional level by
creating, implementing, and supporting institutional priorities for development
and management of patient-focused programs. At the program level, clinical
managers and staff can provide feedback to the team about the best and most
timely way to integrate health promotion interventions with routine patient care.
And at the one-to-one teaching level, clinical managers can support and protect
allotments of time for developing their staff's competencies in teaching patients.

The Joint Commission (2008) requires an interdisciplinary approach to
patient health promotion; each discipline's practice standards explicitly state
its role in patient and family education and health promotion. Commitment to
the use of an interdisciplinary approach helps staff in each discipline to understand the unique role of each team member and address patients' learning needs
more effectively through the use of consistent and evidence-based information
and practices, creating continuity and quality care experiences for patients and
families.

## Commitment to Quality Performance, Improvement, and Continual Evaluation

The principles of education from the literature that yield the most promising
effects on behavior and clinical outcomes include (1) individualization of instruction in order to provide explicit feedback on learning or clinical progress; (2)
reinforcement of learning; (3) tailoring of education to the needs, interests, and
abilities of the learner; (4) use of multiple communication channels, including
information that describes and manages expectations in the care experience; and
(5) creating capacity for the patient and family members to take action or remove
barriers to action (Mullen & Green, 1985, 1990; Padgett, Mumford, Hynes, &
Carter, 1988; Mumford, Hynes, & Carter, 1988; Giloth, 1990; Smith, 1989;
Mason, 2001). Professionals involved with patient-focused health promotion pro
grams in medical settings are committed to continual evaluation of behavioral
and clinical outcomes. In addition, improving and sustaining such programs relies
increasingly on identifying the key components of an intervention that are effective. A challenge is to continue to conduct these efforts and also link with national
initiatives to support institutional or agency efforts in these areas and increase the
visibility of those who have knowledge and experience in incorporating patient,
family, and staff feedback in program development.

# RESOURCES FOR PROGRAMS IN HEALTH CARE ORGANIZATIONS

The growth and expansion of patient-focused health promotion programs in health care organizations can best be seen in the range of health promotion initiatives during the last twenty-five years. This section lists a selection of resources and tools for patient-focused health promotion programs in health care organizations. Those who may find these resources and tools to be useful are not limited to individuals who work with patients in health care organizations; many of these resources may be of use to programs that focus on staff health promotion, patient safety, reduction of medical error, staff safety, community outreach, or consumer rights.

## Crossing the Quality Chasm

In 1996, the Institute of Medicine (IOM) started a three-phase assessment to improve the quality of the nation's health care. The first phase documented the serious and pervasive nature of problems with the quality of health care in the United States, resulting in a burden of harm that is staggering when their collective impact is considered. As a result, the IOM created a framework that defined the nature of the problem as overuse, misuse, and underuse of health care services (National Academy of Sciences, 2006).

During the second phase, spanning 1999 to 2001, the Committee on Quality of Health Care in America laid out a vision of how the health care system and the related policy environment must be radically transformed in order to close the chasm between what we know to be good quality care and what actually exists in practice. The reports released during this phase—*To Err Is Human: Building a Safer Health System* (Kohn, Corrigan, & Donaldson, 2000), and *Crossing the Quality Chasm: A New Health System for the 21st Century* (Institute of Medicine, Committee on Quality of Health Care in America, 2001)—stress that reform on the margins would be inadequate in addressing the system's ills.

*To Err Is Human* put the spotlight on how tens of thousands of Americans die each year from medical errors and effectively put the issue of patient safety and quality on the radar screen of public and private policymakers. *Crossing the Quality Chasm* described broader quality issues and defined six aims—care should be safe, effective, patient-centered, timely, efficient, and equitable—and ten rules for redesign of care delivery.

The third phase of the IOM's quality initiative focuses on operationalizing the vision of a transformed health system described in *Crossing the Quality Chasm*. In addition to the IOM, many others are working to create a more patient-responsive health system, including clinicians, health care organizations, employers, consumers, foundations, researchers, government agencies, and quality organizations. This collection of efforts focuses on reform at three overlapping levels of the system: the environmental level, the level of the health care organization, and the level of the interface between clinicians and patients.

This work has helped to shape national health policies to improve the lives of millions of people in the United States. It represents a merging of the fields of health and medicine and lends support to health promotion advocacy at the state and national level by identifying some of the challenges and barriers to patient-focused health promotion programs as well as potential solutions.

## Center for the Advancement of Collaborative Strategies in Health

The Center for the Advancement of Collaborative Strategies in Health (2004), at the New York Academy of Medicine, helps partnerships, funders, and policymakers realize the full potential of collaboration to solve complex problems related to health or any other area. Working closely with people and organizations involved in collaboration, the center conducts research studies, policy analyses, and joint learning activities to identify and explore key challenges associated with collaborative problem solving. Collaboration between many groups of individuals and organizations is key to effective patient-focused health promotion programs. To help such collaborative efforts the center has developed a number of practical tools and training programs based on the knowledge it obtains. These include collaboration formation guides, a small-group discussion guide, partnership self-assessment, and medical and public health case studies. These can help health promotion program staff to

- Document what partnerships can accomplish when people who are directly experiencing problems are meaningfully engaged in problem solving.
- Generate much more precise information than is currently available about the how-to of successful stakeholder-driven (for example, patient-driven) collaboration.
- Identify the special leadership and management skills that are needed to promote meaningful stakeholder (for example, patient or other program participant) engagement and to learn how to teach those critical skills to others.
- Use valid and reliable measures for assessing whether a collaborative problem-solving process is on the right track.

- Develop products—such as case studies, evidence-based practice guides, funders' guides, and training programs—that will highlight the value and optimal uses of community-driven collaboration and help interested partnerships and funders put such a problem-solving process into practice.

## The Institute for Healthcare Improvement

The Institute for Healthcare Improvement (IHI) is an independent not-for-profit organization helping to lead the improvement of health care throughout the world. Founded in 1991 and based in Cambridge, Massachusetts, IHI works to accelerate improvement by building the will for change, cultivating promising concepts for improving patient care, and helping health care systems put those ideas into action. It aims to improve the lives of patients, the health of communities, and the joy of the health care workforce by focusing on an ambitious set of goals adapted from the Institute of Medicine's six improvement aims for the health care system: safety, effectiveness, patient-centeredness, timeliness, efficiency, and equity. IHI works with health professionals throughout the world to accelerate the measurable and continual progress of health care systems toward these objectives, leading to breakthrough improvements that are meaningful in the lives of patients. IMI provides model programs, materials, and conferences related to patient care and health promotion. Two examples of IHI initiatives focused on patient care and health are Triple Aim and the 100,000 Lives Campaign.

Triple Aim is an initiative of the Institute for Healthcare Improvement that is operating at twelve sites in order to better understand new models that can improve the individual patient experience and the health of entire communities at a reasonable per-capita cost (Institute for Healthcare Improvement, n.d. b). The focus of the first phase of the initiative was studying effective strategies at participating sites and exchanging key findings for possible further action. After the first phase of the Triple Aim initiative, systems are in place at each of the twelve sites to

1. Improve the health of the population
2. Enhance the patient experience
3. Reduce (or at least control) the per-capita cost of care

The Institute for Healthcare Improvement and its partner organizations came together to launch the 100,000 Lives Campaign, a national effort to reduce preventable deaths in 3,100 U.S. hospitals from January 2005 through June 2006. In December 2006, following the success of the 100,000 Lives Campaign, the IHI established the 5 Million Lives Campaign, the largest improvement initiative undertaken by the health care industry in recent history (Institute for Healthcare Improvement, n.d. a).

## Department of Veterans Affairs and Health Promotion Centers of the U.S. Army, Navy, and Marine Corps

Three important models for health promotion program staff in health care organizations can be found in the U.S. armed services. All three can provide resources and materials for individuals in health care organizations who are planning, implementing, and evaluating patient-focused health promotion programs as well as large comprehensive programs such as those at the M.D. Anderson Cancer Center discussed earlier in the chapter (Exhibit 13.1).

First, the Veterans Administration (VA) has implemented a VA-wide employee wellness initiative as part of the National Center for Health Promotion and Disease Prevention of the U.S. Department of Veterans Affairs. The initiative is sponsored by the National Quality Council and focuses on activities designed to enhance the health and well-being of VA employees. Resources for employee wellness and for clinicians, as well as campaigns for weight loss and healthy veterans, are the focus of a few of the programs within this initiative.

Second, the Navy and Marine Corps Public Health Center (NMCPHC) provides leadership and expertise to ensure mission readiness through disease prevention and health promotion in support of national military strategy. In 1964, the idea for a comprehensive Navy occupational health program originated at what was then the Navy's Bureau of Weapons. The bureau recognized the need for an occupational health program that would encompass all fleet readiness and training ordinance field activities. Today, the center serves the Navy and the Marine Corps through a wide range of health and medical services that include clinical epidemiology, health promotion, and preventive medicine programs. Furthermore, the center offers industrial hygiene, occupational medicine, and environmental medicine programs.

Third, the U.S. Army Center for Health Promotion and Preventive Medicine (USACHPPM), established at the beginning of World War II and placed under the direct jurisdiction of the Army surgeon general, today has a mission to provide worldwide technical support for the implementation of preventive medicine, public health, and health promotion and wellness services in all areas of the U.S. Army and the Army community, anticipating and rapidly responding to operational needs in a changing world environment. The USACHPPM provides worldwide scientific expertise and services in clinical and field preventive medicine, environmental health, occupational health, health promotion and wellness, epidemiology and disease surveillance, toxicology, and related laboratory sciences. It supports readiness by keeping soldiers fit to fight, while also promoting wellness among their family members and the federal civilian workforce. Professionals represented include chemists, physicists, engineers, physicians, optometrists, epidemiologists, audiologists, nurses, industrial hygienists, toxicologists, entomologists, health educators, and many others, as well as professionals in related subspecialties.

## National Patient Safety Foundation

The National Patient Safety Foundation (NPSF) is an independent nonprofit organization that, since its founding in 1997, has been diligently pursuing one mission: to improve the safety of patients (National Patient Safety Foundation, 2008). The NPSF remains the sole organization in the field with this singular focus. The NPSF also occupies a unique position by virtue of its inclusive, multistakeholder approach. From patient and family membership on the foundation's board to the structure of its programs, which engage patients and families as co-producers and co-evaluators of safety initiatives, the NPSF fosters collaboration in order to accelerate improvements in patient safety.

Recognizing that health literacy is a critical component in improving the safety of the health care system, the NPSF joined forces in 2007 with the Partnership for Clear Health Communication, the country's leading nonprofit organization dedicated to improving health literacy. Understanding that communication breakdowns are the leading source of medical errors, NPSF promotes health literacy throughout its work by creating, identifying, and disseminating new knowledge; convening stakeholder groups and multidisciplinary projects; and disseminating patient safety tools and programs that advocate for strengthening patient, family, and clinician partnerships.

The NPSF sponsors a number of health promotion patient-focused initiatives. These include a patient and family resource guide, *Patientsafety-L*; a moderated Listserv (online discussion forum using e-mail) devoted to thoughtful conversation toward the development of a safer health care system; Patient Safety Awareness Week (PSAW), a national education and awareness-building campaign for improving patient safety at the local level; and the Universal Patient Compact. The compact is a statement of principles for partnership established by NPSF; it defines the elements of true and effective partnering between patients and providers. It also provides a framework for shaping a health care organization's efforts to make the commitment to integrating patients and families into care teams.

## American Hospital Association

The American Hospital Association (AHA) is a national organization that represents and serves all types of hospitals, health care networks, and their patients and communities (American Hospital Association, 2008). The AHA offers its broad range of members and regional networks resources, research, and advocacy in health care fields. Close to 5,000 hospitals, health care systems, networks, and other providers of care, as well as 37,000 individual members, make up the AHA today. Founded in 1898, the AHA provides education for health care leaders and is a source of information on health care issues and trends. It ensures that members' perspectives are heard and that their needs are addressed in national health policy development, legislative and regulatory debates, and judicial matters. The association also has a patient care partnership that works for protection and inclusion of the patient's voice as services are provided. As part of this initiative the AHA promotes "A Patient's Bill of Rights," which informs individuals about the rights and responsibilities they should expect during a hospital stay. In addition, the AHA is a rich source of pilot-tested and endorsed resources that can be used in any health care setting. AHA's advocacy efforts encompass the legislative and executive branches of government. Its strong advocacy agenda is also supportive of patient-focused health promotion in health care organizations. AHA advocacy activities are described further on the organization's Web site (www.aha.org/aha/about/index.html).

### Institute for Family-Centered Care

The Institute for Family-Centered Care, a nonprofit organization founded in 1992, takes pride in providing essential leadership to advance the understanding and practice of patient- and family-centered care (Institute for Family-Centered Care, 2008a). By promoting collaborative, empowering relationships among patients, families, and health care professionals, the institute facilitates patient- and family-centered change in all settings where individuals and families receive care and support. The institute also serves as a central resource for policymakers, administrators, program planners, direct service providers, educators, design professionals, and patient and family leaders. The institute provides a range of tools, trainings, publications, materials, and conferences related to family-centered patient education and health promotion.

## CHALLENGES FOR PROGRAMS IN HEALTH CARE ORGANIZATIONS

Opportunities for health promotion programs in health care organizations are increasing. Patient-focused and employee-focused initiatives (that is, workplace health promotion programs, discussed in Chapter Fourteen) are probably the two areas that have the most potential for development and career opportunities. Health promotion programs that are implemented through community outreach (discussed in Chapter Fifteen) are another promising area. Some may find it surprising that the areas of patient safety, medical error reduction, and food services fall within the purview of health promotion and health education programming. When working in a health care organization, however, it is critical to take a broad view of efforts to join the fields of medicine and public health in order to promote the health of patients, families, staff members, and community members.

Health care organizations differ from other settings in that their core mandate is restoring, maintaining, and promoting health through the application of resources and the collaboration of staff members from the fields of medicine and public health. As part of this mandate, health care organizations are subject to many regulations, restrictions, and guidelines that are not found in other settings and that govern their policies and procedures. Working in a medical environment requires an understanding of these regulations as well as their practical, day-to-day implementation. For example, the privacy provisions of the federal Health Insurance Portability and Accountability Act of 1996 (HIPAA) apply to health information that is created or maintained by health care providers who engage in certain electronic transactions, health plans, and health care clearing-houses. The HIPAA privacy rule creates, for the first time, national standards to protect individuals' medical records and other personal health information. In addition, it

- Gives patients more control over their health information
- Sets boundaries on the use and release of health records
- Establishes appropriate safeguards that health care providers and others must implement in order to protect the privacy of health information
- Holds violators accountable through civil and criminal penalties that can be imposed when patients' privacy rights are violated
- Strikes a balance when the public good requires disclosure of some forms of data—for example, to protect public health

For patients and families, the HIPAA privacy rule means being able to make informed choices when seeking care or reimbursement for care because they know how personal health information can be used. The HIPAA privacy rule

- Enables patients to find out how their information may be used and about certain disclosures of their information that have been made
- Limits release of information to the minimum reasonably needed for the purpose of the disclosure

- Gives patients the right to examine and obtain a copy of their own health records and request corrections
- Empowers individuals to control certain uses and disclosures of their health information

Another example of a unique health concern in health care organizations is the risk of exposure to blood-borne pathogens, including *Hepatitis B virus*, *Hepatitis C virus*, and HIV. Nurses and other health care providers and, in some settings, housekeeping personnel are examples of workers who may be at risk of exposure. In response to these concerns, environmental and employee safety programs operating in health care organizations promote safe practices for handling needles and large amounts of diverse hazardous wastes that must be properly packaged, transferred, and disposed of in order to protect both the persons handling it and the environment.

A key challenge of working in a health care setting is dealing with multiple stakeholders—patients and families; medical professionals; administrators of health service institutions; insurance companies; large employers; and government-sponsored research, regulatory, and policymaking entities —and their diverse and dynamic priorities and recommendations on how to manage and improve the care experience. Professional conflicts and priorities can divert attention from the priorities of patients and families who are using the health care system. Who can best deliver health promotion services? Many patients want their physician to provide patient and family education and health promotion activities; however, physicians do not have the time and may not have the expertise to provide these services. Likewise, nurses who are often placed in the role of patient or family educator and health promotion expert might also experience tension between these responsibilities and their clinical responsibilities and time commitments. Furthermore, many medical professionals are not trained to deliver health promotion services. Their expertise is often more narrowly focused on diagnosis and treatment of illness. Likewise, the time and physical clinical space that are needed to support people who are engaged in health promotion programs are different from the time and space needed for patients and families who are having routine medical checkups, medical tests, or medical procedures.

Collaborations across professions that support patients, families, and medical staff have proven to be effective in providing health promotion services and programs in health care organizations. Working as a sole individual, group, or organization is often too intensive—in time, money, required knowledge or skills, or other resources—to be effective in delivering services. Furthermore, without collaboration, programs often cannot be sustained. Collaboration provides credibility for health promotion services and helps counter the argument that these programs, though universally viewed as worthwhile, take too much time or are too expensive. However, initial investments of time or resources may be necessary; for example, some patients and families who are accustomed to being passive recipients of care will require time and training to learn new skills and strategies in order to become active participants in health promotion programs. The time it takes to build these partnerships and acquire appropriate knowledge and skills for collaboration will eventually be repaid several times over. When administrators, clinicians, consumers, and families have a shared understanding of and respect for what each brings to the health care experience, the stage is set for mutually beneficial relationships. With shared priorities and goals, time will most likely not be wasted on repetitive, ineffective, or counterproductive activities. The possibility of misunderstanding, dissatisfaction, and even medical error will be greatly diminished.

When health promotion programs focus on the staff of health care organizations, the logistics can be challenging. Many health care organizations operate twenty-four hours a day, seven days a week. They are open and available all the time. While continual service is good for the health care consumer, it requires that health promotion services that target individuals working in health care settings reflect the realities of the around-the-clock schedule. Although safety and health policies and procedures can be implemented regardless of time of day, innovation is required to engage staff in health promotion activities when they work varied schedules and in diverse environments. Further complicating work with health care professionals is the fact that they spend their professional lives as caregivers in often complex health care organizations. The competing responsibilities and effects of caregiving may affect clinicians' ability to attend to their own health needs (SOPHE Medical Care Special Interest Group, personal communication, 2008).

Champions are needed to support health promotion programs in health care organizations. Champions, among other roles, serve on the committees and task forces that design and support these programs; they can be managers, clinicians, or support staff who are already interested in or knowledgeable about health promotion programs. When possible, choose staff members who are already viewed as opinion leaders by their peers for these roles. Providing staff with opportunities to share their positive experiences and to engage in problem-solving discussions in areas of concern is also a helpful strategy in developing and implementing programs, particularly in relation to the around-the-clock operation of many health care organizations. Finally, involving staff in the process of measuring changes and improvements, as well as structuring plans for the dissemination of information and the spread of innovations, will encourage participation in and support of health promotion programs.

Another challenge in health care organizations is building and sustaining health promotion programs in the workplace setting. An employee wellness program can strengthen and support a healthy environment in a medical care setting and can help individuals and teams take better care of themselves and each other. Most employees spend more than half their waking hours at work, and in a medical care setting, they are focused more on taking care of others than themselves. Employee wellness programs can focus on the daily choices that employees make about their health and well-being that can also have significant effects on their work life. Programs can provide help and support to employees and their family members and challenge them to maintain a culture of prevention. Finally, sustaining health promotion programs in a medical care setting requires building the credibility of programs through evaluation and reporting back to stakeholders. Frequent and varied program communication and program materials targeted both to health care organization employees who are program participants and to program staff need to be an ongoing part of program operations.

## CAREER OPPORTUNITIES IN HEALTH CARE ORGANIZATIONS

Career opportunities in health promotion reflect the diversity of programs and services that have been developed over the last twenty-five years in health care organizations. The traditional places for careers and employment in the health care field are hospitals, clinics, and home health agencies, and these venues continue to provide career options. An increasing number of health care organizations now offer varied pathways to a career in health promotion. At the same time, career connections and opportunities in a number of other organizations and fields related to health and medicine are now more plentiful and available. Workers in health promotion programs include physicians, nurses, health educators, counselors, and psychologists as well as individuals trained in the allied health professions who have developed expertise and have the experience and interest to pursue positions in the field. Job titles for such positions include health educator, patient educator, or health promotion specialist, but also dietitian, tobacco educator, family educator, patient relations coordinator, program specialist, or public health officer, among many others.

Following are brief descriptions of organizations that offer opportunities for health promotion careers:

- **Hospitals, clinics, and home health care agencies**. Traditional settings for medical care services often emphasize patient education, medical decision making, staff health promotion, and programs on sustaining a high quality of life. In addition, educators may be called on to work with facilities planners to develop a healing environment or a learning environment for a facility.

- **Consumer groups and interest groups**. Interest groups are voluntary associations with specific and narrowly defined goals. Probably the most common among the health-related interest groups are those focused on a particular health condition, such as the American Cancer Society, the American Diabetes Association, and the American Heart Association. All these groups have large health promotion program operations that work at both the national and local levels. Likewise, professional and trade associations work as interest groups, as do activist groups like those in the ecology movement. Some interest groups may represent one segment of the public (such as retired people or students), or they may represent a value (for example, they may be pro-choice), at which point they shade into ideological or moral crusades.

- **U.S. government**. The U.S. government offers numerous career opportunities for health education specialists, from entry-level to senior positions. The Department of Health and Human Services, as would be expected, employs many health educators both at its headquarters in Washington, D.C., and throughout the nation in state and regional offices. Operating divisions such as the Centers for Medicare and Medicaid Services, the National Institutes of Health, the Centers for Disease Control and Prevention, the Administration on Aging, the Agency for Healthcare Research and Quality, and the Food and Drug Administration have relied on health educators for decades. In addition, the Department of Defense and the Veterans Administration have well-organized health care systems that employ health educators. Refer to http://www.usajobs.opm.gov for specific job announcements.

- **Medical technology units or companies**. Medical technology is the diagnostic or therapeutic application of science and technology to improve or manage health conditions. Technologies can encompass any means of identifying the nature of health conditions in order to allow intervention with devices or with pharmacological, biological, or other methods for the purpose of increasing life span or improving quality of life. All of these units and companies use Web sites to provide information, feedback, personal coaching, and support of people's health promotion activities related to a particular medical condition.

- **Professional associations in medicine and health**. A professional association is an organization, usually nonprofit, whose purpose is to further a particular profession and to protect both the public interest and the interests of the professionals. Almost all health and medical professions have associations. Many are involved in development and monitoring of professional education programs, updating of professional skills, and professional certification. Many are committed to the health and well-being of their members and therefore offer health promotion services and programs. Health promotion organizations in medical care settings include the American Public Health Association's Public Health Education and Health Promotion Section (www .apha.org/membergroups/sections/aphasections/phehp); the Cancer Patient Education Network (www.cancerpatienteducation.org); the Health Care Education Association (http://www.hcea-info.org); the American Academy of Family Practitioners (http://www.aafp.org/online/en/home.html); and the Society for Public Health Education (www.sophe.org).

- **Publishers of educational materials for patients and family members**. Information—whether print, multimedia, or electronic—is at the core of health promotion programs. Education and health publishers recruit staff members with knowledge and expertise in health.

- **Health insurance or managed care organizations**. The insurance industry provides protection against financial losses resulting from medical and health problems. By purchasing insurance policies, individuals and businesses can receive reimbursement for losses due to medical expenses and loss of income due to disability or death. Increasingly, the health insurance industry has embraced health promotion programming as a vehicle for lowering health risks and medical care costs. Many health insurance benefit packages include health promotion programs and opportunities. Often companies will provide incentives for their employees to participate in such activities, as a strategy to lower overall health insurance costs. Many opportunities are available for health promotion professionals to work with health insurance companies in the planning, implementation, and evaluation of employee health promotion programs.

- **Health and medical career education programs**. Colleges, universities, and training programs prepare and train people to work in health care organizations. Universities have schools of medicine, nursing, public health, and allied health, as well as programs in school health, community health, health education, and health promotion. Many other institutions prepare individuals to work as medical assistants and medical support staff. Careers as professors and instructors in these institutions require advanced degrees; however, there are increasing numbers of opportunities for individuals with health promotion training and experience to work in professional preparation programs.

## SUMMARY

Opportunities for health promotion programs in health care organizations reflect a recent blending of medicine and public health and the pivotal role of medical care organizations and facilities in the health and well-being of individuals. Today, a range of health promotion programs operate in health care organizations. Health professionals involved in such programs range from physicians, health educators, and nurses to medical social workers and allied health professionals. These programs are focused on patients, patient safety, employee health, workplace safety, and community outreach. Unique to health care organizations are health promotion programs that historically have been patient-focused and associated with patient education to help people make informed medical and health decisions and develop skills needed to participate in their health care. In today's world, individuals are more involved in their own health care decisions. This increased involvement reflects the increase in health promotion programs and in managed care that has resulted in shorter hospital stays in response to pressure for cost containment and has increased demand for outpatient and in-home services.

## FOR PRACTICE AND DISCUSSION

1. Visit a doctor's office, a community health clinic, or a local hospital. Examine the health promotion materials and information (for example, brochures, posters, handouts, videos, Internet services) that are available for patients. Which are most helpful? What materials and information are missing that you believe are needed?
2. Think about the ways in which technology is currently being used to promote health to consumers and staff in health care organizations. Using your cell phone as a technology platform, describe how you might create a new service to promote the health of the consumers and staff of health care organizations.
3. Discuss strategies that you think might work to increase the voice of consumers in patient-focused health promotion programs at a large urban outpatient clinic.
4. Hospitals and medical clinics are often perceived as places of pain and suffering. In particular, children are often afraid of getting shots, even if the shots will help them, because the shots hurt (a perceived negative consequence and barrier to participation). Design a health promotion program that could be used in a health care organization to address this negative perception that children have about medical care.

5. A hospital is advertising a new job, seeking an individual to plan, implement, and evaluate patient-focused health promotion programs. Prepare a list of interview questions that the hospital's human resource director could use to evaluate the job candidates.

## KEY TERMS

Commitment to quality performance, improvement, and evaluation

Community outreach

Evidence-based practices

Health promotion programs

Interdisciplinary, collaborative approach

Medical decision making

Patient and family education

Patient- and family-centered care

Patient safety

Privacy of patient health information

Regulations, restrictions, and guidelines

## REFERENCES

Agency for Healthcare Research and Quality. (2008). *U.S. Preventive Services Task Force*. Retrieved January 22, 2008, from http://www.ahrq.gov/clinic/uspstfix.htm.

American Academy of Family Practice. (2009). *Patient-centered medical home*. Retrieved November 1, 2009, from http://www.aafp.org/online/en/home/membership/initiatives/pcmh.html.

American Diabetes Association. (2009). *Clinical practice recommendations*. Retrieved November 1, 2009, from http://professional.diabetes.org/CPR_search.aspx.

American Hospital Association. (2008). *American Hospital Association*. Retrieved October 24, 2008, from http://www.aha.org/aha_app/index.jsp.

Barry, M., Mulley, A., Fowler, F., & Wennberg, J. (1988). Watchful waiting vs. immediate transurethral resection for symptomatic prostatism. *Journal of the American Medical Association, 259*, 3010–3017.

Breckon, J., Harvey, J. R., & Lancaster, R. B. (1998). *Community health education: Settings, roles, and skills for the 21st century*. Gaithersburg, MD: Aspen.

Cancer Patient Education Network. (2002). *Guidelines for establishing comprehensive cancer patient education services*. Retrieved August 21, 2008, from http://www.cancerpatienteducation.org/resources.cfm?action=viewCategory&section=1&category=13.

Center for the Advancement of Collaborative Strategies in Health. (2004). *Pathways to collaboration: A knowledge building workgroup*. Retrieved August 21, 2008, from http://www.pathwaystocollaboration.net/index.html.

Davenport-Ennis, N., Cover, M. T., Ades, T. B., & Stovall, E. (2002). An analysis of advocacy: A collaborative essay. *Seminars in Oncology Nursing, 18*(4), 290–296.

Giloth, B. E. (1990). Promoting patient involvement: Educational, organizational and environmental strategies. *Patient Education and Counseling, 15*, 29–38.

Holmes-Rovner, M., Nelson, W. L., Pignone, M., Elwyn, G., Rovner, D. R., O'Connor, A. M., et al. (2007). Are patient decision aids the best way to improve clinical decision making? Report of the IPDAS symposium. *Medical Decision Making, 27*, 599.

Indian Health Service. (2008). *Patient and family education protocols and codes* (14th ed.). Retrieved November 1, 2009, from http://www.ihs.gov/nonmedicalprograms/healthed/index.cfm?module=initiative&option=protocols&newquery=dsp_NatlPatientEd_Protocols.cfm.

Institute for Family-Centered Care. (2008a). *FAQ.* Retrieved February 28, 2008, from http://www.familycenteredcare.org/faq.html.

Institute for Family-Centered Care. (2008b). *Partnering with patients and families to design a patient and family-centered health care system: Recommendations and promising practices.* Retrieved November 1, 2009, from http://www.familycenteredcare.org/tools/downloads.html.

Institute for Healthcare Improvement. (n.d. a). *Protecting 5 million lives from harm: Some is not a number; soon is not a time.* Retrieved August 21, 2008, from http://www.ihi.org/IHI/Programs/Campaign/Campaign.htm?TabId=1.

Institute for Healthcare Improvement. (n.d. b). *The Triple Aim.* Retrieved August 21, 2008, from http://www.ihi.org/IHI/Programs/StrategicInitiatives/TripleAim.htm.

Institute of Medicine, Committee on Quality of Health Care in America. (2001). *Crossing the quality chasm: A new health system for the 21st century.* Washington, DC: National Academies Press.

Johnson, J. (2000). The health care institution as a setting for health promotion. In B. D. Poland, L. Green, & I. Rootman (Eds.), *Settings for health promotion: Linking theory and practice* (pp. 175–216). Thousand Oaks, CA: Sage.

Joint Commission. (2008). *Joint Commission.* Retrieved October 24, 2008, from http://www.jointcommission.org.

Joint Commission. (2009). *Joint Commission: 2010 accreditation requirements.* Retrieved November 1, 2009, from www.jointcommission.org/Standards.

Kohn, K., Corrigan, J., & Donaldson, M. (2000). *To err is human: Building a safer health system.* Washington, DC: National Academies Press.

Lasker, R. D. (1997). *Medicine and public health: The power of collaboration.* New York: New York Academy of Medicine.

Mason, D. (2001). Promoting health literacy: Patient teaching as a vital nurse function. *American Journal of Nursing, 101*(2), 7.

Mullen, P. D., & Green, L. W. (1985). Educating patients about drugs. *Promoting Health, 6*, 6–8.

Mullen, P. D., & Green, L. W. (1990). Educating and counseling for prevention: From theory and research to principles. In R. B. Goldbloom & R. S. Lawrence (Eds.), *Preventing disease: Beyond the rhetoric* (pp. 474–479). New York: Springer-Verlag.

Mumford, E., Hynes, M., & Carter, R. (1988). Meta-analysis of the effects of education and psychosocial interventions on management of diabetes mellitus. *Journal of Clinical Epidemiology, 41*(10), 1007–1030.

National Academy of Sciences. (2006). *Crossing the quality chasm: The IOM health care quality initiative.* Retrieved November 1, 2009, from http://www.iom.edu/About-IOM.aspx.

National Action Plan on Breast Cancer. (2000). [Home page.] Retrieved March 1, 2008, from http://www.4woman.gov/napbc.

National Patient Safety Foundation. (2008). *National Patient Safety Foundation.* Retrieved October 24, 2008, from http://www.npsf.org.

O'Connor, A., Rostom, A., Fiset, V., Tetroe, J., Llewellyn-Thomas, H., Entwistle, V., et al. (1999). Decision aids for patients facing health treatment or screening decisions: Systematic review. *BMJ, 319,* 731–734.

Padgett, D., Mumford, E., Hynes, M., & Carter, R. (1988). Meta-analysis of the effects of education and psychosocial interventions on management of diabetes mellitus. *Journal of Clinical Epidemiology, 41*(10), 1007–1030.

Smith, C. E. (1989). Overview of patient education: Opportunities and challenges for the twenty-first century. *Nursing Clinics of North America, 24*(3), 583–587.

Squyres, W. (1982). The professional health educator in HMOs: Implications for training and our future in medical care. *Health Education Quarterly, 9*(1), 74–77.

# CHAPTER FOURTEEN

# HEALTH PROMOTION PROGRAMS IN WORKPLACE SETTINGS

LAURA LINNAN

KIMBERLY L. PEABODY

JENNIFER WIELAND

## LEARNING OBJECTIVES

■ Discuss the health and non-health benefits to staff and administration of offering health promotion programs and services at the workplace

■ Describe the history of workplace health promotion, highlighting seminal events and figures over the past three decades

■ Discuss the challenges and opportunities of offering health education programs and services in the workplace, given new technology and shifting demographics

■ Describe current tools, resources, and approaches for effective workplace health promotion programs

■ Describe administrative, clinical, and programming careers in workplace health promotion

The authors acknowledge Garry Lindsay and Jennifer Childress for their support in the preparation of this chapter.

Mᴏʀᴇ ᴛʜᴀɴ 60 ᴘᴇʀᴄᴇɴᴛ of U.S. adults over age eighteen are employed, and they spend a majority of their waking hours at work (Bureau of Labor Statistics, 2008a). Thus the workplace is an important place to reach the U.S. adult population with health information and services. Workplace programs often run concurrently or are complementary with other health promotion programs. For example, one component of a coordinated school health program is health promotion for staff (Exhibit 14.1). Likewise, workplace programs are operated by federal, state, and local governments for their employees. And health care organizations and community health organizations as well as local health departments operate workplace programs for their employees while these organizations are involved in delivery of health promotion programs for the populations they serve (for example, hospitals may offer patient-focused as well as employee health promotion programs).

The workplace environment exerts an independent influence on the health of employees as well. Specifically, the physical and social environment at work; the pace of work; and exposures to noise, chemicals, repetitive movement, hazardous conditions, harassment, or abuse represent realities of work-related experiences that influence employee health. When work conditions promote health and include opportunities to access health-related information or services, screening tests, and resources, employees are more productive and are better positioned to achieve and maintain positive health outcomes and high quality of life. For these reasons, health promotion in the workplace represents a clear public health priority.

## WORKPLACE HEALTH PROMOTION—1970 TO THE PRESENT

Most historical reviews of health promotion efforts at work sites in the United States begin in the 1970s, when a handful of employers developed executive fitness programs to keep their top management team fit for duty (Reardon, 1998). Attempts to avoid premature death of key executives and the use of fitness programs as a company perk to help recruit and retain top executives were the impetus for these programs. As evidence grew of the positive health outcomes experienced by executives and the related cost benefits to the company's bottom line, health promotion programs were expanded beyond fitness programming to general wellness and were offered to the entire workforce.

Concurrent with the fitness-to-wellness shift of the mid-1980s was a programmatic evolution from a treatment focus to a prevention focus. Executive fitness programs typically included a physical examination in order to identify leaders who were at high risk for cardiovascular disease—the leading cause of premature death (Murray & Lopez, 1996)—so that they could be referred into intensive treatment programs that focused on physical activity and diet. As a broader shift toward disease prevention as the recognized priority occurred, workplace health promotion interventions changed as well (Reardon, 1998). It was not practical or affordable to offer complete physicals and personal trainers for the entire work-force at a work site. Moreover, multi-session, clinic-oriented treatment programs for high blood pressure, high blood cholesterol, smoking cessation, and weight loss were staff-intensive and required too much time away from work, so certain groups of employees remained unable to participate. Employers and those who provided services to employers (including voluntary health agencies, private vendors, and health insurers) began to develop minimal-intensity interventions that were less costly to create and deliver yet attracted larger numbers of employees and were more practical for implementation throughout a work site (Reardon, 1998). For example, intensive, multi-session classes on smoking cessation were replaced with self-help or other Web-based cessation programs, clean air campaigns to reduce exposure to smoke, and contests to motivate individuals to quit smoking with minimal help. Delivery and evaluation of minimal-intensity, prevention- and treatment-oriented intervention programs began in the 1990s and is likely to continue as employers attempt to make the best use of the time, resources, and expertise invested and to reach the largest number of employees with effective (and cost-effective) health promotion programs.

The early 1990s represented a time of unprecedented growth for work site health promotion on the national scene; even as the U.S. economy stagnated, research on work site health promotion programs was funded at greater levels (Stokols, Pelletier, and Fielding, 1996). During this time period, the link between employee health and organizational health gained increased attention as employers realized that the social and physical environment of a work site and work-related policies have both direct and indirect influences on employee health. For example, employers learned that creating a smoke-free work environment (through a policy change) not only increased the number of attempts to quit and actual cessation rates among smokers but saved them cleaning and insurance costs as well. Discounting low-fat food choices in vending machines, making healthier food options available in the cafeteria, and developing nutrition education programs also created a work environment in which employees were more aware of and more likely to make healthy food choices.

As work site health promotion moves into the twenty-first century, two trends are noteworthy. First, the focus on organizational health has been maintained and extended to include a re-integration of employee health protection with employee health promotion efforts (Sorensen & Barbeau, 2006). Originally, labor unions helped secure safe work conditions and health insurance coverage for workers, yet over time, worker safety and health promotion have mostly operated on separate tracks (Sorensen & Barbeau, 2006). Health promotion experts focused on encouraging employees to make lifestyle or behavioral changes, while health protection experts addressed employee health by creating safe work conditions and limiting

## EXHIBIT 14.1
## Workplace Health Promotion at Lincoln Industries: Go! Platinum Program

**Location**: Lincoln, Nebraska
**Type of industry**: Manufacturing
**Number of employees**: 450
**Company belief statement**: "Wellness and healthy lifestyles are important to our success."
**Program vision**: "Lincoln Industries Wellness encompasses the body, mind, and spirit. We support our people in making smarter, healthier lifestyle choices. We encourage balance between work, home, and personal goals. We believe that supporting our people's health and wellness interests is a sound investment in our company, and the most important asset of the company is the people."

### Comprehensive Program Components

*Health Interventions*

- Free on-site, on-the-clock tobacco cessation and weight management interventions for employees and their family members
- More than ten major health interventions

*Supportive Social and Physical Environment*

- Tobacco-free campus
- Wellness mentors
- Recognition of wellness (incentives include free trip to Colorado to climb 14,000-foot mountain)

hazardous exposures. However, the National Institute for Occupational Safety and Health recently sponsored a series of national meetings to facilitate the re-integration of safety and health promotion as a means of promoting worker health (National Institute for Occupational Safety and Health, 2008b).

A second recent trend is the increasing demand for greater accountability for the effects of work site health promotion and health protection efforts (Stokols, Pelletier, & Fielding, 1996). Specifically, identifying ways to maximize employer investment in employee health has taken center stage. Productivity, absenteeism, and job performance are increasingly monitored in addition to health and safety outcomes. Being specific about the return on investment and cost-effectiveness of intervention efforts is becoming an essential component of work site health promotion and evaluation efforts.

To support the efforts of employers, the U.S. Chamber of Commerce and Partnership for Prevention have united to share employers' success stories about

*Linkage to Related Programs*

- Health reimbursement account with credits for being tobacco-free
- Wellness presented in concert with all other company benefits and business strategies at the onset of employment

*Integration of Health Program into Organizational Structures*

- Wellness objectives, set by all employees, tied to overall performance and pay
- Departmental wellness champions
- Company-sponsored wellness events
- Wellness integrated into Lincoln's strategic plan, business initiatives, and employee development

*Work Site Screening Programs*

- Mandatory quarterly health screenings and individual coaching

*Results*

- Go! Platinum received the top national wellness program award in 2003 and 2006.
- Health care costs are 50 percent below national average.
- Workers compensation costs average less than 1 percent of payroll.

**CEO statement**: "Too often, companies look at wellness as just another benefit. We have fully integrated wellness into every aspect of our company's culture. It's a source of pride and reflects how we care for one another. As a result, wellness has become a critical element of our success."

improving the health and productivity of their workforce. *Leading by Example: Leading Practices for Employee Health Management* provides examples and strategies for improving employee health from employers of every size (U.S. Chamber of Commerce & Partnership for Prevention, 2007). In addition, the U.S. Department of Health and Human Services created the Innovation in Prevention Award, which showcases creative initiatives by organizations that have implemented effective health promotion programs in prevention of chronic disease.

One such organization is Lincoln Industries, a midsize manufacturing company, which was recognized in *Leading by Example* and was an Innovation in Prevention Award recipient for its efforts in promoting healthy lifestyles in its community (Partnership for Prevention, 2005). Exhibit 14.1 provides a case example of Lincoln Industries, identifying its remarkable achievements in creating a culture of wellness and health.

## RESOURCES AND TOOLS

An increasing number of resources are available to help those who wish to plan, implement, and evaluate health promotion programs at work sites. Most of these resources have been developed in the last twenty-five years in order to address a wide range of health issues and problems.

### Wellness Council of America

The Wellness Council of America (www.welcoa.org) was established as a national nonprofit organization in the mid-1980s through the efforts of a number of forward-thinking business and health leaders and has since helped influence the face of workplace wellness in the United States (Wellness Council of America, 2008). With membership in excess of 3,200 organizations, the Wellness Council of America is dedicated to improving the health and well-being of all working Americans. The company's mission is to serve business leaders, workplace wellness practitioners, public health professionals, and consultants of all kinds by promoting corporate membership, producing leading-edge work site wellness publications and health information, conducting training sessions that help work site wellness practitioners create and sustain results-oriented wellness programs, and creating resources that promote healthier lifestyles for all working Americans.

### Healthier Worksite Initiative

In 2002, the Centers for Disease Control and Prevention (CDC) developed the Healthier Worksite Initiative (HWI) for its own employees, with the vision of making the CDC a work site where healthy choices are easy choices and sharing the lessons learned with other federal agencies (Centers for Disease Control and Prevention, 2007). In the years since its inception, HWI has worked on a number of demonstration projects, policies, and environmental changes that affect the entire CDC workforce. Lessons learned from these projects, ideas for new and revised policies to enhance health initiatives, and step-by-step instructions for implementing similar programs at other work sites form the basis of the HWI Web site (www.cdc.gov/nccdphp/dnpa/hwi/index.htm). In line with the HWI's mission to serve as a model and resource for other federal work sites, the Web site was developed as a comprehensive one-stop shop for planners of workforce health promotion programs.

## Partnership for Prevention

Partnership for Prevention (www.prevent.org) is a membership organization of businesses, nonprofit organizations, and government agencies that are advancing policies and practices to prevent disease and improve the health of all Americans. The organization seeks to increase investment in disease prevention and health promotion and to make prevention a national priority. Partnership for Prevention programs seek to increase the priority given to prevention in health-related policy and in the U.S. health care system by analyzing leading-edge scientific research in order to identify effective polices and practices that should be adopted to accelerate progress toward better health for all Americans. Partnership for Prevention also convenes diverse health care stakeholders and facilitates dialogue among them in order to assess critical issues, find mutually agreeable solutions, and set priorities for action in the public sector and the private sector. In addition, Partnership for Prevention educates decision makers in every sector about innovative prevention policies and practices, provides analytical tools to aid implementation of health promotion programs, and advocates for the adoption of these approaches (Partnership for Prevention, 2007).

## The Guide to Community Preventive Services

To highlight the importance of work sites in promoting health, the Centers for Disease Control and Prevention (2008) created a task force on community preventive services that focuses on work site health promotion as a topic for systematic review. The systematic reviews on various aspects of work site health promotion are intended to give employers and organizations an evidence base to help them determine which available approaches are effective in promoting healthy lifestyles, preventing disease, and increasing the number of people who receive appropriate preventive counseling and screening. These reviews will provide recommendations on workplace-specific policies and activities in order to help employers choose health promotion program components that have proven effective in changing the behavior and improving the health of employees. Topics to be addressed include interventions at the work site (for example, offering on-site health education classes or posting signs to encourage stair use), interventions that are made available to employees at other locations (for example, reducing out-of-pocket costs for gym memberships or flu shots), and interventions that are incorporated into employees' benefits plans (for example, providing vouchers for nicotine patches or exercise classes). Several of the reviews are nearly completed: incentives and competitions to increase smoking cessation; smoke-free policies to reduce tobacco use; point-of-decision prompts to increase stair use; and assessment of health risk with feedback. When completed, the results of these reviews will be made available on the Community Guide Web site (www .thecommunityguide.org/worksite).

## Guide to Developing a Workplace Injury and Illness Prevention Program with Checklists for Self-Inspection

The California Occupational Safety and Health Administration created the *Guide to Developing a Workplace Injury and Illness Prevention Program with Checklists for Self-Inspection* (State of California, 2005). This online manual is designed to help employers provide better workplace protection for their employees and to reduce losses resulting from accidents and injuries. The material on the site is based on principles and techniques that have been developed by occupational safety and health professionals nationwide. Necessary elements in implementing an injury and illness prevention program include

- Management commitment and assignment of responsibilities
- System for communicating with employees about safety
- System for ensuring employee compliance with safe work practices
- Scheduled inspections and an evaluation system
- Accident investigation
- Procedures for correcting unsafe or unhealthy conditions
- Safety and health training and instruction
- Record keeping and documentation

## Making Your Workplace Drug Free

At work sites across the country, employers are looking for practical ways to address alcohol and other drug abuse. Employers also are concerned about meeting the health needs of their employees and controlling the costs of health care and workers compensation. Most important, employers are asking for clear, simple steps for planning effective drug-free workplace programs. *Making Your Workplace Drug Free: A Kit for Employers* offers guidance, specific strategies, and easy-to-follow steps for creating a drug-free workplace program or for enhancing an existing one (U.S. Department of Health and Human Services, Public Health Service, Substance Abuse and Mental Health Services Administration, Center for Substance Abuse Prevention, n.d.). It was designed for owners and managers in businesses of all sizes, but especially in smaller businesses. The kit suggests low-cost approaches for a health program geared toward preventing alcohol and other drug abuse. The kit should be especially helpful for employers who don't have much time to develop a program. They will find what many employers have said they need: immediate, practical answers and easy-to-use materials. The advice and issues addressed in this kit came from employers who already have successful programs for creating a drug-free workplace, as well as from employers who would like to start one. Line staff and supervisors also contributed to the development of the kit.

## Employee Health Services Handbook

The U.S. federal government promotes and supports health promotion and disease prevention activities for its employees. Agencies are encouraged to adopt health policies and programs that reduce the risk of premature morbidity, mortality, and disability; foster healthy lifestyles; and support a healthy working environment. Work sites are effective and convenient places for employees to receive employee health education and services. In the federal government, these programs are now widely established and are well accepted as a valuable resource for enhancing workforce effectiveness. The U.S. Office of Personnel Management, in cooperation with the Department of Health and Human Services, provides policy and guidance on federal civilian employee health and assistance programs. The *Employee Health Services Handbook* (U.S. Office of Personnel Management, n.d.) provides policy guidance to assist agency managers and program administrators in developing and administering comprehensive employee health services programs. The handbook uses a question-and-answer format to address the most common administrative issues, divided into the following areas: administering employee health programs; providing physical fitness programs; administering employee assistance programs; federal program resources; and a list of employee health resources available on the Internet.

## Essential Elements of Effective Workplace Programs and Policies for Improving Worker Health and Wellbeing

*Essential Elements of Effective Workplace Programs and Policies for Improving Worker Health and Wellbeing* is a resource document developed in 2008 by the National Institute for Occupational Safety and Health (NIOSH) (2008a) with substantial input from experts and interested individuals. The National Institute for Occupational Safety and Health is the federal agency responsible for conducting research and making recommendations for the prevention of work-related injury and illness.

This document, a key part of the NIOSH WorkLife Initiative, is intended as a guide for employers and employer-employee partnerships wishing to establish effective workplace programs that sustain and improve worker health. The *Essential Elements* document identifies twenty components of a comprehensive work-based health protection and health promotion program and includes both guiding principles and practical direction for organizations seeking to develop effective workplace programs.

The WorkLife Initiative is intended to identify and support comprehensive approaches to reduce workplace hazards and promote worker health and well-being. The premise of this initiative, based on scientific research and practical experience in the field, is that comprehensive practices and policies that take into account the work environment—both physical and organizational—while also addressing the personal health risks of individuals, are more effective in preventing disease and promoting health and safety than is each approach taken separately.

## The Canadian Healthy Workplace Council

The Canadian Healthy Workplace Council (www.healthyworkplacemonth.ca/home) consists of a number of leading Canadian practitioners and organizations whose members are dedicated to promoting a comprehensive and integrated approach to workplace health in order to improve and sustain the health of Canadian organizations, their work environments, and their employees.

The council works to accomplish its mission through

- Advocating nationally, provincially, and locally for healthy workplaces through members' speeches and articles, involvement in local workplace health networks, and other related activities
- Serving in an advisory capacity to various organizations on workplace health issues
- Adjudicating the Canadian Workplace Wellness Pioneer Award that is presented annually at the Health, Work & Wellness Conference

The council recently released a call to action for stakeholders from across the spectrum of workplace health. Recognizing that a critical mass of governments, organizations, and workplace health practitioners are pursuing healthy workplace goals, the council believes the time is right for a *coordinated action agenda to create healthy workplaces*. The goals are a more integrated public policy and wider diffusion of best practices in workplaces.

The council invites stakeholders to consider, discuss, and provide feedback on the following approach to developing a coordinated healthy workplace action agenda:

- Create a shared vision of a healthy, safe, and productive workplace that achieves individual, organizational, and societal goals and that is accepted by all stakeholders.
- Enable stakeholders from all levels of government, employers, unions, professional associations, researchers, and nongovernmental organizations (NGOs)

to share information, identify priority actions, and implement these actions in the most effective manner possible.

• Identify opportunities for a more horizontal approach to public policy across jurisdictions, levels of government, and policy areas to achieve healthy workplace goals.

## CHALLENGES

Over the past three decades, evidence has shown that work site health promotion programs can improve employee health behaviors and health status; increase morale, job satisfaction, and quality of life; and improve productivity (Chapman-Walsh, Jennings, Mangione, & Merrigan, 1991; Stokols, Pelletier, & Fielding, 1996; DeJoy & Southern, 1993). Thus, employers have many important reasons to consider offering these programs. In addition to embracing opportunities to improve their own health and safety, employees indicate that they are motivated to participate in work site wellness programs when they are involved in identifying health problems and in planning or developing programs to address their needs and interests (Gates, Brehm, Hutton, Singler, & Poeppelman, 2006; Lassen, Bruselius-Jensen, Somer, Thorsen, & Trolle, 2007; Rasmussen et al., 2006; Hunt et al., 2007) Employees report that they favor the use of e-mail and Web-based interventions to make participation easier and more convenient (Franklin, Rosenbaum, Carey, & Roizen, 2006) and that they are more likely to participate in a program that includes personal coaching, tailored interventions, or incentives (Denelsbeck, 2006).

Health promotion programs developed at work sites have taken an approach similar to that of health promotion programs developed at schools (Chapter Twelve), which provide a range of services, have an ecological health perspective, and forge collaborations. Typically a comprehensive work site health promotion program consists of (1) health education programs, (2) a supportive social and physical environment, (3) linkage to related programs such as employee assistance programs, (4) integration of health promotion into the organizational structure of the work site, and (5) health screening and appropriate follow-up services. The Lincoln Industries program shown in Exhibit 14.1 exemplifies a comprehensive work site health promotion program, and more examples of work sites that have developed and implemented such programs can be obtained from Partnership for Prevention (www.prevent.org). Healthy People 2020 objectives for the nation aim to increase to at least 75 percent the number of employers who offer a comprehensive work site health promotion program.

Although many reasons motivate employers and employees to support work site health promotion programs, it is useful to understand the key challenges or barriers to offering these programs, especially given the fact that few employers offer a comprehensive work site health promotion program. According to the results of the 2004 National Worksite Health Promotion Survey, only 6.9 percent of employers offer a comprehensive program and small work sites are significantly less likely to offer their employees any type of health promotion program, service, policy, or environmental support (Linnan et al., 2008). The most common barriers or challenges to offering health promotion programs reported by employers of all sizes and industry types were lack of interest among employees, lack of staff resources, lack of funding, and lack of management support (Linnan et al., 2008). Few differences by work site size were apparent, but larger employers also cited concerns about lack of participation among high-risk employees.

Even when work site health promotion programs are offered, employees often face challenges to participating in such programs. First, not all employees have equal access to programs at work. Grosch, Alterman, Petersen, and Murphy (1998) found that laborers, men, and minorities report less access to health promotion programs at work; however, when access to programming is equal, these same groups of workers report the highest levels of participation. Concerns about lack of privacy at work, negative peer pressure, competing work or time demands, or lack of support from an immediate supervisor are typical reasons why employees do not participate in health promotion programs at their work site. These challenges can be anticipated and addressed when health promotion is supported by all levels of management (Linnan, Weiner, Graham, & Emmons, 2007) and when programs are developed through a systematic planning process.

When designing, implementing, and evaluating a work site health promotion program, it is necessary to ensure that the program is evidence-based and tailored to the particular workplace and its employees. Work conditions can be toxic and may be detrimental to employee health. Integrating work site health programs into the organizational structure and culture of a workplace makes adoption and long-term sustainability of health promotion programs more likely and contributes directly to a healthier and more productive workforce.

While striving to offer comprehensive work site health promotion programs, it is also important to be aware of changes in the national social and political scene that influence the extent to which work site health promotion programs are offered: changes in the demographic characteristics of the workforce, changes in the nature of work, and changes in the health care environment.

There are several important demographic changes to consider. First, the U.S. population is aging. By 2050, one in five Americans will be over the age of sixty-five (Toossi, 2002). This trend has important implications, as some of these older Americans will remain in the workforce past the traditional retirement age. It is important to consider who these older workers will be, how long they will continue to work, and whether enough young workers are joining the workforce to replace those who do leave. Second, women continue to outnumber men in the U.S. population. By 2050, women will outnumber men by 6.9 million (compared with 5.3 million in 2000) (Toossi, 2002). In addition, the percentages of working women overall and of working women with children are increasing (Juhn & Potter, 2006). Perhaps the most dramatic population-based changes involve an increase in the prevalence of nonwhite workers. In 2000, non-Hispanic whites represented 69.4 percent of the population, whereas projections for 2050 indicate that whites will represent just 50.1 percent of the population (Toossi, 2002). Moreover, both the Hispanic and Asian American populations are expected to triple by 2050. The largest source of new workers in the United States is expected to be Hispanic workers; this portion of the labor force may grow as much as 33 percent in the decade from 2002 to 2012, compared with just 9 percent growth for all other workers combined (see Figure 14.1) (Bureau of Labor Statistics, 2004).

What do these demographic shifts mean for health promotion efforts at work sites? Employers will be called on to develop promotions and services that are culturally and programmatically appropriate for a diverse set of workers. For example, an aging workforce may require programs and services to prevent or treat arthritis or other chronic health conditions that are more prevalent in older workers. The changing labor force will dictate the need for tailored programs and services for a variety of demographic subgroups.

**FIGURE 14.1    Projected Percentage Growth in U.S. Labor Force from 2002 to 2012, by Ethnic Origin**

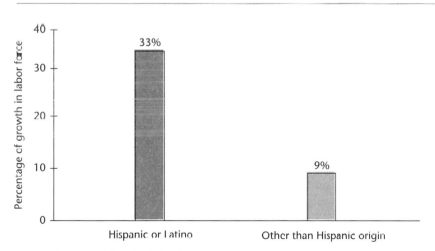

*Source*: Bureau of Labor Statistics, 2004.

A second important trend that will affect work site health promotion programs is the changing nature of work. Work in the United States has changed from primarily farming, manufacturing, or production work to service-oriented work. For example, nearly 40 percent of the workforce in 1900 were in farm-related jobs, while less than 3 percent of workers were in farm-related jobs in 1995 (National Research Council, 1999). Moreover, one in six workers is currently employed in service occupations (National Research Council, 1999). Advances in technology have contributed to these changes, and technological advances will continue to create demands for different types of workers with different skills (National Research Council, 1999). For example, some service industry work requires low levels of education or skills, while the technology industry typically requires much higher or more specific skill sets. As U.S. companies are transformed by technologically demanding tasks, it is likely that an increasing number of employees will work part of the day from home or locations away from traditional workplace settings.

How will these changes in the nature of work affect health promotion efforts at work sites? Health promotion programs and services will need to target workers at nontraditional work sites, with adaptations for workers who are not based in a single organizational setting or who have less direct contact with their co-workers. For example, "work site" health promotion programs may need to be delivered as Web-based programs, via cell phone, or through other types of personal data or communication devices.

A third important trend in the larger social context that influences work site health promotion is the changing health care environment. Health care is becoming increasingly expensive, and in 2006, the annual premium that a health insurer charged an employer for a health plan covering a family of four averaged $11,500 (National Coalition on Health Care, 2008). The average health insurance premium increase is outpacing wage and earnings increases (Kaiser Family Foundation, 2007); for example, wages and salaries increased by 39 percent between 1996 and 2005, yet employers' health insurance costs rose 97 percent (California HealthCare Foundation, 2007). Furthermore, employer-sponsored health insurance in the United States is eroding. In 2005, 60 percent of all employees were offered health benefits, down from 69 percent in 2000, and small employers were less likely than large employers to offer their employees health benefits (Linnan & Birken, 2006). Low-wage, minority workers (especially Latinos) and workers employed in small firms are significantly less likely to have employee benefits and are most likely to be uninsured (Fronstin, 2006). Finally, employees in the growing service sector are less likely than employees in manufacturing or public sector jobs to have health benefits (Stanton & Rutherford, 2004).

What do these changes in the health care environment mean for those who are developing comprehensive work site health promotion programs? First, the results of the 2004 National Worksite Health Promotion Survey indicate that many employers rely on their health insurers to provide the health promotion and disease management programs that are offered to their employees (Linnan et al., 2008). Because fewer employers overall are offering health insurance benefits—and because other workers may be underinsured with policies that require high co-payments or deductibles—efforts are needed to prevent a further drop in the number and variety of health promotion programs offered. Second, it is clear that small businesses will require special consideration. The majority of U.S. workers are employed in small businesses, and few small businesses offer either health promotion programs or health insurance benefits for their employees (Linnan & Birken, 2006). Thus large groups of workers are uninsured and lack access to health promotion programs, services, or policies at work. This lack of access to health insurance and health programs represents a public health challenge that must be addressed.

Despite the larger social, political, and economic realities that represent challenges to offering work site health promotion programs, there are several important opportunities to explore ways of expanding work site programs and activities. First, it is critically important to continue to conduct national employer surveys in order to monitor the status of work site health promotion offerings (and their change over time). Second, it would be extremely useful to add a parallel survey of employees, using a nationally representative sample of workers, to investigate access barriers and participation in work site health promotion programs among all types of workers. Third, investigating case studies of employers who offer successful comprehensive programs is a worthwhile endeavor, particularly if examples from small and medium-size businesses are included, given the challenges currently facing those employers and their employees.

Monitoring changes in the U.S. health care system will be important as well. Due to the high cost of health care and treatment, employers may be priced out of health insurance; therefore, true partnerships with health insurers should be developed, particularly with insurers that provide incentives for prevention programs. If universal health care or health insurance becomes available to all employees, we are hopeful that more health promotion programs, services, and environmental supports will be made available at work sites. Ongoing efforts to integrate safety promotion and health promotion as well as a genuine recognition of the influence of the work environment on employee health are needed. Work pace, work demands, and exposure of employees to violence, harassment, discrimination, noise, repetitive strains, hazards, or chemicals can represent significant work toxins. Ideally, employers would address these potentially harmful environmental conditions; however, in the absence of employer leadership, employee groups or unions typically take up this fight. Employee involvement in wellness committees is needed at a time when union membership has dropped to only 12 percent of U.S. workers (Bureau of Labor Statistics, 2008b).

In addition to changing workforce characteristics, the changing nature of work, and a changing health care environment, there are fundamental challenges to implementing comprehensive work site health promotion programs that should be acknowledged from both employer and employee perspectives. One challenge that employers perceive is a lack of interest among employees, especially high-risk employees, in participating in health promotion programs at work (Linnan et al., 2008). This challenge can be addressed by offering high-quality programming that is accessible to all employees regardless of shift status, income, or job category. When the strategic planning process identifies programming needs and interests and when high-quality programs are delivered with respect for individual privacy, at a convenient time, and at an affordable cost, there is evidence that employees will participate (Gates, Brehm, Hutton, Singler, & Poeppelman, 2006; Lassen, Bruselius-Jensen, Somer, Thorsen, & Trolle, 2007; Rasmussen et al., 2006; Hunt et al., 2007). Understanding who participates in health promotion programs is fundamentally important, and evaluation efforts should collect and report these data.

Sharing initial success stories of wellness programs with employers and employees will help secure ongoing support. Research suggests that some employers, especially small business owners, believe that safety is an important employer responsibility but that health promotion is not as important (Eakin, 1992). Helping key decision makers in organizations understand the fundamental connections between health, chronic disease, productivity, absenteeism, and risk factors is important yet challenging. Even though evidence of the effects, cost-effectiveness, and return on investment associated with health promotion programs is growing, cultivating a prevention-oriented mind-set remains a challenge when competing demands for profitability and productivity are prioritized.

Employees face many challenges that inhibit their full participation in work site health promotion programs. As work pace and work demands increase domestically and globally and as boundaries between work and family are blurred by technology such as cell phones, PDAs, and twenty-four-hour wireless access to the Internet, employees may find it difficult to focus on personal health issues. Moreover, employees may be suspicious or skeptical of health promotion programs that are sponsored by employers. Health educators who are responsible for planning and delivering health promotion programs at work sites should not minimize these concerns but, rather, should address them with a spirit of collaboration and trust building. Wellness committee members can be extremely helpful in the trust-building process. If employees are actively involved in the planning and delivery of health promotion programs, they can encourage full employee participation and serve as program champions. It is also important to share employees' success stories about changing their health behavior (when permission is given to do so). Moreover, as employees witness management-approved changes in health-promoting policies and environmental supports (for example, measured walking trails, new fitness equipment for employees, introduction of a salad bar in the cafeteria), they see evidence that their organization is attempting to create a culture that supports employee health.

To meet the stated challenges, there are many opportunities for health educators to utilize their skills in planning, implementing, and evaluating comprehensive work site health promotion programs. Understanding ecological approaches in which interventions are delivered at multiple levels will be extremely helpful. Traditional group classes and self-help programs must be complemented with policy changes and organizational and environmental supports. Cross-processing of health promotion and safety efforts, along with integration of wellness efforts into the organizational culture of a work site, gives the best chance for effectiveness and long-term sustainability of these programs. As employers and employees become more environmentally conscious, *green* intervention strategies may become more prevalent at work. For example, offering vouchers or incentives for bicycling to work might also promote physical activity. Local farmers may provide healthy, locally grown food products to employees directly or as part of cafeteria offerings. Future work site health and safety programs are likely to become more environmentally and ecologically conscientious, with an eye toward sustainability for both the organization and the planet.

Trained individuals with expertise in planning, developing, implementing, and evaluating health promotion programs at work sites currently come from a variety of fields and specialties, including exercise physiology, health education, public health, health promotion, nutrition, and organizational development. Given that dedicated staff is the single biggest predictor of having a comprehensive work site health promotion program, it may be time to consider specialized training programs for those who want to manage work site programs in health promotion (Peabody & Linnan, 2007).

## CAREER OPPORTUNITIES

Over the past three decades, workplace-based health promotion programs have multiplied (Office of Disease Prevention and Health Promotion, 1999). Thus employers are expected to continue to have a high demand for well-trained health educators who are able to plan, implement, and evaluate comprehensive and effective health promotion programs at work sites. Various career paths are available to someone who is interested in health promotion at work sites. Potential employers for those considering a career in work site health are companies with existing work site wellness programs, insurance companies, for-profit vendors of health promotion programs, government agencies, voluntary health agencies, or research institutions (Peabody & Linnan, 2007).

Obviously, companies that are in the process of establishing work site health programs will be interested in hiring individuals with basic competencies in program planning and evaluation. Managed care organizations or insurance companies such as the Blue Cross and Blue Shield Association, Kaiser Permanente, and United Health Care hire individuals to work on program development and evaluation for their insured clients (or their own employees). Evidence suggests that employers rely heavily on managed care organizations to provide health promotion programs for their employees, a trend that has continued over time (Office of Disease Prevention and Health Promotion, 1992, 1999; Linnan et al., 2008).

Another major employer of work site health professionals is for-profit vendors of health promotion programs, disease management programs, or services such as Weight Watchers at Work or MediFit. Work site health professionals employed by vendors can be involved in program development, sales, customer relations, or evaluation. Government agencies at federal, state, and local levels also employ work site health promotion professionals, usually to conduct work site health promotion programs for their employees or constituents. The National Institutes of Health and the Centers for Disease Control and Prevention both offer wellness programs for their employees.

Voluntary health agencies such as the American Heart Association, American Cancer Society, American Lung Association, and American Red Cross all hire work site health professionals to develop, implement, and evaluate work site health promotion programs. Jobs with these organizations may be at the local, state, regional, or national level. For example, field staff from the American Cancer Society (2006) are hired to implement Active for Life, a work site health promotion program that encourages people to become more physically active in order to reduce their risk of cancer and other chronic diseases. Other voluntary health organizations offer a wide range of workplace-based health promotion programs and provide training programs for those who are interested in offering such programs.

Some health promotion professionals may be more interested in joining a research team that manages or delivers work site health promotion programs. In recent years, funding for workplace-based health promotion research has increased. In 2004, the Centers for Disease Control and Prevention funded twenty workplace-based research projects in twenty-two states in order to build evidence of program effectiveness as well as increase the likelihood that these programs can be disseminated broadly.

The preparation needed to enter a career in work site health promotion can be obtained through various forms of academic training or advanced, specialized training. Health professionals who work in this field may have undergraduate or graduate training in many fields, including nutrition, health education, health promotion, public health, social work, exercise science, and psychology. It can be advantageous to pursue one degree (undergraduate or master's) that provides generalist training (for example, in public health, work site health promotion, or health education) and a second degree that provides content expertise (for example, in dietetics, psychology, sports medicine or athletic training, kinesiology, or exercise physiology) that moves beyond the generalist training. For example, an individual with an undergraduate degree in health education (generalist) and a master's degree in exercise physiology (specialist) broadens her career options in several directions. Pursuing graduate-level training is a highly desirable option if one intends to remain in the field of work site health promotion. Typical degrees to pursue include degrees in health education, business, public administration, public health, exercise physiology, or nutrition. In addition, some colleges and universities offer undergraduate and graduate degree programs in work site health promotion (see, for example, East Carolina University, 2009) or a master's degree with a concentration in work site health and productivity (see, for example, University of Tennessee at Chattanooga, 2009).

## SUMMARY

Workplaces remain an important setting for reaching U.S. adults with health and safety programming and services. Interventions to address worker health must address the concerns of individual employees, interactions between employees and co-workers or supervisors, the physical and social environment at the work site, policies within the workplace, and the larger social context in which workplaces are embedded. In this chapter, we have acknowledged the importance of workplace health promotion and provided direction for developing a comprehensive program. We also discussed how factors in the larger social context, such as changing workforce demographics, the changing nature of work, and a changing health care environment, create challenges and opportunities for promoting worker health and safety in the future. Finally, we offered an overview of ways in which those who are interested can pursue a wide range of career opportunities in work site health promotion.

## FOR PRACTICE AND DISCUSSION

1. List five ways that you would overcome some of the barriers to employee participation that are discussed in the chapter.
2. Small employers are much less likely than large employers to offer any type of work site wellness program. Name three strategies for encouraging small employers to offer health promotion programs for their employees.
3. Think about the growing diversity at most workplaces and the fact that Hispanics are a growing percentage of the U.S. population. Name at least

## EXHIBIT 14.2
## Job Description for the Director of a Corporate Health Promotion Center

The **Corporate Health Promotion Center Director** manages and leads the operations and the programs of the corporate wellness center, including monthly and quarterly budgets; daily operations of the center and full-time and part-time staff; health education, physical activity, nutrition, physical health screening, and behavioral health programs and classes; employee wellness programs and services; and all special events. The director will provide the Corporate Chief Operating Officer and board of directors with regular updates and status reports from the center. She or he will lead the planning, implementation, and evaluation of all new and existing center health promotion programs. Collaborates with the Corporate Medical Director on overseeing employees' pre-employment physicals and drug screenings and on creating a healthy, safe, violence-free, and drug-free work environment. Collaborates with Food Services Director on employee food and nutrition services.

### Position Requirements

- B.S. degree in health promotion, health education, public health, wellness, exercise physiology, allied health, nursing, or related field.
- Master's degree in related field is preferred.
- Eight to ten years of experience in the health and wellness industry; experience in promoting corporate wellness is a must.
- Minimum of five years of experience with supervision and a proven track record of hiring, scheduling, training, evaluation, and other supervisorial duties.
- CHES, CPH, or ACSM (American College of Sports Medicine) credential preferred.
- CPR, AED (automated external defibrillator), and First Aid certifications.
- Experience in budgetary and fiscal management.
- Direct experience in high-quality customer service delivery and development.
- Advanced skills in computer technology.

The director must possess a wide range of professional and personal skills and abilities. The director must understand the basic concepts and workings of a corporate wellness environment.

four challenges that low-wage Hispanic employees might encounter in using a workplace-based fitness center. What strategies might you adopt to overcome these barriers?

4. Debate this question: Should employers have access to employee medical information?

The position calls for a person with a strong background in administration, planning, organization, and supervising, as well as the ability to teach others. The director must be willing and able to explore creative and new approaches in health promotion programming that will aid in achieving budgetary goals.

## Position Responsibilities

1. Manage all operations of the Corporate Health Promotion Center, including but not limited to customer service, employee health needs assessment, corporate health capacity assessment, program development, enrollment, scheduling, communication, corporate wellness initiatives, and staffing to ensure efficient and effective operations and delivery of thriving programs and services.

2. Manage all staffing and training needs of Corporate Health Promotion Center staff, including but not limited to administration, paperwork, use of technology systems, part-time staffing, staff recruitment, staff expectations, staff in-service training sessions, volunteer instructors, staff cultural competence, group exercise scheduling, and user utilization reports.

3. Develop, implement, and evaluate evidence-based programs and class offerings that are current with industry standards and address a diverse population of needs (for example, cultural diversity; different stages of change in regard to health behaviors; and different site locations, job responsibilities, and employee schedules).

4. Provide a cohesive approach to customer service and training that directly affects the end user's commitment and personal growth. Build a culture of corporate health promotion and service delivery that is responsive to employees' health issues and needs.

5. Chair the Corporate Health Promotion Center's advisory committee. Recruit and retain high-quality, culturally diverse internal (employee) and external committee members with health promotion expertise and practical experience.

6. Oversee development and administration of the Corporate Health Promotion Center's budget. Develop and monitor budget in order to meet fiscal objectives.

7. Link the Corporate Health Promotion Center with internal corporate health initiatives through the Human Resources Department and community partnerships and coalitions.

8. Develop and implement the overall strategy for marketing programs and services that are responsive to the needs of employees and their family members, retention goals, and the need to recruit new employees into health programs.

9. Encourage and demonstrate the corporate core values of caring, honesty, respect, and responsibility at all times. Positively take part in all other duties assigned.

5. Review the job description for a work site health promotion program director in Exhibit 14.2. What surprises you about the job? Discuss the requirements and responsibilities of the position. Develop a plan to obtain the necessary education, training, credentials, and experience to meet and exceed the position requirements and feel confident in your ability to get and do the job.

## KEY TERMS

Comprehensive work site
  health promotion

Employee assistance
  programs (EAPs)

Health protection

Health risk appraisal

Policy and environmental
  change

Return on investment

Screening program

Wellness

Wellness committee

## REFERENCES

American Cancer Society. (2006). *Active for Life*. Retrieved, October 26, 2009, from http://www.cancer
  .org/docroot/PED/content/PED_1_5X_Active_For_Life.asp.

Bureau of Labor Statistics. (2004). Labor force. *Occupational Outlook Quarterly*, 42–48.

Bureau of Labor Statistics. (2008a). *The employment situation: January 2008*. Retrieved February 1, 2008,
  from http://www.bls.gov/news.release/empsit.nr0.htm.

Bureau of Labor Statistics. (2008b). *Union members in 2007*. Retrieved January 25, 2008, from http://
  www.bls.gov/news.release/union2.nr0.htm.

California HealthCare Foundation. (2007). *Snapshot: Employer health insurance costs in the United
  States*. Retrieved January 28, 2008, from http://www.chcf.org/documents/insurance/
  EmployerHICostsUS.pdf.

Centers for Disease Control and Prevention. (2007). *About us*. Retrieved August 22, 2008, from http://
  www.cdc.gov/nccdphp/dnpa/hwi/about_us/index.htm.

Centers for Disease Control and Prevention. (2008). *Worksite health promotion*. Retrieved August 22, 2008,
  from www.thecommunityguide.org/worksite.

Chapman-Walsh, D., Jennings, S. E., Mangione, T., & Merrigan, D. M. (1991). Health promotion vs.
  health protection? Employees' perceptions and concerns. *Journal of Public Health Policy*, *12*,
  148–164.

DeJoy, D. M., & Southern, D. J. (1993). An integrative perspective on worksite health promotion.
  *Journal of Medicine*, *35*(12), 1221–1230.

Denelsbeck, S. (2006). Engaging employees in health and wellness: The healthy Pfizer program.
  *American Journal of Managed Care*, *12*(Suppl.), SP40–SP43.

Eakin, J. M. (1992). Leaving it up to the workers: Sociological perspective on the management
  of health and safety in small workplaces. *International Journal of Health Services: Planning,
  Administration, and Evaluation*, *22*(4), 689–704.

East Carolina University. (2009). *The College of Health & Human Performance: Department of Health Education
  and Promotion*. Retrieved October 28, 2009, from http://www.ecu.edu/cs-hhp/hlth/worksite
  .cfm.

Franklin, P. D., Rosenbaum, P. F., Carey, M. P., & Roizen, M. F. (2006). Using sequential e-mail messages to promote health behaviors: Evidence of feasibility and reach in a worksite sample.
  *Journal of Medical Internet Research*, *8*(1), e3.

Fronstin, P. (2006). *Workers' health insurance: Trends, issues, and options to expand coverage*. Retrieved January
  28, 2008, from http://www.cmwf.org/usr_doc/Fronstin_workershltins_908.pdf.

Gates, D., Brehm, B., Hutton, S., Singler, M., & Poeppelman, A. (2006). Changing the work environment to promote wellness: A focus group study. *AAOHN Journal: Official Journal of the American Association of Occupational Health Nurses, 54*(12), 515–520.

Grosch, J. W., Alterman, T., Petersen, M. R., & Murphy, L. R. (1998). Worksite health promotion programs in the U.S.: Factors associated with availability and participation. *American Journal of Health Promotion, 13*(1), 36–45.

Hunt, M. K., Barbeau, E. M., Lederman, R., Stoddard, A. M., Chetkovich, C., Goldman, R., et al. (2007). Process evaluation results from the Healthy Directions–Small Business Study. *Health Education & Behavior, 34*(1), 90–107.

Juhn, C., & Potter, S. (2006). Changes in labor force participation in the United States. *Journal of Economic Perspectives, 20*(3), 27–46.

Kaiser Family Foundation. (2007). *Employer health benefits: 2007 summary of findings*. Retrieved January 30, 2008, from http://www.kff.org/insurance/7672/upload/Summary-of-Findings-EHBS-2007.pdf.

Lassen, A., Bruselius-Jensen, M., Sommer, H. M., Thorsen, A. V., & Trolle, E. (2007). Factors influencing participation rates and employees' attitudes toward promoting healthy eating at blue-collar worksites. *Health Education Research, 22*(5), 727–736.

Linnan, L., & Birken, B. E. (2006). Small businesses, worksite wellness, and public health: A time for action. *North Carolina Medical Journal, 67*(6), 433–437.

Linnan, L., Bowling, M., Bachtel, J., Lindsay, G., Blakey, C., Pronk, S., et al. (2008). Results of the 2004 National Worksite Health Promotion Survey. *American Journal of Public Health, 98*(8), 1503–1509.

Linnan, L., Weiner, B., Graham, A., & Emmons, K. (2007). Manager beliefs regarding worksite health promotion: Results from the Working Healthy Project 2. *American Journal of Health Promotion, 21*(6), 521–528.

Murray, C.J.L., & Lopez, A. D. (1996). *The global burden of disease*. Cambridge, MA: Harvard University Press.

National Coalition on Health Care. (2008). *Facts on the cost of health care*. Retrieved January 26, 2008, from http://www.nchc.org/facts/cost.shtml.

National Institute for Occupational Safety and Health. (2008a). *Essential Elements of Effective Workplace Programs and Policies for Improving Worker Health and Wellbeing*. Retrieved November 10, 2009, from http://www.cdc.gov/niosh/worklife/essentials.html.

National Institute for Occupational Safety and Health. (2008b). *NIOSH program portfolio: WorkLife initiative*. Retrieved November 1, 2009, from http://www.cdc.gov/niosh/programs/worklife.

National Research Council. (1999). *The changing nature of work: Implications for occupational analysis*. Washington, D.C.: National Academies Press.

Office of Disease Prevention and Health Promotion. (1992). *Healthy worksites: Directory of federal initiatives in worksite health promotion*. Washington, DC: U.S. Government Printing Office.

Office of Disease Prevention and Health Promotion. (1999). *Healthy worksites: Directory of federal initiatives in worksite health promotion*. Washington, DC: U.S. Government Printing Office.

Partnership for Prevention. (2005). *Leading by example: Leading practices for employee health management*. Retrieved October 26, 2009, from http://prevent.org/content/view/30/57.

Partnership for Prevention. (2007). *About us*. Retrieved August 22, 2008, from http://www.prevent.org/content/view/108/5.

Peabody, K., & Linnan, L. (2007). Careers in worksite health promotion. *Eta Sigma Gamma: The Health Education Monograph Series, 23*(2), 18–21.

Rasmussen, K., Glasscock, D. J., Hansen, O. N., Carstensen, O., Jepsen, J. F., & Nielsen, K. J. (2006). Worker participation in change processes in a Danish industrial setting. *American Journal of Industrial Medicine, 49*(9), 767–779.

Reardon, J. (1998). The history and impact of worksite wellness. *Nursing Economics, 16,* 117–121.

Sorensen, G., & Barbeau, E. M. (2006). Integrating occupational health, safety, and worksite health promotion: Opportunities for research and practice. *La Medicina del Lavoro, 97*(2), 240–257.

Stanton, M. W., & Rutherford, M. K. (2004). Employer-sponsored health insurance: Trends in cost and access. *Research in Action* (Issue 17; AHRQ Pub. No. 04-0085). Rockville, MD: Agency for Healthcare Research and Quality.

State of California. (2005). *Guide to developing a workplace injury and illness prevention program with checklists for self-inspection.* Retrieved November 1, 2009, from https://www.dir.ca.gov/dosh/dosh_publications/IIPP.html.

Stokols, D., Pelletier, K., & Fielding, J. (1996). The ecology of work and health: Research and policy directions for the promotion of employee health. *Health Education Quarterly, 23,* 137–158.

Toossi, M. (2002). A century of change: The U.S. labor force, 1950–2050. *Monthly Labor Review, 125*(5), 15–28.

University of Tennessee at Chattanooga. (2009). *Master of science degree in health and human performance with a concentration in worksite health and productivity.* Retrieved October 28, 2009, from http://www.utc.edu/Academic/HealthAndHumanPerformance/worksitehpdegree.php.

U.S. Chamber of Commerce & Partnership for Prevention. (2007). *Leading by example: Leading practices for employee health management.* Retrieved January 28, 2009, from http://www.prevent.org/LBE/LBE_USCC_FullBook.pdf.

U.S. Department of Health and Human Services, Public Health Service, Substance Abuse and Mental Health Services Administration, Center for Substance Abuse Prevention. (n.d.). *Making your workplace drug free: A kit for employers.* Retrieved August 22, 2008, from http://ncadi.samhsa.gov/govpubs/workit/folder.aspx.

U.S. Office of Personnel Management. (n.d.). *Employee health services handbook.* Retrieved August 22, 2008, from http://www.healthierfeds.opm.gov/healthierfedsmanual.asp#top.

Wellness Council of America. (2008). *WELCOA overview.* Retrieved August 22, 2008, from http://www.welcoa.org/presskit/index.php.

# CHAPTER FIFTEEN

# PROMOTING COMMUNITY HEALTH

## Local Health Departments and Community Health Organizations

MICHAEL T. HATCHER

DIANE D. ALLENSWORTH

FRANCES D. BUTTERFOSS

---

### LEARNING OBJECTIVES

- Describe the history of health departments and the history of voluntary health organizations in the United States

- Describe the functions of your state or local health authority and the impact of its structure on its staffing, the services provided, and the percentage of the population served

- Identify tools and resources to plan, implement, and evaluate health promotion programs in local health departments

- Discuss the challenges of engaging a community in public health promotion efforts, campaigns, and services

- Describe administrative, clinical, and program careers in local or state health departments

**C**ONDUCTING COMMUNITY health promotion programs, in most situations, means working with the local public health department and community health organizations. These are organizations that are focused on the community and that operate many, if not most, of the community health promotion programs. They have the mobility and flexibility to go to parks, day camps, after-school programs, housing projects, street corners, stores, malls, or any location within a specific geographic area. Compared with health promotion programs at schools, workplaces, and health care organizations, community health promotion programs are less constrained by organizational structures, rules, and procedures. Community programs are more fluid and flexible, reflecting the social, economic, and cultural makeup of a community. Often, community health promotion programs start with an individual or a group of individuals who have a health concern. These grassroots groups often blossom into organizations, form coalitions and partnerships with health departments and other community organizations, or become part of existing community health organizations. This chapter explores the two predominant types of organizations that operate community health promotion programs: local health departments and community health organizations.

## BRIEF HISTORY OF LOCAL HEALTH ORGANIZATIONS

Local health departments and community health organizations have their roots in public health. Life expectancy was less than fifty years in 1900. The crude death rate at the beginning of the twentieth century was 17.2 deaths per 1,000 people per year, and the infant mortality rate was approximately 120 per 1,000 births. The top three causes of death in 1900 were infectious diseases. By the end of the twentieth century, life expectancy had increased to seventy-seven years, while the annual death rate had dropped to 8.7 per 1,000 and the annual infant mortality rate had dropped to 6.9 per 1,000. Heart disease, cancer, and stroke were the top causes of death at the beginning of the twenty-first century (Ward & Warren, 2007).

A number of public health innovations were responsible for the shift in causes of mortality from infectious disease to chronic disease during the past century. The top ten public health achievements during the twentieth century, as identified by the Centers for Disease Control and Prevention (CDC), were (1) vaccines; (2) control of infectious diseases through sanitation and antimicrobial therapy; (3) motor vehicle safety (improved engineering and seat belt use); (4) safer workplaces;

(5) recognition of tobacco as a health hazard; (6) fewer deaths from heart disease and stroke as a result of smoking cessation; (7) blood pressure control and better treatments for high blood pressure; (8) safer and healthier food, which has virtually eliminated nutritional deficiency diseases; (9) healthier mothers and babies as a result of family planning and contraceptive services; and (10) fluoridation of drinking water to prevent tooth decay (Centers for Disease Control and Prevention, 1999).

Local health departments promoted public health innovations at the community level. Although a few local health departments were established during the colonial period in cities that experienced severe health problems from infectious disease, it was not until a major epidemic of typhoid fever in 1910 and 1911 that a federal recommendation prompted the organization of local health departments. By the mid-1930s, more than a quarter of the counties in the United States provided public health services (Novick, 2001). Even today, the extent of public health services varies within and between states. Only a few states have no local public health departments that serve a defined population. In other states, counties and cities have local health departments (Leep, 2006). The services provided by local health departments have expanded over the past century to include prevention of epidemics and the spread of disease, protection against environmental hazards, prevention of injuries, promotion of healthy behaviors, disaster response and recovery assistance, and ensuring the quality and accessibility of health services. Local health departments have the authority to protect, promote, and enhance the health of people living in a specific geographic area. States give this authority to the government of a county, city, or municipality, which oversees the local public health department. Tax dollars fund local health departments, and their staff members are government employees.

At the same time that local health departments were developing, the first voluntary health organizations were formed. These organizations were designed to address specific health problems and were run primarily by volunteers. For example, the National Association for the Study and Prevention of Tuberculosis was established in 1902, and the American Cancer Society was founded in 1913. The March of Dimes, another voluntary health organization, had great success in the twentieth century in focusing action on polio and was instrumental in eliminating the disease from the United States. Following that success, the organization now has a focus on birth defects.

From these early organizations, a large number of diverse health organizations have developed over the past hundred years. Today, many are large, well-run national organizations with a professional staff. Many small local organizations also have a professional staff and solid funding. Illustrations of the types of community health organizations that address local health concerns such as diabetes, physical activity, substance abuse, injury prevention, and clean water are found in Exhibit 15.1. As Chapter One discusses, community health organizations go by many names but their common bond is their operation by community members and a focus on a local health problem. Many community organizations are nonprofit and as such are not owned by an individual; by law, they are governed by boards of directors who have responsibility for their operation. They are recognized as exempt from paying federal, state, and local taxes, in accordance with section 501(c)(3) of the U.S. Internal Revenue Code (26 U.S.C. 501(c)). Tax-exempt status also has implications for how organizations conduct advocacy efforts (see Chapter Seven). Health care organizations such as hospitals and medical clinics (discussed in Chapter Thirteen) may have the same organizational structure as community organizations (nonprofit) but have a broader mission that includes medical treatment.

## EXHIBIT 15.1
## Types of Community Health Organizations

- Health and mental health programs (treatment and counseling)
- Environmental health programs (clean food, water, and air)
- Voluntary health agencies (for example, associations focused on cancer or heart or lung diseases)
- Human service or social service programs (for example, child protection, homeless shelters)
- Community primary care clinics
- Recreation and fitness programs
- Nutrition programs
- Health coalitions and collaborations
- Safety and disaster preparedness programs
- Faith-based organizations and their programs
- Youth development programs
- Senior service programs
- Neighborhood policing and safety programs
- Labor unions' health programs
- Urban planning agencies (built environment and land use issues)
- Brownfield programs (industrial site redevelopment)
- Community health foundations

# LOCAL HEALTH DEPARTMENT SERVICES

The size of the population served by a local health department influences the size of the department's staff and the scope of the services provided by the department. For example, the profile of local health departments produced by the National Association of County and City Health Officials (NACCHO) indicates that the number of residents served by local health departments ranges from fewer than 1,000 to nearly 10 million (Leep, 2006). Most local health departments (62 percent) serve less than 50,000 residents, and 60 percent of local health departments employ fewer than twenty-five full-time employees (Leep, 2006). Collectively these small departments provide public health services to about 10 percent of the U.S. population. In contrast, 6 percent of local health departments serve populations of more than 500,000, and collectively these large departments provide services to approximately 54 percent of U.S. residents (Leep, 2006). Overall, only 14 percent of local health departments employ more than 100 full-time employees (Leep, 2006). The median staffing level for departments that serve populations of under 25,000 is eight employees, while departments that serve populations of 1 million or more have a median of 491 employees (Leep, 2006).

Services offered by local health departments range from health surveillance to preventive services, clinical services, disease control, food and water safety, environmental protection and pollution hazards mitigation, waste disposal, vector control (for example, mosquito-control programs to reduce mosquito-borne diseases in human health), policy initiatives, regulatory and enforcement services, and education. NACCHO has identified seventy-five public health services and related activities that local health departments perform. The most common health services provided by local health departments are adult and child immunizations, communicable disease surveillance, tuberculosis screening and treatment, food service inspections, food safety education, and environmental health surveillance (Leep, 2006). Specific findings from the NACCHO study are provided in Table 15.1. This table outlines eighteen services provided across small and large local health departments, including the eight services offered most often by departments and twelve others that are less frequently offered. All of the services have implications for health promotion. The scope of services delivered generally increases with population size. However, even in small health departments, health promotion activities are a priority. For example in Larimer County, Colorado, which covers 2,640 square miles that include farmland, ranch lands, forests, and mountains, the health department makes health promotion a priority even on a tight budget (for example, see Exhibit 15.2).

TABLE 15.1  Services of Local Health Departments,
by Size of Population Served (percentages)

| Services and Activities | All Departments | Population of Fewer Than 25,000 | Population of More Than 500,000 |
|---|---|---|---|
| Adult immunizations | 91% | 88% | 91% |
| Child immunizations | 90 | 84 | 92 |
| Communicable disease surveillance | 89 | 81 | 96 |
| Tuberculosis screening | 85 | 77 | 90 |
| Food service regulation | 76 | 66 | 75 |
| Food safety education | 75 | 64 | 76 |
| Environmental health surveillance | 75 | 64 | 83 |
| Tuberculosis treatment | 75 | 64 | 88 |
| Tobacco use prevention | 69 | 60 | 87 |
| Obesity prevention | 56 | 46 | 79 |
| Unintended pregnancy prevention | 51 | 44 | 62 |
| Chronic disease surveillance | 41 | 34 | 65 |
| Injury prevention | 40 | 33 | 61 |
| Behavioral risk factor surveillance | 36 | 28 | 57 |
| Substance abuse prevention | 26 | 20 | 44 |
| Violence prevention | 25 | 20 | 48 |
| Injury surveillance | 24 | 17 | 49 |
| Mental illness prevention | 14 | 11 | 28 |

*Note:* Some local health departments that served populations of between 25,000 and 500,000 provided more services than departments that served populations below 25,000 and above 500,000 did.

*Source:* Leep, 2006.

The structure of a local health department typically includes a local board of health and a health commissioner (Figure 15.1). Laws may prescribe who can be a health commissioner (for example, a physician, dentist, or someone who holds a doctorate in public health). If the health commissioner is not a physician,

## EXHIBIT 15.2
## Health Promotion Programs in a Small Local Health Department

Health District of Northern Larimer County, Colorado
The health district's health promotion services focus on four main areas:

- **Heart disease screenings**. Heart disease can be prevented. Our team of nurses offers free blood pressure screening and low-cost cholesterol tests in a variety of locations in the community.
- **Nutrition services**. Registered dietitians offer individual nutrition counseling, a weight management class called Healthy Weighs, and a variety of cooking classes throughout the year.
- **Smoking cessation services**. Our trained counselors can help people to quit smoking, using a no-pressure approach and proven techniques. We offer individual counseling as well as classes for those who want to quit in a group setting. We offer free nicotine replacement patches, gum, and lozenges to district residents who enroll in the program.
- **Adult immunizations**. We provide low-cost vaccinations for influenza in the fall. Tetanus and pneumonia vaccinations are available year-round.

*Source:* Health District of Northern Larimer County, n.d.

FIGURE 15.1  Organizational Chart of a Local Health Department

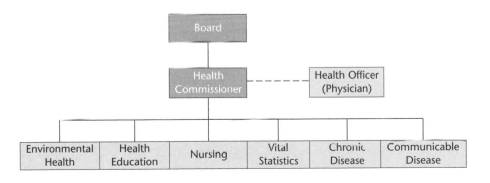

then the department will probably have a health officer who is a physician support the department through a consulting relationship. The health commissioner is appointed by the board of health, the members of which are themselves appointed by officials in the city or county government or, in some situations, elected by the general public. Staff members of local health departments have education and experience in medical and health-related fields. Local health departments are funded by local, state, and for some services, federal tax dollars. The funding levels of health departments vary and determine the range and intensity of department programs and services.

One source of guidance for health promotion in local health departments was the development in 1995 of the ten essential public health services (EPHS) by the Public Health Functions Steering Committee of the U.S. Department of Health and Human Services (2008). The ten EPHS (outlined in Exhibit 15.3)

---

## EXHIBIT 15.3
### Ten Essential Public Health Services

1. Monitor health status of the population to identify and solve community health problems
2. Diagnose and investigate health problems and health hazards in the community
3. Inform, educate, and empower people about health issues
4. Mobilize community partnerships and action to identify and solve health problems
5. Develop policies and plans that support individual and community health efforts
6. Enforce laws and regulations that protect health and ensure safety
7. Link people to needed personal health services and ensure the provision of health care when otherwise unavailable
8. Ensure a competent public health and personal health care workforce
9. Evaluate effectiveness, accessibility, and quality of personal and population-based health services
10. Conduct research to discover new insights and innovative solutions to health problems

*Source:* Adapted from U.S. Department of Health and Human Services, Public Health Functions Steering Committee, 2008.

now define public health practice and are performed within local health departments in collaboration with their community partners. Many of the EPHS are invisible to the public and are only recognized when a problem develops (for example, when an outbreak of disease occurs). However, effective performance of the EPHS facilitates health promotion efforts and is crucial in safeguarding the health of a community.

The EPHS reflect one of the greatest opportunities facing local health departments. Tackling the health implications of modern lifestyles such as tobacco use, consumption of high-calorie, high-salt foods, and physical inactivity, as well as the threat of globally spreading infectious diseases, requires the availability of a well-trained public health workforce. Having fewer public health nurses means fewer screenings and fewer immunizations. Not having enough epidemiologists makes it harder to respond to food-borne outbreaks or to track emerging infectious diseases like drug-resistant staph infections (MRSA). Hurricane Katrina made clear the importance of local health department workers in responding to natural disasters. Given the growing complexity of public health challenges, more specialists need to be trained in additional public health subdisciplines. Furthermore, in the era of globalization, the U.S. public health workforce needs to be adequately prepared to prevent and handle health threats that often arise from beyond U.S. borders.

## COMMUNITY HEALTH ORGANIZATION SERVICES

Community health organizations are typically nonprofit organizations that have been created by individuals in a community to address a specific health issue. They may be local affiliates of a national organization or organizations unique to the community. The issues addressed by community health organizations are numerous. Community health organizations are usually started in order to raise money for research, educate professionals, serve individuals affected by a disease or health problem, and advocate for beneficial government policies and procedures; however, almost all have disease prevention and health promotion as part of their mission.

The numbers and types of community health organizations engaged in health promotion programs are also directly related to the population size and the diversity of the health needs of the community. Compared with the focus of a local health department, the focus of a community health organization is generally more tailored and fitted to a priority population. This tighter focus on a particular population provides an opportunity to develop in-depth expertise on the health concern or the target population of the organization.

## EXHIBIT 15.4
## Services of a Community Health Organization That Promotes the Health of Senior Citizens in the Community

**Health risk assessments**: assessments that evaluate the health status of an individual comparing chronological age to health age.

**Routine health screening**: screenings for certain diseases or conditions, which may include hypertension, glaucoma, high cholesterol, cancer, impaired vision, impaired hearing, memory problems, diabetes, and inadequate nutrition.

**Fitness activities**: organized activities that promote the physical health of older adults. These activities incorporate cardiovascular exercise, muscle toning, and agility improvement.

**Nutrition counseling**: provision of individualized advice and guidance on options and methods for improving their nutritional status to those at nutritional risk because of their health or nutritional history, their dietary intake, their use of medications, or chronic illness. Services are performed by a health professional in accordance with state law and policy.

**Education for individuals or groups**: programs to promote better physical or mental health by providing accurate health information and instruction to participants or caregivers in a group or individual setting, overseen by an individual with health-related expertise or experience.

For example, Exhibit 15.4 lists the services of a community organization that is focused on the mission of positively influencing the experience of aging in the community. The organization's goals are for individuals aged sixty and older to

- Stay active and healthy
- Maintain independence
- Pursue interests
- Make new friends

Recently funders of community health programs (for example, United Way, foundations, and local government) have placed more emphasis on community

**Health promotion programs**: programs relating to management of chronic disabling conditions (including osteoporosis and cardiovascular disease), alcohol and substance abuse reduction, smoking cessation, weight loss and control, and stress management.

**Home injury control services**: screening of high-risk home environments and provision of educational programs on injury prevention (including fall and fracture prevention) in the home environment.

**Medication management**: oversight of medications by a registered nurse for older adults who have been assessed as requiring management of their medications.

**Informational programs concerning Medicare benefits**: educational programs on availability, benefits, and appropriate use of preventive health services covered by Medicare.

**Senior center**: an attractive center that provides a wide variety of activities and programs (for example, arts and crafts, social engagement and sponsored outings, and exercise) for seniors.

**Adult day care**: the time demands of caring for an older adult require many family care providers to make sacrifices in their professional and personal lives. At some point, they simply need some help. Adult day care programs provide assistance in caring for a dependent adult family member.

health program outcomes; this has been accompanied by changes in policy and an increase in general public concern about accountability. Pressure for results has intensified, and organizations are increasingly being asked to demonstrate that specified goals have been achieved. For example, the U.S. Government Performance Results Act (Office of Management and Budget, 1993) specifies that organizations funded by the federal government must set program outcome goals and publicly report on progress toward achieving those goals. Community health organizations are asked to demonstrate outcomes, including the achievements of their health promotion programs, and report those outcomes during their annual budget cycles. While much of the pressure to measure outcomes comes from fiscal accountability requirements, the primary reason to evaluate outcomes is to learn how programs are performing and to manage them effectively to achieve the health mission.

## RESOURCES AND TOOLS

A number of unique resources can help health promotion specialists in planning, implementing, and evaluating community health promotion programs. Most of the organizations listed in this section provide tools, technical assistance, and other resources needed to address the range of issues that health promotion specialists are asked to address in their work at health departments and community organizations.

### National Association of County and City Health Officials

The National Association of County and City Health Officials (NACCHO) represents approximately 3,000 local health departments. NACCHO supports local health efforts by calling for strong national policy, developing useful resources and programs, promoting health equity, and supporting effective local public health practice and health system performance. NACCHO provides assistance in four key areas: (1) The community health program helps local health departments conduct health promotion and preventive disease initiatives within communities. (2) The environmental health program helps promote human health by building safe environments that address the relationship between people's health and their environments. (3) The public health infrastructure and systems program helps local health departments perform their core governmental functions and EPHS. (4) The public health preparedness program enhances local health departments' readiness to respond to emergencies. As part of NACCHO's services it has created a Web toolbox of public health-related tools. This toolbox is a free service available for public use, intended to promote and advance public health objectives including health promotion (http://www.naccho .org/toolbox).

### Association for Community Health Improvement

The Association for Community Health Improvement (http://www.community hlth.org/communityhlth/join.html) evolved in 2002 as the successor to three national community health initiatives: the Community Care Network Demonstration Program, the ACT National Outcomes Network, and the Coalition for Healthier Cities and Communities. These three initiatives had compatible missions and had made complementary contributions to community health since the mid-1990s. Each organization was approaching the end of its individual grant cycle and saw the merger of initiatives as a way to sustain their organizational efforts, which included

- Building health care delivery and preventive health systems that ensure accessibility and are accountable to local needs
- Planning and measuring progress toward defined community health goals
- Applying broad community engagement efforts in resolving systemic challenges to community health and social well-being

The association adopted the key tenets of these initiatives and blended them with additional commitments to effective community health practice to create a unified professional association that now serves as a hub of networking and continual learning. The association is a program of the Health Research and Education Trust. This organization provides professional conferences and publications focused on health promotion practices in health care organizations and community settings.

## Community Tool Box

The Community Tool Box (CTB) is the world's largest online resource for free information on essential skills for building healthy communities (http://ctb .ku.edu/en). The CTB provides over 7,000 pages of practical step-by-step guidance on specific community-building skills, along with key tasks, examples, and support for developing and performing sixteen core public health competencies that promote community health and development. Creation of the CTB has been ongoing since 1994. The University of Kansas hosts the CTB team within the Work Group for Community Health and Development. The national and international partners of the CTB team have identified what community users need to know to build healthier and more equitable communities.

## Area Health Education Centers

The mission of Area Health Education Centers (AHECs) is to improve the supply, distribution, diversity, and quality of the health care workforce in medically underserved communities (http://bhpr.hrsa.gov/ahec). The long-term educational strategy of the AHECs is to form academic and community partnerships in order to train health care providers at sites and in programs that are responsive to state and local health manpower needs. Programs to interest K–12 students in health careers and recruit them for those careers are emphasized. AHECs link the resources of university health science centers with local planning, educational, and clinical resources. This network of health-related institutions provides multidisciplinary educational services to students, faculty, and local practitioners. Ultimately, this work can improve health care access and delivery by increasing the number of health professionals in medically underserved areas. Area Health

Education Centers work extensively in the planning, implementation, and evaluation of health promotion programs, emphasizing community collaborations and the elimination of health disparities.

Fifty-three AHEC programs and 221 affiliated AHECs operate in forty-five states and the District of Columbia. The states of Kansas, Michigan, North Dakota, and South Dakota and the Commonwealth of Puerto Rico do not have federally funded AHECs or AHEC programs. AHECs include nonprofit 501(c)(3) organizations, community colleges, hospitals, and health centers.

## Office of Rural Health Policy

The Office of Rural Health Policy (ORHP) promotes better health care service in rural America (http://ruralhealth.hrsa.gov). It was established by Congress in 1987 and located in the Health Resources and Services Administration (HRSA), which is part of the U.S. Department of Health and Human Services (DHHS). Congress charged the office with informing and advising DHHS on matters affecting rural hospitals and health care, coordinating activities within DHHS that relate to rural health care, and maintaining a national information clearinghouse. The office is a champion of health promotion initiatives in rural America. It works at federal, state, and local government levels and with private sector associations, foundations, health care providers, and community leaders in seeking solutions to rural health care problems and promoting health. In particular, the ORHP

- Helps shape rural health policy
- Works with state offices of rural health
- Promotes rural health research
- Funds innovative rural health programs
- Provides support to the National Advisory Committee on Rural Health and Human Services
- Acts as a voice for the concerns of rural hospitals, clinics, and other rural health care providers
- Acts as a liaison with national, state, and local rural health organizations
- Works with minority populations in rural areas
- Sponsors the National Clearinghouse of Rural Health Information
- Conducts ORHP's program evaluation

## National Public Health Performance Standards Program

The National Public Health Performance Standards Program (NPHPSP) is a partnership initiative that was formed by national public health organizations in order to work collaboratively to establish national performance standards (http://www.cdc.gov/od/ocphp/nphpsp). The standards identify the optimal level of performance for state and local public health systems (that is, all organizations that contribute to public health in a given area) and local governing boards. The NPHPSP provides a framework for assessing the capacity and performance of a public health system and seeks to ensure that strong effective public health systems are in place to deliver EPHS. The standards provide a foundation for state and local health departments to plan, implement and evaluate health promotion programs. The four program goals are (1) providing performance standards for public health systems and encouraging their widespread use; (2) engaging and leveraging national, state, and local partnerships to build a stronger foundation for public health preparedness; (3) promoting continuous quality improvement of public health systems; and (4) strengthening the scientific basis for improvement of public health practice. The CDC sponsors the program.

## Public Health Foundation

The Public Health Foundation (PHF) is dedicated to achieving healthy communities through research, training, and technical assistance (http://www.phf.org). The PHF is a national nonprofit organization that creates new information and helps public health agencies and other community health organizations access and more effectively use information in order to manage and improve performance, understand and use data, and strengthen the competencies of the public health workforce. The foundation is a resource and support for the creation of innovative health promotion programs for diverse populations and settings. It has also created TRAIN, a Web-based learning resource for health professionals (https://www.train.org/DesktopShell.aspx) that allows users to find current local, regional, and national training opportunities, many of them offered via the Internet.

## U.S. Environmental Protection Agency

The mission of the Environmental Protection Agency (EPA) is to protect human health and the environment (http://www.epa.gov). The EPA provides national leadership in environmental science research and education and in environmental risk assessment, develops and enforces regulations associated with environmental laws enacted by Congress, and is responsible for setting national standards for a variety of environmental programs. The EPA delegates responsibility for issuing permits, monitoring compliance, and enforcing regulations to state and tribal governments. When national standards are not met by a regulated organization, the EPA can issue sanctions and take other steps to compel an offending organization to achieve the desired levels of environmental quality. The EPA provides grant funds to state governments, nonprofits, and academic institutions to support the high-quality research that is needed to improve the scientific basis for decisions on national environmental issues and to help the EPA achieve its mission and goals.

The EPA is one of the first resources to consult when planning, implementing, and evaluating an environmental health promotion program. It is a source for funding, resources (for example, professional conferences and materials), current research, and legislative updates and regulations. The EPA and its partners (local, state, and federal agencies, laboratories, and research institutions) work to assess community-level environmental contamination and human health risk, identify and understand the toxicity of chemicals in ecosystems, and improve the science and technology of risk assessment and the management of current and emerging environmental health issues. The agency works with over 10,000 industries, businesses, nonprofit organizations, and state and local governments on over forty voluntary pollution prevention programs and energy conservation efforts, such as water and energy conservation, greenhouse gas and toxic emissions reduction, solid waste reuse, and control of indoor air pollution.

## Public Health Training Centers

Public Health Training Centers (PHTCs) are partnerships between accredited schools of public health, related academic institutions, and public health agencies and organizations. They are designed to improve the nation's public health system by strengthening the technical, scientific, managerial, and leadership competence of current and future public health professionals. PHTCs are a source for resources (for example, professional conferences and materials), current research, and legislative updates and regulations. On the basis of the recommendations of the Institute of Medicine report *Who Will Keep the Public Healthy? Educating Public Health Professionals in the 21st Century* (Institute of Medicine, 2003), PHTCs assess the learning needs of the public health workforce and provide training to meet those needs. This training serves as a foundation for improving the public health infrastructure as well as achieving the health objectives of Healthy People 2020. Currently, forty-five states, the District of Columbia, and the U.S. Associated Pacific Islands are covered by PHTC activity. To accommodate the general training needs of the public health workforce, approximately 60 percent of the PHTCs' training and training tools are offered as distance education.

## Centers for Public Health Preparedness

The CDC established the Centers for Public Health Preparedness (CPHP) in 2000 to strengthen emergency preparedness and preparedness for terrorism by linking academic expertise to state and local health agency needs (http://emergency .cdc.gov/cotper/cphp). The Centers offer funding, resources (for example, professional conferences and materials), current research, and legislative updates and regulations. They bring together community colleges, four-year colleges, and universities with a common focus on public health preparedness, establishing a national network of education and training resources. Of these institutions, twenty-seven are accredited schools of public health.

The CPHP's goals are to

- Strengthen public health workforce readiness through lifelong learning programs
- Strengthen state and local preparedness for terrorism and capacity for emergency public health response
- Develop an academic network to support national preparedness for terrorism and emergency response and to share expertise and resources across state and local jurisdictions

## Children's Safety Network

The Children's Safety Network (CSN), funded by the Maternal and Child Health Bureau of HRSA, seeks to prevent injuries and violence among children and adolescents by strengthening the staff and organizational capacity for injury prevention of state maternal and child health (MCH) programs (http://www .childrenssafetynetwork.org). It is a source for funding, resources (for example, professional conferences and materials), current research, and legislative updates and regulations. CSN also works with national organizations and federal agencies that are responsible for promoting child and adolescent health and safety. CSN capacity development includes

- Implementing activities to strengthen MCH performance measures related to injuries and violence
- Integrating injury prevention into MCH activities
- Building partnerships among MCH programs and injury prevention programs
- Implementing proven strategies to prevent injuries—including injuries related to motor vehicles, violence, and recreational activities and injuries sustained in homes, schools, and workplaces—in a broad range of settings

- Developing core components of an effective injury prevention program: data, interventions, infrastructure, technical support and training, and public policy. Information about these components is available from the Web site of the State and Territorial Injury Prevention Directors Association (http://www .stipda.org).
- Training and educating injury prevention professionals.
- Increasing recognition of the value of injury prevention among state and national policymakers.
- Providing technical assistance by telephone, mail, and e-mail and through site visits. Each public health region is assigned a CSN state outreach specialist who focuses on the specific injury prevention needs of states within those regions.

### United Way

Over 1,300 United Ways operate in the United States via a coalition of local nonprofit organizations that pool efforts in fundraising support (http://www .liveunited.org). The focus of United Way is identifying and resolving pressing community issues, as well as making measurable changes in communities through partnerships with schools, government agencies, businesses, organized labor, financial institutions, community development corporations, voluntary and neighborhood associations, the faith community, and others. The issues that United Way offices address are determined locally, out of respect for the diversity of the communities served. United Way organizations raise money in numerous ways—most notably, through workplaces, where employees can authorize automatic payroll deductions for United Way. Exhibit 15.5 shows the services that the United Way of the Capital Region in Pennsylvania offers in order to help community health organizations promote the health of community members.

## CHALLENGES

Health promotion in communities depends on effective community engagement. Engaging community members and organizations in community health promotion work presents many challenges. Lack of trust or respect often exists among local health departments and community health organizations that may have experienced few direct benefits from their community-level participation. The unequal distribution of information, formal education, income,

**EXHIBIT 15.5**
**Services for Community Health Organizations Offered by United Way of the Capital Region**

United Way of the Capital Region (UWCR) provides a variety of services and financial support to nonprofits in Dauphin, Cumberland, and Perry counties in Pennsylvania. These services help nonprofits improve the efficiency and effectiveness of their programs and services.

- **United Way funding**. UWCR is best known for providing financial support to nonprofits through its annual fundraising campaign and grant programs. It directs funding to local programs and services that address critical needs and demonstrate a measurable difference in the lives of community members. Presently, UWCR offers three funding streams to nonprofits: annual allocations, venture grants, and community impact initiative grants. Venture grants and community impact initiative grants are open to any nonprofit that offers services in the Capital Region. Annual allocations are open only to previously selected and approved programs.
- **Training and technical assistance**. UWCR assists nonprofits with training, outcome measurement, recruitment of volunteers and new board members, in-kind donations of equipment and supplies, and creation of community groups to address emerging needs.
- **Research on community needs**. UWCR conducts research and assesses the evolving health and human service needs of the Capital Region on an ongoing basis—for example, it conducts a community needs and assets study. This research helps UWCR to target United Way resources toward the most pressing needs of the community, as well as to promote awareness of these issues.
- **Volunteer Center**. The Volunteer Center is a UWCR program that offers many services to nonprofits. The Center serves as a clearinghouse for volunteer activities in the Capital Region and as an advocate for volunteerism. In addition, the center supports the recognition of volunteers and coordinates access to in-kind donations.

*Source:* Adapted from United Way of the Capitol Region, 2009.

and power in communities reflects underlying social inequalities of economic class, race or ethnicity, age, and gender. These may, in turn, affect whether community members feel they will have influence over decisions and whether they want to engage and participate in community-based activities. Differences in community organizations' perspectives, priorities, assumptions, values, beliefs, and languages also may make engagement difficult and conflict more likely. Finally, because of resource competition or turf issues between community groups (Israel, Schultz, Parker, & Becker, 1998), challenges may arise over the extent to which community organizations represent and reflect the "real" community. Ultimately, participation is influenced by whether community members believe that the benefits of participation outweigh the costs. Overcoming the challenges to community engagement depends on successful community assessment and community self-empowerment, as well as attention to the general conclusions about community building that are detailed in this section. In order to bring about desired changes, community engagement efforts should address multiple levels of the social environment and health determinants within the community rather than only individual behaviors.

Ongoing action planning can identify specific community and system changes that influence or compel widespread behavior changes and make community health improvements more likely (Roussos & Fawcett, 2000). Health behaviors are influenced by culture. To ensure that engagement efforts are culturally and linguistically appropriate, they must be developed from an understanding and respect for the culture of the community being served.

While a sense of empowerment cannot be externally imposed on a community, engendering the ability to take action, influence, and make decisions on critical issues is crucial for successful engagement efforts. Coalitions and partnerships, when adequately supported, can be useful vehicles for mobilizing community assets for decision making and action on health issues.

Community mobilization and self-determination frequently need nurturing. Before individuals and organizations can gain control and influence and become partners in decision making and action on community health issues, they frequently need training to develop additional knowledge, leadership skills, and resources in order to exert their power.

Health professionals and community leaders can use their understanding of perceived costs associated with health issues in order to develop appropriate incentives for participation. Such incentives might include fostering a sense of community, choosing relevant issues, and making the process and organizational climate of participation open and supportive of community members' right to have a voice in the process. Based on the social science literature and the principles discussed in this section, Exhibit 15.6 summarizes some specific factors that can positively influence the success of community engagement efforts, and Table 15.2 highlights specific barriers to community participation and some suggestions for how to overcome them.

## EXHIBIT 15.6
## Factors That Contribute to the Success of Community Engagement Efforts

*Environment*

- A history of collaboration or cooperation exists in the community.
- The collaborating group (and its member agencies in the group) is seen as a leader in the community.
- The political and social climate is favorable.

*Membership*

- Partners have mutual respect, understanding, and trust.
- Partners represent an appropriate cross-section of the community.
- Engagement is seen as being in partners' self-interest—the benefits of engagement offset the costs.
- Partners have the ability to compromise.

*Process and Structure*

- Partners feel ownership—that is, share a stake in both the process and the outcome.
- Every level of each organization in the collaborating group participates in decision making.
- The collaborating group has flexibility.
- Roles and guidelines are clear.
- Partners can sustain collaboration in the midst of changing conditions.

*Communication*

- Open and frequent interaction, information, and discussion occur.
- Informal and formal channels of communication exist.

*Purpose*

- Goals are clear and appear realistic to all partners.
- Partners have a shared vision.
- The purpose is unique to the effort (that is, it is different, at least in part, from the mission, goals, or approaches of the member organizations).

*Resources*

- The effort has sufficient funds.
- The effort has a skilled convener.

**TABLE 15.2  Barriers to Community Engagement and Potential Solutions**

| Problem | Solution |
|---|---|
| Organization is cautious about engaging. | Be clear about opportunities and incentives for participation. |
| Organization faces administrative challenges (for example, staff are unavailable to answer phone or work irregular hours). | Be consistent and patient in communication with organization. |
| | Be flexible; meet staff when and where they are available. |
| Organization needs help with capacity building. | Suggest ways to help the organization maximize strengths and work around its challenges. |
| | Offer to share effective practices that have worked for your program or organization. |
| | Walk through organization's processes or procedures step by step in order to highlight areas of inefficiency. |
| Organization lacks access to information. | Invite the organization into community partnership and networking opportunities. |
| | Introduce the organization's staff to new and different sources of information. |
| Organization has language barriers or uses words in ways that differ from your organization's uses. | Provide translation services. |
| | Ask clarifying questions, and define your terms carefully. |
| Organization is protective of its programs and perceives other programs as potentially taking money, volunteers, or other resources away from an already limited capacity. | Discuss how the new activity or partnership will support the organization's mission and use its resources to benefit the community. |
| | Ensure that the organization has both the benefits and the responsibilities of full partnership. |

# CAREER OPPORTUNITIES

Local health departments and community health organizations are where people work and develop careers in community health promotion programming. Government agencies and community organizations operate under different personnel rules. Civil service or other personnel hiring rules bind government agencies at the local, state, and federal levels to prescribed hiring practices. Historically, the civil service has used job classifications and competitive examinations to fill vacant positions. Civil service or other government personnel systems have formal procedures for announcing and filling position vacancies. Vacancy announcements describe a job, including the title, salary, duties, qualifications and requirements, closing date, and application procedures. There is no universal format for vacancy announcements. Each government personnel system independently manages its vacancy announcement and hiring practices. Typically, vacancy announcements include a section with directions called "How to Apply." Because application procedures vary across government agencies, it is essential to follow the directions provided within each vacancy announcement. Failure to do so could result in rejection of an application.

Jobs in community health organizations often have less rigorous application processes and may require only submission of a résumé. Many types of community organizations hire individuals who are skilled in health promotion. Exhibit 15.7 lists examples of community organizations that typically advertise health promotion positions. The job title may not fully describe the responsibilities and tasks involved in a position, so it is important to read the job description closely and talk with the agency's human resource officer, the person who will supervise the position, and people in similar jobs. Some jobs require staff members to work in an office, clinic, or storefront, while other jobs require staff members to visit people at their homes or work sites. Local or overnight travel is required in some jobs. Public speaking, preparing health communication materials, maintaining electronic correspondence, and working with people in small and large groups are common and important parts of working in community health promotion settings.

Careers in local health departments and community health organizations are demanding. Although the work is rewarding, community organizations and health departments often have difficulty recruiting and retaining well-qualified staff. Geographic locations, budget constraints, low salaries, demanding workloads, and complex work tasks may create challenges, but staff members often have opportunities to develop, implement, and sometimes direct programs early in their career. There is a lot of work at the local level, and it provides excellent career development opportunities. To retain and develop staff, directors and supervisors in community organizations and health agencies provide supervision that is informative, instructive, and supportive. They offer flexible schedules, staff development and training events (for example, participation in conferences, professional associations, and online learning), and opportunities for leadership.

Other factors that may help a person obtain employment opportunities and a successful career in health departments or community organizations are having cultural competence, having personal values that align with the mission of a perspective employer, and having networking skills. Individuals who work in community health promotion interact and serve people of diverse cultural and ethnic backgrounds. Such interactions require knowledge, skill, and appreciation

## EXHIBIT 15.7
## Community Health Organizations That Post Health Promotion Jobs

- Community health centers
- Faith-based organizations or groups based in places of worship such as churches, synagogues, or mosques (for example, Catholic Charities, Council of Jewish Women)
- Community action and consumer advocacy organizations
- Local housing and homeless coalitions
- Organizations that focus on children and families (for example, Boys Clubs, Girls Clubs)
- Organizations that address birth defects and developmental impairments (for example, March of Dimes)
- Senior service and senior advocacy groups (for example, AARP chapters)
- Mental health, drug, and alcohol programs (for example, MADD)
- Organizations that address the health needs and protect the rights of people of color (for example, local chapters of the NAACP and Council of La Raza)
- Organizations that address the health needs and protect the rights of women (for example, YWCA, Big Sister Association)
- Organizations that address the health needs and protect the rights of gays and lesbians (for example, Gay Men's Health Crisis, AIDS Action)
- Disability rights organizations (for example, National Alliance for the Mentally Ill)
- Health service organizations and health reform advocacy organizations
- Organizations that address specific diseases or groups of diseases (for example, American Cancer Association, American Heart Association, and American Lung Association)
- Primary care clinics
- Hospitals
- Hospital and health care organization associations (for example American Hospital Association, American Health Care Association)
- Professional societies (for example, associations for pediatricians, nurses, health educators, nurse midwives, or physician assistants)
- Immigrant or migrant worker health rights groups (for example, Migrant Health Network)
- Regional rural health associations
- Agricultural extension offices
- Local affiliates of national organizations (such as AARP, NAACP, or YMCA)

of the assets, strengths, and differences among people of different cultures and ethnicities. Staff members of community organizations often become community leaders who serve as champions and advocates for the communities they serve. Having a passion for serving others and empathy for community members who need assistance builds support for health programs and those who work in them. Likewise, networking skills that help to build relationships with stakeholders and funders can create opportunities that contribute to effective programs and successful professionals. These three attributes contribute to health promotion professionals' being recognized, valued, and recruited for their work capabilities.

## SUMMARY

Communities are the site for many health promotion programs. Programs focus on individuals, families, and populations that reside in the community or on the environment in order to ensure safe and healthy living conditions. Local health departments and community health organizations employ people to plan, implement, and evaluate community health promotion programs. Local health departments and their partners perform the ten essential public health services (EPHS). Community health organizations focus their efforts on the unique needs and service gaps within communities. The key to effective community health promotion programs in these settings is community engagement and empowered community actions. Careers in community-level health promotion are demanding but offer many opportunities to develop as a health promotion professional. To get the most out of early job opportunities, seek out organizations that provide informative, instructive, and supportive supervision and offer continuing education opportunities.

## FOR PRACTICE AND DISCUSSION

1. Visit your local health department. What health issues are being addressed, and how is the department working to promote those health issues among local citizens?
2. Rural communities are often less able than urban communities to offer access to public health services for their community members. Name three strategies for enabling rural communities to develop and offer access to public health services.

3. Forming a coalition takes a lot of work, time, and energy. Can you identify times in your life when you felt that working with other people was problematic and that you would rather have worked alone (for example, on a class team project in which team members did not share the work evenly). If working with people can be difficult, why do you think that forming and supporting health coalitions is so important? Why not just let each person take care of himself or herself?

4. Think about the ways in which technology is currently being used to promote health for your family and friends in the community where you attended high school. Using your cell phone as the technology platform, create a new health promotion service to improve the health of your family and friends in that community.

5. Visit a local organization that is working to promote the health of community members. What is the organization's focus (for example, cancer, heart disease, alcoholism, violence)? Who participates in the organization's programs, and what are the programs? How does the organization know whether the programs are effective?

## KEY TERMS

Barriers to community
engagement

Civil service

Community empowerment

Community engagement

Community health
organizations

501(c)(3)

Local health departments

Ten essential public health
services (EPHS)

United Way

## REFERENCES

Centers for Disease Control and Prevention. (1999). Ten great public health achievements—United States, 1900–1999. *Morbidity and Mortality Weekly Report, 48*(12), 1–3.

Health District of Northern Larimer County. (n.d.). *Health promotion services*. Retrieved November 15, 2009, from http://www.healthdistrict.org/services/healthpromotion.htm.

Institute of Medicine. (2003). *Who will keep the public healthy? Educating public health professionals in the 21st century*. Washington, DC: National Academies Press.

Israel, B. A., Schultz, A. J., Parker, E. A., & Becker, A. B. (1998). Review of community-based research: Assessing partnership approaches to improve public health. *Annual Review of Public Health, 19*, 173–202.

Leep, C. J. (2006). *2005 National Profile of Local Health Departments*. Retrieved June 3, 2009, from http://www.naccho.org/topics/infrastructure/profile/upload/NACCHO_report_final_000.pdf.

Novick, L. F. (2001). Defining public health: History and contemporary developments. In L. F. Novick & G. P. Mays (Eds.), *Public health administration: Principles for population-based management* (pp. 3–33). Gaithersburg, MD: Aspen.

Office of Management and Budget. (1993). *Government Performance Results Act of 1993*. Retrieved June 10, 2009, from http://www.whitehouse.gov/omb/mgmt-gpra/gplaw2m.html.

Roussos, S., & Fawcett, S. (2000). A review of collaborative partnerships as a strategy for improving community health. *Annual Review of Public Health, 21*, 369–402.

United Way of the Capitol Region. (2009). *United Way of the Capitol Region*. Retrieved November 15, 2009, from http://www.uwcr.org/site/nonprofits.

U.S. Department of Health and Human Services, Public Health Functions Steering Committee. (2008). *Public health in America*. Retrieved November 3, 2008, from http://www.health.gov/phfunctions/public.htm.

Ward, J. W., & Warren, C. (2007). *Silent victories: The history of public health in twentieth-century America*. New York: Oxford University Press.

# Glossary

**Access.** People's ability to receive high-quality health services and care easily and in a timely and culturally sensitive fashion.

**ACHA-National College Health Assessment.** The American College Health Association's annual assessment of students at four hundred institutions of higher education. Students are assessed in the areas of smoking, contraception, mental health, relationship difficulties, sexual behaviors, exercise, preventive health practices, perceptions of drug and alcohol use, and health links to academic performance.

**Action (or behavioral) objectives.** Needed changes in actions or behaviors of the target population. Behavioral objectives are developed during program planning and are often assessed as part of the impact evaluation.

**Action plan.** A document that guides an organization's development of a health promotion program, including a mission statement, overall program goal, measurable objectives, marketing plan, evaluation plan, budget, and timeline.

**Adaptation.** The degree to which an intervention undergoes change in its implementation to fit needs of a particular delivery situation.

**Advisory boards.** Groups of key stakeholders who come together to provide program support, guidance, and oversight. These groups look different across settings. Some are formal, with bylaws, regular meeting schedules, member responsibilities, and budgets. Others are informal, perhaps without any meetings but with, instead, a loose network of individuals who will offer advice and information when called on by program staff. Advisory board members are people who have a genuine interest in the setting or program and who communicate well with others. On an advisory board, it is important to have a diverse group of constituencies and organizations represented. Also see *Wellness committee*.

**Advocacy.** The process by which individuals or groups attempt to bring about social or organizational change on behalf of a particular health goal, program, interest, or population. Advocacy activities can be political (for example, lobbying for specific legislation) or social (for example, speaking out on behalf of those without a voice). Viewed broadly, advocacy is part of being a professional in a health field.

**Advocacy agenda.** A document that defines a health promotion program's advocacy efforts and articulates its advocacy strategies, answering five key questions: What health problem does the program address? Who needs to take action? What message does this target audience need to hear? Whom does the audience need to hear the message from? What actions will you use to make your point?

**Appropriations.** Legislation that designates funding for a program.

**Audience segmentation.** The division of a target population into subgroups that share similar qualities or characteristics, such as geographic, demographic, or psychographic traits (for example, attitudes, beliefs, self-efficacy) behaviors; or readiness to change. The goal is to segment the intended audience according to characteristics that are relevant to the health behavior that needs to be changed and then to organize a program's efforts around these groups of similar individuals.

**Authorizations.** Legislation that sets policies or programs.

**Balance sheet.** A summary of an organization's balances (also called a *statement of financial position*); assets and liabilities are listed as of a specific date, such as the end of a financial year. A balance sheet is often described as a snapshot of an organization's financial condition.

**Barriers to community engagement.** Barriers that block citizens' participation in health promotion programs. From an organization's point of view, barriers may involve administrative, informational, or programmatic conflicts with a community or problems in obtaining access to a population.

**Behavior.** Any overt action, conscious or unconscious, with a measurable frequency, intensity, and duration.

**Bias.** Bias occurs when a sample is selected in a manner (for example, by a convenience sample) that results in people being left out who have unique characteristics (in terms of, for example, race or ethnicity, health beliefs or behaviors, or socioeconomic status) and that causes the final survey responses to be uncharacteristic of the overall target population.

**Bill.** A proposed law presented for approval to a legislative body.

**Board members' fundraising responsibilities.** These responsibilities involve the elements of program fundraising suited to board member interests, skills, and capabilities. Responsibilities might include providing input on a fundraising plan, identifying and cultivating new funding prospects, asking peers for donations, or accompanying staff members on key visits to funders.

**Budget.** A financial document used to project future income and expenses. The budgeting process is used by an organization to estimate whether the organization can continue to operate with its projected income and expenses.

**Capacity assessment.** Part of a needs assessment at a particular site that determines what resources—for example, health promotion materials, technology, staff, programs, funding, and services—are available as well as what gaps and needs in resources need to be filled in order to address the identified health concerns and problems. A key element of a capacity assessment is empowerment of potential program participants, staff, and stakeholders to mobilize forces to address and solve the health problems or concerns that have been identified in the needs assessment.

**Cash flow statement.** A financial statement that shows how changes in balance sheet and income accounts affect cash and cash equivalents; it analyzes the cash flows into operating, investing, and financing activities.

**CDC evaluation framework.** A six-step evaluation framework for health promotion programs that is promulgated by the Centers for Disease Control and Prevention. The six steps are as follows: (1) engage stakeholders, (2) describe the health promotion program, (3) focus the evaluation design, (4) gather credible evidence, (5) justify conclusions, and (6) ensure use of the results and share lessons learned.

**Certified Health Education Specialist (CHES).** A health educator who has successfully completed the competency-based exam given by the National Commission for Health Education Credentialing, Inc.

**Certified in Public Health (CPH).** A credential created in 2005 to ensure that graduates of institutions accredited by the Council on Education for Public Health have the knowledge and skills to be successful in the field of public health.

**Champion.** An important program stakeholder (also called *advocate*) who provides the leadership, passion, and emotion for a program. A champion knows the setting, the health problem, and the target population affected by the health problem. In the process of planning, implementing, and evaluating a program, champions often provide access to the organization. They know the history of the health issue and what has worked well in solving it as well as what has not worked. (Champions are also often called *key informants*, because they hold this key information about an organization, community, or issue.)

**Change.** The process or the result of individuals' and environments' altering, modifying, transforming, or transiting from one health status, condition, or phase to another, which health promotion programs need to accommodate.

**Channels.** The media or routes through which a health message is transmitted to its intended audience. For example, interpersonal channels include one-to-one communication; community channels reach a group of people within a distinct geographic area or a group that shares common interests or characteristics; mass media channels, which can reach large audiences quickly, include the Internet, television, radio, newspapers, magazines, outdoor or transit advertising, and direct mail.

**Characteristics of an effective health education curriculum.** Fourteen characteristics, identified by the Centers for Disease Control (CDC), that emphasize the teaching of functional knowledge (that is, essential health concepts), shape personal values and group norms for healthy behavior, and develop essential skills that students need in order to adopt and maintain healthy behaviors. These characteristics provide importance guidance for the development and evaluation of effective health education curricula and guided the revision of the National Health Education Standards.

**Circular evaluation model.** The idea that evaluations start at the beginning of a health promotion program, occurring in parallel with planning and implementation in order to provide a continual feedback loop of information that will help to improve and shape the program. Through dialogue and reflection, the information contributes to decision making and planning, which in turn leads to action. The action then prompts a new cycle of information feedback.

**Civil service.** Employment in federal, state (or provincial), and local governmental agencies that are responsible for the public administration of the government in a country.

**Client fees.** The amounts (also known as *fees for services*) that individuals pay to receive a service or participate in a program . Often services are offered at no cost to recipients because the organization collects revenue from other sources to cover the costs of offering the service or program. Increasingly, however, individuals are being asked to pay some fee for their participation. Organizations with client fees have policies that regulate the fee amounts as well as safeguards to ensure that fees are not a barrier to receiving services.

**Climate.** The social atmosphere of a setting or a learning environment, in which individuals have different experiences depending on the protocols set up by the staff and administrators.

**Coalition.** An organization of individuals representing a variety of interest groups who come together to share resources and to plan and work together.

**Collaboration.** The mutually beneficial association of two or more parties who are working to achieve a common goal.

**Collaborations and cooperative agreements.** Legal instruments, distinct from contracts, between two or more organizations that are substantially involved in carrying out specific funded activities. Typically, the organizations use their complementary strengths and resources to address a health need that otherwise might go unmet.

**Commitment to quality performance, improvement, and evaluation.** An element of effective patient-focused health promotion programs in health care organizations.

**Communication objectives.** The achievements the program staff hope to accomplish with the communications of a health promotion program.

**Communication theory.** A community-level (or setting-level) health promotion theory that focuses on (1) message production, which involves both the creation of a message and the way the message is delivered, and (2) investigation of media effects, the impacts that a health message has on one or more levels (for example, individual, group, or society).

Effective message production requires that messages be tailored to the target audience with respect to content, context, design and production, and amount and type of channels.

**Communities.** One of the four major settings for health promotion programs, communities are usually defined as places where people live—for example, neighborhoods, towns, villages, cities, and suburbs. However, communities are more than physical settings; they are also groups of people who come together for a common purpose. The people do not need to live near each other. Thus, people are members of many different communities at the same time (families, cultural or racial groups, faith organizations, fans of sports teams, hobby enthusiasts, motorcycle riders, hunger awareness groups, environmental organizations, animal rights groups, and so on). These community groups often have their own physical locations (for example, community recreation centers; golf, swimming, or tennis clubs; temples, churches, or mosques; buildings; or parks). These affinity groups are all within communities and part of communities, and at the same time, they are their own community. Health promotion programs frequently seek out people both in the physical environment of the neighborhood where they live and within the affinity groups that they identify with as their community.

**Community empowerment.** A multidimensional social process that helps people gain control over their own lives. It is a process that fosters power (that is, the capacity to implement actions or change) in people for use in their own lives, in their communities, and in their society through acting on issues that they define as important.

**Community engagement.** The participation of members of a community in assessing, planning, implementing, and evaluating solutions to problems that affect them. Levels of engagement can range from being consulted about a proposed course of action to determining the allocation of resources of a health project or being involved in the delivery of a health promotion program. Depending on a program's objectives, the issue, and the community whose engagement is sought, some approaches might be more suitable than others.

**Community health organizations.** Organizations rooted in local community members' health concerns, issues, and problems. These organizations work at the grassroots level and often operate a range of health promotion programs that target community members. Most are nonprofit organizations, exempt from paying federal, state, and local taxes in accordance with Section 501(c)(3) of the U.S. Internal Revenue Code. As such, they are not owned by an individual; by law, they are governed by a board of directors that has responsibility for the organization's operation. The term *community health organization* is synonymous with the terms *community agency*, *program*, *initiative*, *human services*, and *project*.

**Community mobilization.** Individuals' action that is organized around specific community issues. Community mobilization focuses on community-based strategies to improve health outcomes. The result is empowered communities moving forward to create change and solve problems.

**Community organizing.** Efforts to involve individuals at a site in activities ranging from defining needs for prevention of health problems to obtaining support for prevention programs. Organizing involves working with and through constituents to achieve common goals, and it emphasizes changing the social and economic structures that influence health.

**Community outreach.** Sponsored public health initiatives that use scientific advances and technology to prevent health problems and, in some cases, eliminate them by addressing them early. Community outreach was first implemented by health care organizations such as hospitals and independent clinics; today, local health departments and community health organizations also engage in community outreach.

**Community readiness model.** A model for developing a health promotion program. The model is used to assess and build a community's capacity to take action on social issues. It provides a framework for assessing the social contexts in which individual behavior takes place and for taking account of a community's culture, resources, and level of readiness to more effectively address an issue. The model consists of nine stages that can be used as a guide to assess community readiness and to determine the intervention (or interventions) that best align with each stage.

**Comprehensive work site health promotion.** Health promotion in which workplace programs are offered in order to improve employee health, decrease health care costs, reduce absenteeism, and increase productivity. A comprehensive approach includes five key elements: health education programs, a supportive social and physical environment, integration of health promotion into organizational structure, linkage to related programs, and work site screening programs.

**Concept.** A building block or primary element of a theory.

**Concept development.** The process of using the health communication plan and formative research to generate ideas that can be tested and used in the development of promotional materials.

**Consensus building.** A process for achieving general agreement among program participants and stakeholders about a particular problem, goal, or issue of mutual interest.

**Construct.** A defining element of a theory that has been adopted, developed, and tested over time.

**Content validity.** The extent to which a measure (for example, a needs assessment survey) represents and reflects all the content areas that it attempts to measure.

**Coordinated school health program.** A widely used eight-component model (created by the Centers for Disease Control and Prevention) for school health programs that promotes students' health and learning.

**Core competencies.** The eight professional competencies identified in the Galway Consensus Conference Statement as requirements for engaging in the practice of health promotion.

**Counseling, psychological, and social services.** Services that focus on behavioral health and are one component of a coordinated school health program.

**Cross-cultural staff training.** Training that focuses on staff awareness and skills in relation to program participants' cultural, linguistic, and social environment and is an overarching strategy that improves organizations' and programs' effectiveness in planning, implementing, and evaluating health promotion programs and eliminating health disparities.

**Cultural competence.** The ability to interact effectively with people of different cultures. Cultural competence comprises four components: (1) awareness of one's own cultural worldview, (2) attitude toward cultural differences, (3) knowledge of different cultural practices and worldviews, and (d) cross-cultural skills. Developing cultural competence results in an ability to understand, communicate with, and effectively interact with people across cultures.

**Cultural sensitivity.** The acknowledgment that cultural differences affect individuals' health status and health care.

**Culturally appropriate.** Conforming to a culture's acceptable expressions and standards of behavior and thoughts. Interventions and educational materials are more likely to be culturally appropriate when representatives of the intended target audience are involved in planning, developing, and pilot-testing them.

**Delphi technique.** A primary data collection method that was originally conceived as a way to obtain the opinions of experts without necessarily bringing them together face to face. The technique is now used with groups of stakeholders with knowledge and expertise about a health concern or area. A group is guided through a series of qualitative data collections in which initial data are collected from the group and then used to determine subsequent data collection questions with the purpose of clarifying the health needs of a target population.

**Diffusion of innovations model.** A community-level (or setting-level) health theory that focuses on the dissemination of new ideas and their adoption by people in a systematic manner. In addition, it is a tool for analyzing social change.

**Direct lobbying.** Communication with a legislator or his or her staff member that conveys a viewpoint about specific legislation.

**Disability.** A factor that can be a determinant of health disparities.

**Diversity.** Individual differences along the dimensions of race, ethnicity, gender, sexual orientation, socioeconomic status, age, physical abilities, religious beliefs, political beliefs, health or disease status, or other conditions or ideologies. The concept of diversity encompasses acceptance and respect and an understanding that each individual is unique.

**Ecological health perspective.** A perspective that emphasizes the interaction between and the interdependence of factors within and across levels of a health problem. It highlights people's interaction with their physical and sociocultural environments, and it identifies three levels of influence for health-related behaviors and conditions: (1) the intrapersonal or individual level; (2) the interpersonal level; and (3) the community or setting level, which includes institutional or organizational factors, community factors, and public policy factors.

**Education.** A factor that can be a determinant of health disparities.

**Education entertainment.** The blending of core communication theories and fundamental entertainment pedagogy to guide the preparation and delivery of health communications.

**Electioneering.** The persuasion of voters in a political campaign.

**Elevator speech.** A concise statement, usually fifteen or so seconds long, that highlights program features such as mission, goals, setting, and outcomes.

**Employee assistance programs (EAPs).** Services provided free of charge to employees by an employer through outside agencies in order to allow confidential assessment, referral, and short-term counseling for personal problems.

**Environmental factors.** A cause of racial and ethnic disparities. Examples include exposure to toxins, viral or microbial agents, poor or unsafe physical and social environment, inadequate access to nutritious food and exercise, and community norms that do not support protective behaviors.

**Equity.** Equal opportunity and treatment for members of minority groups.

**Ethnicity.** This factor can be a determinant of health disparities.

**Evaluation costs.** The expense of conducting an evaluation, which is related to the complexity of the program being evaluated and the program's internal resources and expertise.

**Evaluation design.** The characteristics of an evaluation that must be carefully chosen in order to achieve the evaluation's purpose and meet the needs of the users who will receive the results. Evaluation design should also focus on developing answerable questions and reasonable methods and on reaching agreement on the roles and responsibilities of those conducting the evaluation. An evaluation may be designed to use qualitative methods, quantitative methods, or a combination of the two.

**Evaluation ethics.** Ethics that relate to safeguarding and protecting program participants' rights.

**Evaluation highlights.** An overview of an evaluation and of its significant findings.

**Evaluation report.** A report on the outcome of a health program evaluation. It typically consists of a cover page, executive summary, introduction, the evaluation questions, methods and results, and findings and recommendations.

**Evidence-based interventions.** Programs that have been evaluated as effective in addressing a specific health-related condition, in the context of a particular ethnicity or culture. These programs identify the target populations that benefited from the program, the conditions under which the program works, and sometimes the change mechanisms that account for their effects. They use various tested strategies that target a disease or behavior. A defining characteristic of evidence-based interventions is their use of health theory both in developing the content of the interventions (for example, activities, curriculum, or tasks) and evaluation (for example, measures and outcomes).

**Evidence-based practices.** Commonly used activities and strategies in health promotion programs that are based on sound science and theory; a logic model matches the science and theory to the intended outcomes of interest for a particular target population at a setting.

**Face validity.** How functional a measure (for example, a needs assessment survey) appears to be. Does it seem to be a reasonable way to gain the desired information? Does it seem well designed? Does it seem as though it will work reliably?

**Family and community involvement.** A component of a coordinated school health program; it requires involving and engaging family members and community members in promoting the health of school-age children and adolescents.

**Fidelity.** The extent to which the delivery of a health intervention conforms to the curriculum, protocol, or guidelines for implementing that intervention. Intervention fidelity is rated from high to low. A high-fidelity intervention is one that is delivered almost exactly as intended by the people who created it. A low-fidelity program is one that is delivered quite differently than intended by the people who created it.

**Fiscal management.** The maintaining of sound records and procedures in order to safeguard and maximize a program's money, assets, and resources, which protects the program's sustainability and allows it to operate with economy, effectiveness, and efficiency.

**Fiscal year.** The dates that establish a program's funding year. Some grants or contracts begin on January 1 and end on December 31, so the funding cycle aligns with the calendar year. Other funding, particularly that associated with schools or universities, begins on July 1 and ends on June 30. Still other funds may have a start date based on the day the award was made—March 1, October 1, or any other month.

**501(c)(3).** A section of the U.S. tax code that exempts certain types of organizations from federal taxation of income. Organizations apply to the Internal Revenue Service and, if they qualify under Section 501(c)(3), they are declared tax-exempt. Organizations that qualify for 501(c)(3) status are primarily schools, colleges, universities, religious organizations, and charitable organizations (for example, community health organizations). Many health promotion programs are part of 501(c)(3) or government agencies.

**Focus group.** A qualitative data collection technique in which a small group of individuals meet to share their views and experiences in regard to some topic. The ideal group size depends, in part, on the skills of the facilitator.

**Formative evaluation.** The gathering of information and materials to aid program planning and development. This type of evaluation can be used to understand needs assessment data that were gathered during the program planning process.

**Formative research (or consumer research).** Research focused on the intended audience: who they are, what is important to them, what influences their behavior, and what will enable them to engage in the desired behavior. Formative research may also determine the intended audience's readiness to change, the social or cultural factors that might affect the program, how best to reach the audience, the audience's preferred communication channels, and the audience's preferred learning styles, language, and tone.

**Foundations.** Entities that are established as nonprofit corporations or charitable trusts with the principal purpose of making grants to unrelated organizations or institutions or to individuals for scientific, educational, cultural, religious, or other charitable purposes.

**Fundraising.** The process of soliciting and gathering money or in-kind gifts by requesting donations from individuals, businesses, charitable foundations, or governmental agencies. Some organizations have staff members who are dedicated solely to fundraising.

**Fundraising field.** This field advances philanthropy through advocacy, research, education, and certification programs. It fosters development and growth of fundraising professionals and promotes high ethical standards in the fundraising profession. The field has its roots in the belief that in order to guarantee human freedom and social creativity, people must have the right to freely and voluntarily form organizations to meet perceived needs, advocate causes, and seek funds to support these activities.

**Fundraising professionals.** Individuals who advance philanthropy through responsibilities that include writing grant proposals, researching requests for proposals from foundations and corporations, overseeing and implementing fundraising plans and strategies, and establishing structures for effective fundraising.

**Galway Consensus Conference Statement.** A product of the 2008 Galway Consensus Conference to promote global exchange and understanding in regard to eight domains of core competency in the professional preparation and practice of health promotion and health education specialists.

**Gantt chart.** A visual depiction of the schedule for completing a program's objectives—that is, a timeline for program implementation.

**Gender.** A factor that can be a determinant of health disparities.

**Geographic information system (GIS).** A technique used in needs assessment data analyses and reporting. A GIS uses computer software to capture, store, analyze, manage, and present data that are linked to location, allowing people to view, understand, question, interpret, and visualize data in ways that reveal relationships, patterns, or trends in the form of maps, reports, and charts. A GIS helps to answer questions and solve problems by presenting data in a way that is quickly understood and easily shared.

**Geographic location.** A factor that can be a determinant of health disparities.

**Goal.** A statement of a program's direction and intent. Program goals clarify what is important in a health promotion program and state the end results of the program. A goal includes the program's target population and, in general, uses action words such as *reduce*, *eliminate*, or *increase*.

**Grant-writing process.** A fundraising endeavor that involves assembling information in accordance with funders' guidelines. The process requires identifying potential grant sources; formulating a plan for gathering and organizing grant information before beginning to write; producing, reviewing, and submitting a proposal; and following up on the proposal submission. Typically, the process must be completed with limited staff and time constraints; thus good time management and organization are essential.

**Grants.** Sums of money that are awarded to finance a particular activity or program. Generally, these grant awards do not need to be paid back.

**Grassroots lobbying.** Any attempt to indirectly influence legislators by motivating members of the public to express their views to legislators and legislative aides.

**Health.** A resource for everyday life, not the object of living. It is a positive concept that emphasizes social and personal resources as well as physical capabilities.

**Health belief model.** An individual-level health theory that attempts to explain and predict health behaviors by focusing on the attitudes and beliefs of individuals.

**Health care organizations.** One of the four major settings for health promotion programs, these organizations provide health care to reduce the impact and burden of illness, injury, and disability and to improve the health and functioning of individuals. Health care organizations include community hospitals, specialty hospitals, community health centers, physician offices, clinics, rehabilitation centers, skilled nursing and long-term care facilities, and home health and other health-related entities.

**Health communication.** The art and technique of informing, influencing, and motivating individual, institutional, and public audiences in regard to important health issues. Health communication is a multifaceted and multidisciplinary approach to reaching different audiences and sharing health-related information with the goal of influencing, engaging, and supporting individuals, communities, health professionals, special groups, policymakers, and the public in championing, introducing, adopting, or sustaining a behavior, practice, or policy that will ultimately improve health outcomes.

**Health communication plan.** A plan that guides and develops information exchange between and among a health program's staff, stakeholders, and participants, so that program communications deliver clear messages that are received and acted on with behavior that is consistent with the program's goals and objectives.

**Health disparities.** Differences among populations in health status, behavior, and outcomes due to gender, income, education, disability, geographic location, sexual orientation, and race or ethnicity.

**Health education.** A discipline with a distinct body of knowledge, a code of ethics, a skill-based set of competencies, a rigorous system of quality assurance, and a system of credentialing health education professionals. Health education is one component of a coordinated school health program.

**Health Education Curriculum Analysis Tool.** A tool designed to help school districts, schools, and others analyze health education curricula on the basis of the National Health Education Standards and the Centers for Disease Control and Prevention's characteristics of an effective health education curriculum. It includes questions for analyzing the overall characteristics of a curriculum as well as the specific health-related behaviors, functional knowledge, skills, and subskills addressed in the curriculum.

**Health insurance.** Insurance that provides protection against the costs of hospital and medical care or against lost income arising from an illness or injury. The majority of Americans have group health insurance coverage through their employer or the employer of a family member. Most health insurance benefits are defined by an employer's agreement with a health insurance company. Increasingly, health insurance companies are offering employers a range of products and services, depending on the needs of the employees. Health insurance coverage purchased by an employer is offered to eligible employees (and often to employees' family members) as a benefit of working for that company.

**Health literacy.** The capacity of an individual to obtain, interpret, comprehend, and assess health information and services in order to make informed health decisions and take health-enhancing actions in regard to healthy behaviors, self-care, or disease management.

**Health promotion.** The planned change of health-related lifestyles and life conditions through any combination of health education and related organizational, economic, or environmental supports for behavior of individuals, groups, or sites that is conducive to health.

**Health promotion for staff.** A component of a coordinated school health program; it involves promoting the health of a school's faculty and staff.

**Health promotion policies.** Operating rules for health promotion programs that specify people's rights and responsibilities as well as spell out the rights and responsibilities of the organization in regard to its stakeholders (for example, students, employees, clients, or members).

**Health promotion programs.** Programs that provide planned, organized, and structured activities and events over time that focus on helping individuals make informed decisions about their health. In addition, health promotion programs promote policy, environmental, regulatory, organizational, and legislative changes at various levels of government and organizations. Health promotion programs are often designed to take advantage of their pivotal position within settings such as schools, workplaces, health care organizations, or communities, combining interventions in an integrated, systemic manner in order to effectively reach children, adults, and families. Two common program types, found in health care organizations and in communities, are patient-focused programs and employee programs.

**Health protection.** The provision of safe work conditions, particularly through limiting hazardous exposures.

**Health risk appraisal.** An assessment of employees' or other beneficiaries' health risks, interest in participating in specific programs, and readiness to change unhealthy lifestyle habits. A health risk appraisal may also be called a *health assessment questionnaire* or *health improvement questionnaire.*

**Health services.** A component of a coordinated school health program; it focuses on physical health.

**Health status.** The overall evaluation of an individual's degree of wellness or illness with a number of indicators, including morbidity, impairments, mortality, functional status, and quality of life.

**Health-promoting universities.** An initiative that applies the principles of K–12 coordinated school health programs to colleges and universities. Program goals include improving the health of students, university personnel, and the wider community as well as integrating health into a university's culture, structure, and processes.

**Healthy People 2020.** A strategic plan for public health practitioners and policymakers that sets measurable objectives at the national level.

**Healthy school environment.** A component of a coordinated school health program; it involves creating and sustaining a healthy, safe, and drug-free school environment.

**Hook.** In advocacy, something that gets people's attention and raises their awareness of an issue. Providing a hook or a sound bite allows programmers to frame a health issue in a way that increases the chance that people will discuss the issue in appropriate terms.

**Ideas.** Abstract entities that are building blocks or primary elements of a theory.

**Impact evaluation.** An evaluation that measures the immediate effects of a health promotion program and the extent to which program goals that could lead to the program's ultimate desired outcome (for example, changes in self-efficacy that could lead to a desired behavior change) were attained. The primary question in an impact evaluation is what has been the immediate effect on the program's participants?

**Implementation challenges.** Challenges often encountered when moving through a program's implementation stages, especially program installation, initial implementation, and full operation.

**Implementation stages.** The phases in the process of creating a health promotion program, moving from exploration of the idea through long-term program operation.

**Income.** This factor can be a determinant of health disparities.

**Income statement.** A statement that shows the financial performance of an organization over a specified time period—typically a year.

**Indicated preventive interventions.** Interventions that target high-risk individuals who have detectable signs or symptoms but have not reached the diagnostic criteria for a particular health problem. An example of an indicated preventive intervention is a smoking cessation program for heavy smokers.

**Individual and behavioral factors.** A cause of racial and ethnic disparities. One example of such a factor is participation in high-risk behaviors such as smoking, not wearing a seat belt, choosing a sedentary lifestyle, and eating poorly.

**Individual-level certification and licensure.** Credentials issued by a recognized professional credentialing body to individuals who meet specified criteria (for example, by passing an examination, gaining professional experience, completing continuing education, or obtaining recommendations) that demonstrate competence in professional skills, the ability to deliver quality services, and ethical practice.

**Infrastructure (operating, core, or hard) funding.** Monies that an organization obtains in order to operate its infrastructure before offering any program, activities, or services. Such monies might pay for the director's salary, staff salaries, rent, janitorial services, clerical staff and bookkeeping, or payroll operations.

**Institute of Medicine obesity evaluation framework.** A framework used to assess progress in a range of childhood obesity prevention efforts across different sectors and settings. The framework recognizes the impact of key contextual factors (for example, environmental, cultural, normative, and behavioral factors) on the potential impact of an intervention. It also categorizes outcomes according to the nature of the change.

**Institute of Medicine's model of preventive intervention.** This model identifies and categorizes preventive interventions for different target populations and different health problems and concerns.

**Institutionalized racism.** Differential access to goods, services, resources, and opportunities by race.

**Intended audience.** The audience for whom the health communication is developed—that is, the intended receivers and users of a health communication. A clear understanding of the intended audience helps program staff to tailor program communication to the health needs of the audience and make the best use of resources for producing the communication.

**Interdisciplinary, collaborative approach.** An element of effective patient-focused health promotion programs in health care organizations.

**Intermediate outcomes.** In a logic model, the results that may or may not be seen after a single activity but that are expected to happen in the future and also to be measured at some point in the future.

**Internalized racism.** The acceptance by individuals of negative messages from others about their worth and abilities as members of a stigmatized race. It manifests as self-devaluation, helplessness, and hopelessness, potentially leading to risky behaviors that can endanger a person's health.

**Interpersonal level.** The facet of the ecological health perspective that focuses on the influences of interpersonal processes and primary groups that provide social identity, support, and role definition (for example, family, friends, and peers).

**Intervention.** Any set of methods, techniques, activities, or processes designed to effect changes in behaviors or the environment.

**Intervention mapping.** A model that provides health promotion program planners with a framework for effective decision making at each stage of intervention planning, implementation, and evaluation. The framework consists of six steps: (1) needs assessment, (2) matrices, (3) theory-based methods and practical strategies, (4) program, (5) adoption and implementation plan, and (6) evaluation plan.

**Intrapersonal level.** The facet of the ecological health perspective that focuses on individual characteristics that influence behavior, such as knowledge, attitudes, beliefs, and personality traits.

*Jakarta Declaration on Leading Health Promotion into the 21st Century.* An agreement signed at the World Health Organization's Fourth International Conference on Health Promotion, which was held in Jakarta in 1997. The declaration reiterated the importance of the agreements made in the *Ottawa Charter for Health Promotion* and added emphasis to certain aspects of health promotion. It gave new prominence to the concept of the health setting as the place or social context in which people engage in daily activities in which environmental, organizational, and personal factors interact to affect health and well-being.

**Key informant.** An individual who possesses unique and important information that can provide insights into the health issues at a site.

**Key informant interviews.** A primary data collection method that uses structured and unstructured interviews to collect qualitative data from key informants.

**Lalonde report.** Titled *A New Perspective on the Health of Canadians*, this report was produced in Canada in 1974. It is considered the first modern government document in the Western world to acknowledge that our emphasis on a biomedical health care system might be misplaced and that governments need to look beyond the traditional health care system (which actually is a sick care system) in order to improve the health of the public.

**Law.** In federal government, a bill that has passed both the U.S. Senate and the U.S. House of Representatives and has been signed by the president (or that Congress has passed by overriding a presidential veto).

**Letter to the editor.** A letter written by an individual citizen to a newspaper editor as a means of sharing his or her opinion and inspiring others to take positive action on an issue of concern. Political leaders and other policymakers rely on editorials in newspapers and blogs to gauge the views of their constituents. The philanthropic actions of community health organizations are often inspired by issues facing the community that were initially brought to the public's attention through letters to the editor. Also see *Op-ed*.

**Linear evaluation model.** A model that embodies the concept that evaluation is the last phase of a health promotion program and is conducted only after a program is complete.

**Local health departments.** Local public agencies that are part of the government's efforts to support healthy lifestyles and create environments that support health. Their many responsibilities include sanitation, disease surveillance, and monitoring of environmental risks (for example, lead or asbestos poisoning) and ecological risks (for example, destruction of the ozone layer or air and water pollution). The staff at a local health department typically include a wide variety of professionals who promote health in the community, such as public health physicians, nurses, public health educators, community health workers, epidemiologists, and sanitarians.

**Logic model.** A visual depiction of the underlying logic of a planned program. It shows the relationships between the program's resources (inputs), its planned activities (outputs), and the changes that are expected as a result (outcomes). Logic models can take many forms, but all are designed to provide a simple graphic illustration of the assumed relationships between the activities that will be initiated and the results anticipated. A logic model reads from left to right. Each column flows into the next, indicating that achieving what is shown in one column depends on achieving what is shown in the column before it. Thus, a logic model shows what a program's planners are assuming will happen as the program progresses.

**Long-term outcomes.** In a logic model, the results that represent the ultimate extension of a program's impact. If the program's activities are effective and achieve both the short-term and intermediate outcomes, the logic model specifies the related long-term results that might be reasonably expected. Most health promotion programs are designed to achieve a long-term outcome that is health-related or disease-related.

**MADD.** See *Mothers Against Drunk Driving*.

**Mastering change.** A process of supporting and engaging people and resources in the context of an evolving and dynamic environment in order to enhance program staff members' and participants' health status, develop networks of people committed to health promotion, and improve health promotion program outcomes and impacts.

**MATCH model.** See *Multilevel approach to community health (MATCH) model*.

**Matching funds, cost sharing, and in-kind contributions.** All these terms refer to monies and resources that are provided by one group or organization to another organization for its operations or programs. Matching funds are monies paid concurrently with the expenditure funds for the operation of a program. Cost sharing applies to monies that have to be spent by the time a program concludes. In-kind contributions are non-cash contributions (for example, materials, equipment, vehicles, or food) used to operate programs or services.

**Media advocacy.** The strategic use of news media and, when appropriate, paid advertising in order to support community organizing to advance a public policy initiative.

**Medical care factors.** These factors can be a cause of racial and ethnic disparities. Examples include lack of access to health care, lack of quality health care, and providers who lack cultural competence.

**Medical decision making.** The process by which individuals and families use medical and health-related information and experience, in conjunction with medical and health professionals, to decide how to address medical and health problems and concerns.

**Message concepts.** Health communication messages intended to present ideas to an audience. Concepts are not the final messages but rather the starting point for developing health communications.

**Mission.** The general focus or purpose of a program. The mission explains why a health promotion program is being established or developed and reflects the program's values. A program's mission is communicated to stakeholders and participants and to the general public via a mission statement.

**Mixed or integrated methods.** The combination of qualitative and quantitative methods in an evaluation.

**Model.** A model draws on two or more health theories to address a specific health problem, event, or situation.

**Mothers Against Drunk Drinking (MADD).** An advocacy group founded by Candy Lightner after her daughter was killed by a drunk driver. MADD used media advocacy to advance a campaign to educate the public about the dangers of drunk driving. MADD's media advocacy has been recognized as the impetus that inspired a change in public policy related to the legal drinking age and reduction in drunk-driving fatalities.

**Multilevel approach to community health (MATCH) model.** A model that guides health professionals in developing, implementing, and evaluating health programs. It is composed of five main phases, which are subdivided into steps. The phases are goal selection, intervention planning, program development, implementation preparation, and evaluation.

**National Health Education Standards.** A framework for state and local initiatives related to school health education curriculum, instruction, and assessment. The performance indicators identify the key concepts, skills, or elements of skills that students need to know or be able to do, as well as the beliefs, values, and norms that students need to espouse in order to demonstrate achievement of each standard.

**National Partnership for Action to End Health Disparities.** A partnership created by the Office of Minority Health in the U.S. Department of Health and Human Services as part of its strategic framework for eliminating health disparities. The partnership identified twenty strategies that health promotion programs should implement in order to eliminate health disparities.

**National Registry of Evidence-Based Programs and Practices (NREPP).** A searchable database of interventions for the prevention and treatment of mental and substance use disorders. NREPP, a service of the Substance Abuse and Mental Health Services Administration in the U.S. Department of Health and Human Services, was developed as a resource to help people, agencies, and organizations implement evidence-based programs and practices in their communities.

**Need.** The difference between "what is" at the present time and "what should be" under more ideal circumstances.

**Needs assessment.** The process of obtaining information about individuals' health needs and a site's available support and resources for the purpose of planning, implementing, and evaluating a program. Making sure that a health promotion program addresses the needs of the people at the site of the program is critical to its success.

**Needs assessment report.** The final product of a needs assessment. It contains an executive summary, acknowledgments, table of contents, demographics of the community or setting (for example, a school or workplace), methods of data collection, the main findings, established priorities, references, and appendixes. The report is often used as a resource during a program's implementation and evaluation.

**Networking.** The action of building alliances to address a health problem or concern; it involves deliberate action to get to know people, resources, and organizations.

**Nonprofit sector.** A sector of the economy that comprises organizations that operate for the benefit of the community and meet the federal criteria for exemption from paying taxes. Any money generated from these organizations' operations is directed back to the community rather than to personal gain or profit. Foundations and charitable organizations are included in this sector and are an important source of funding for health promotion programs.

**NREPP.** See *National Registry of Evidence-Based Programs and Practices.*

**Nutrition services.** A component of a coordinated school health program; it involves providing healthy food services that reflect students' culture and offering nutrition screening and counseling.

**Objectives.** The specific steps (or subgoals) that need to be completed in order to attain program goals. They are specific and measurable targets with a timeline that identifies by when the objective will be attained. An objective statement specifies who, what, when, and where and clarifies by how much, how many, or how often. Each objective makes clear what is expected and is stated in such a way that its achievement can be measured. Types of objectives are process objectives, action objectives, and outcome objectives.

**Office of Minority Health.** An agency established in 1986 by the U.S. Department of Health and Human Services (DHHS). Its mission is to improve and protect the health of racial and ethnic minority populations through the development of health policies and programs that will eliminate health disparities. It advises the DHHS secretary and the Office of Public Health and Science on public health program activities affecting American Indians and Alaska Natives, Asian Americans, Blacks/African Americans, Hispanics/Latinos, Native Hawaiians, and other Pacific Islanders.

**Op-ed.** An abbreviation of *opposite the editorial page* (though it is often believed to be an abbreviation of *opinion editorial*). An op-ed is a newspaper article that expresses the opinions of a named writer who is usually unaffiliated with the newspaper's editorial board. Op-eds are different from editorials, which are usually unsigned and written by members of the editorial board.

**Ordinance.** A local statute or regulation, usually enacted by a city government.

**Ottawa Charter.** An agreement developed at the first International Conference on Health Promotion, held in Ottawa, Canada, in 1986. The charter identifies the prerequisites for health; methods of achieving health promotion through advocacy, enabling, and mediation; and five key strategies: build healthy public policy; create supportive environments; strengthen community action; develop personal skills; and reorient health services.

**Outcome evaluation.** Assessment of the impact or bottom-line results of an intervention; it answers the question, What was the effect or impact of the health programs offered? Outcome evaluation examines the changes in the target population during or after their participation in a health promotion program. Although the ultimate goal of health promotion programs is to improve a population's health status (for example, by reducing lung cancer), funding and time limitations often force program managers to choose outcomes that are proxy measures for long-term outcomes. Some examples of proxies are measures of knowledge gains, attitude changes, skills acquired, or behavior changes. Depending on its design, the outcome evaluation might examine changes in the short term (hours or days after program participation), intermediate term (one to six months), or long term (six months to a few years).

**Outcome objectives.** The specific, measurable long-term accomplishments (targets) of a health promotion program.

**Outreach.** The intentional sharing of information about a health promotion program with specific individuals and groups for the purpose of educating them about the program and for developing support for program participants.

**Partnerships.** Mutually beneficial relationships between organizations, built on trust and commitment and usually intended to extend the reach and effectiveness of a health promotion program. Partner organizations are generally equal in their relationships and agree on their mutual effort's goals and objectives.

**Patient and family education.** The ongoing process of educating patients and family members about an illness in order to improve their coping skills and their ability to make decisions related to the illness. Patient-focused health promotion programs can trace their roots to patient and family education. For years, patients and their families relied on physicians and nurses as their main educational sources; these professionals shared information about a disease, discussed proposed treatments as well as potential side effects of the treatments, and prepared patients and family members for the patient's return to his or her home environment or transfer to another health care setting.

**Patient- and family-centered care.** According to the Institute for Family-Centered Care, this is "an approach to the planning, delivery, and evaluation of health care that is grounded in mutually beneficial partnerships among health care patients, families, and providers" and built on the four core concepts of dignity and respect, information sharing, participation, and collaboration.

**Patient safety.** Patient safety was greatly improved in the 1980s and 1990s when hospital operations were scrutinized and emphasis was placed on efficient service delivery and improved working conditions. Patient safety programs laid the groundwork for health promotion programs in health care organizations.

**PEARL model.** An approach to making decisions about interventions in health promotion programs. The model consists of five exterior feasibility factors that have a high degree of influence in determining how a particular problem can be addressed: propriety, economic feasibility, acceptability, resources, and legality.

**Performance evaluation.** A way for program directors and supervisors to evaluate staff on a continual basis. Such ongoing evaluation starts with staff goals that are formulated in partnership with supervisors and that meet staff, program, and organizational needs. These goals provide the blueprint for staff work, are discussed in regularly scheduled meetings with the primary supervisor, and are adjusted as necessary on the basis of changes at the staff, program, or organizational level. Workplace performance evaluation is often thought to mean year-end reviews that determine raises, bonuses, or even job cuts. While annual reviews play a role in performance evaluation, the focus should be on synthesizing and summarizing staff performance instead of providing a single high-stakes, make-or-break performance rating.

**Personally mediated racism.** Discrimination in which the majority racial group treats members of a minority group as inferior and views the minorities' abilities, motives, and intents through a lens of prejudice based on race. This type of racism is what most individuals think of when they hear the term *racism*.

**Physical education.** A component of a coordinated school health program; it focuses on physical activity.

**Plain language.** Language that audience members can understand the first time they read it or hear it. Presenting health information in plain language (or plain English) is an integral component of improving health literacy.

**Policies.** Operating rules that provide a program's stakeholders (for example, students, employees, clients, and members) with their organizational rights and responsibilities. Policies are the backbone of health promotion programs; they provide program infrastructure. Effective policies clearly state the health values and priorities of the organization and are tailored to the unique requirements and needs of the setting and stakeholders. Program procedures are drawn from program policies.

**Policy and environmental change.** An intervention approach to reducing the burden of chronic diseases that focuses on enacting effective policies (for example, laws, regulations, or formal or informal rules) or promoting environmental change (for example, changes in economic, social, or physical environments).

**Population level.** The facet of the ecological health perspective that focuses on institutional or organizational factors, social capital factors, and public policy factors.

**Power analysis.** An analysis to ensure having an adequate number of people participating in a needs assessment (that is, a survey), in order to be able to generalize the findings from the sample to the population.

**PRECEDE-PROCEED model.** A model that consists of eight phases that guide planners in developing health promotion programs, beginning with more general outcomes and moving to more specific outcomes. The PRECEDE portion of the model focuses on program planning, while the PROCEED portion focuses on implementation and evaluation. Gradually, the process leads to creation of a program, delivery of the program, and evaluation of the program.

**Pretesting.** A way to determine which message or what material best fulfills the requirements of a program's communication plan in order to ensure that the intended audience will understand and act on the materials developed for the program.

**Primary data.** Data obtained directly from individuals at a site, providing new information that will be used to answer specific questions. Primary data are new, original data that did not previously exist, often collected through surveys, interviews, focus groups, or direct observation.

**Primary health promotion.** The use of health promotion programs designed to identify and strengthen protective ecological conditions that are conducive to health, and to identify and reduce various health risks in order to prevent illness.

**Primary prevention.** Taking action prior to the onset (new incidents) of a health problem to intercept its causation or to modify its course before people are involved.

**Priorities.** The intervention points and strategies of a health promotion program that are derived from analyzing the collected data of a needs assessment. Approaches to establishing priorities from data include the nominal group process and the PEARL model.

**Priority population.** A defined group of individuals who share some common characteristics related to the health concern being addressed. Frequently the term *program participants* is synonymous with *priority population*.

**Privacy of patient health information.** A unique challenge that arises for workers in a health care organization. The privacy provisions of the Health Insurance Portability and Accountability Act of 1996 (HIPAA), a federal law, apply to health information created or maintained by health care providers who engage in certain electronic transactions, health plans, and health care clearinghouses.

**Private sector.** A sector of the economy that comprises large and small businesses that are operated to generate profits for owners and shareholders. Businesses pay taxes. In the United States, 65 percent of the workforce has a job in the private sector.

**Process evaluation.** An evaluation intended to learn why and how an intervention worked and for whom it worked best and worst; it answers the question, Were the selected programs, policies, or environmental supports implemented as intended? Process evaluation involves systematically gathering information during program implementation. It is useful for formally monitoring implementation, for identifying necessary changes to a program's implementation, and for overall improvement of a health promotion program or any one of its individual strategies.

**Process objectives.** The specific, measurable outcomes that identify needed changes or tasks in the administration of a program (for example, hiring staff, providing professional development for staff, or seeking additional funding). This type of objective is used to evaluate progress in the implementation of the program (process or formative evaluation).

**Professional preparation program accreditation.** Credentials issued by a recognized professional credentialing body to organizations and programs that set specific criteria that demonstrate the competence of professional staff, high-quality service delivery, and ethical practice.

**Program evaluation.** An evaluation that involves systematically collecting information about a health promotion program in order to answer questions and make decisions about the program. There are several kinds of program evaluation, including *formative evaluation*, *process evaluation*, *impact evaluation*, and *outcome evaluation*.

**Program procedures.** Program supports that are drawn from the program policies; they address program logistics and day-to-day operating details such as program participant rights, protection, recruitment, retention, and recognition. Also see *Standard operating procedures*.

**Program sustainability.** The likelihood that a program will remain viable and available over a period of time.

**Public funds.** Tax dollars that are collected and spent by the government to provide the infrastructure for the systems and organizations that operate state and local health and human services.

**Public sector.** A sector of the economy that comprises federal, state, and local governments that generate money through taxes (for example, personal income, property, business, and sales taxes). Federal, state, and local governments are also sources of legislation, resources, and research. Public schools and colleges are part of the public sector. (Private and parochial schools and college are part of the private or nonprofit sectors.)

**Public service announcements (PSAs).** Noncommercial advertisements broadcast on radio or television in the public interest. PSAs are intended to modify public attitudes by raising awareness about specific issues. The most common topics of PSAs are health and safety. A typical PSA is part of a public awareness campaign to inform or educate the public about an issue such as smoking or compulsive gambling.

**Qualitative data.** Data that are more narrative than numerical, derived more from perceptions than statistical measures (see *Qualitative methods*).

**Qualitative methods.** Methods of research that involve gathering non-numerical data, including program descriptions that often include the perspectives and experiences of the program participants themselves. Qualitative data consist primarily of information gathered from interviews with key informants (for example, policymakers), observations of program intervention activities (for example, nutritious meal preparation), and focus groups with people who may share common values or experiences (for example, a gay and lesbian focus group discussing their experience and knowledge of tobacco use in the GLBT community).

**Quality of life.** The degree to which an individual can enjoy his or her life.

**Quantitative data.** Statistical information and measures, such as percentages, means, or correlations (see *quantitative methods*).

**Quantitative methods.** Methods of research that involve gathering and analyzing numerical data. Various techniques are then used to make sense of numbers or scores in order to interpret the results of a program or intervention. Numerical data might take the form of a summary of demographic variables, pretest and posttest scores, attitude and self-efficacy ratings, or previously existing numerical data.

**Race.** A factor that can be a determinant of health disparities.

**Racism.** The belief that race is the primary determinant of human traits and capacities and that racial differences produce an inherent superiority of a particular race. Three types of racism affect health outcomes: institutionalized racism, personally mediated racism, and internalized racism.

**Random selection.** A technique that involves selecting members of a population in such a way that each member has an equal chance of being selected to participate (to receive a survey questionnaire, for example).

**REACH communities.** Communities that are participating in the Centers for Disease Control and Prevention's Project REACH (Racial and Ethnic Approaches to Community Health), which engages minority groups and communities directly in addressing health issues.

**RE-AIM evaluation framework.** With five dimensions—reach, effectiveness, adoption, implementation, and maintenance—the RE-AIM evaluation framework recognizes the importance of both external validity (reach and adoption) and internal validity (efficacy and implementation) in the evaluation of program interventions. It is useful in estimating public health impact, comparing different health policies, designing policies for increased likelihood of success, and identifying areas for integration of policies with other health promotion strategies.

**Referral.** The process of connecting a person to a health promotion program. Program staff identify where potential program participants are and who can direct these individuals to the program.

**Regulations, restrictions, and guidelines.** Health care organizations are subject to many regulations, restrictions, and guidelines that are not found in other settings and that govern the organizations' policies and procedures. Health workers need to understand these regulations and their practical, day-to-day implementation.

**Reliability.** The ability of an evaluation instrument (for example, a needs assessment survey) to provide consistent results each time it is used.

**Research-Tested Intervention Programs (RTIPs).** A searchable database of evidence-based health promotion interventions, developed as a resource to help people, agencies, and organizations implement research-tested programs and practices in their communities. RTIPs is a service of the National Cancer Institute in the National Institutes of Health, U.S. Department of Health and Human Services.

**Response bias.** Bias that occurs when the people who respond to a survey (for example, as part of a needs assessment) are different in their health beliefs or behaviors from those who do not respond to the survey. The more the beliefs and behaviors of the respondents differ from the beliefs and behaviors of the nonrespondents, the greater the magnitude of the response bias.

**Return on investment.** A financial indicator that evaluates the worth of a project by comparing its benefits (return) with its cost (investment).

**Root causes of health disparities.** Systemic, institutionalized sources of health disparities that have been many decades or even centuries in the making. The relationships among the root causes of health disparities are multidirectional and cyclical, exacerbating one another and calling for intervention at every level.

**RTIPs.** See *Research-Tested Intervention Programs.*


**Sample.** The group of individuals who are the primary data source in a survey or intervention (for example, in a needs assessment). Three considerations are key to obtaining needs assessment results that accurately represent the health-related perceptions, behaviors, and needs of the entire group or community that is being assessed. First is correctly selecting the people who will receive the questionnaire. Second is selecting a large enough sample that the results will represent the entire population. Third is making sure the return rate is high enough (better than 50 percent) to reach this adequate sample size.

**Sampling bias.** Bias that occurs when the sample is selected in a manner that omits people who have unique characteristics (for example, race or ethnicity, health beliefs or behaviors, or socioeconomic status), which results in final survey responses that are uncharacteristic of the population.

**School Health Index.** A self-assessment and planning tool that schools can use to improve local initiatives related to coordinated school health programs. The School Health Index includes modules linked to each of the eight components of coordinated school health programs. Each module contains questions to assess school strengths and weaknesses related to the component (for example, health education) in general as well as with respect to five specific health topics: safety, physical activity, nutrition, tobacco use, and asthma. Each module also includes a planning activity for school personnel to complete once they have conducted the self-assessment process.

**School Health Policies and Programs Study.** An assessment of all eight components of coordinated school health programs, conducted by surveying fifty state departments of education and a national, representative sample of districts and elementary, middle, and high schools. The results provide school and public health practitioners as well as all who care about the health and safety of youths with an analysis of current school health programming.

**School Health Profiles.** A biannual survey conducted by the Centers for Disease Control and Prevention in even-numbered years (between administrations of the Youth Risk Behavior Survey). The School Health Profiles survey assesses secondary school programs, services, and policies related to health education, physical education and physical activity, health services, healthy and safe school environments, and family and community involvement in secondary schools.

**Schools.** One of the four major sites for health promotion programs, include child care centers; preschools; kindergarten; elementary, middle, and high schools; two-year and four-year colleges; universities; and vocational and technical education programs. Young people spend large portions of their lives in schools. Increasingly, postsecondary institutions are also sites where one can find nontraditional students (for example, adults seeking a career change or retired individuals seeking enrichment).

**Screening program.** A program that tests individuals without symptoms for the presence of risk factors. Appropriate follow-up includes personal counseling and monitoring in order to help individuals adopt healthy lifestyles, with supportive management by health professionals where necessary.

**Secondary data.** Data that already exist because they were collected by someone for another purpose. These data may or may not be directly from the individual or population that is currently being assessed. Sources of secondary data can be internal to a setting or organization (for example, student data, employee records) or external to a setting (for example, data from *Healthy People 2020*, vital records, census data, or peer-reviewed journals).

**Secondary health promotion.** The use of health promotion programs that help people identify, adopt, and reinforce specific protective behaviors and to improve early detection and reduction of existing health problems.

**Secondary prevention.** Interrupting problematic behaviors among those who are engaged in unhealthy decision making and perhaps showing early signs of disease or disability.

**Selective preventive interventions.** Interventions that target individuals or a subgroup of the population whose risk of developing illness or disorders is significantly higher than average. Examples include an education program for construction workers on wearing earplugs or protective devices when operating noisy machinery or grief counseling sessions provided to students who are experiencing a traumatic loss.

**Settings.** The sites of health promotion programs In 1997, the *Jakarta Declaration on Leading Health Promotion into the 21st Century* gave new prominence to the concept of the health setting as the place or social context in which people engage in daily activities in which environmental, organizational, and personal factors interact to affect health and well-being.

**Sexual orientation.** A factor that can be a determinant of health disparities.

**Short-term outcomes.** In a logic model, effects that can be expected to happen as an immediate result of each of the planned activities.

**SMART.** An approach to writing program objectives developed by the Centers for Disease Control and Prevention. The mnemonic SMART indicates that objectives should be specific, measurable, achievable, realistic, and time-bound.

**Social cognitive theory.** An interpersonal-level health theory that defines human behavior as an interaction of personal factors, behavioral factors, and environmental factors. Social cognitive theory is the most frequently used paradigm in health promotion. It is based on the reciprocal determinism between behavior, environment, and person; their constant interactions constitute the basis for human action.

**Social marketing.** A strategy that uses commercial marketing techniques to influence the voluntary behavior of target audience members for a health benefit. Social marketing promotes a behavior change to a targeted group of individuals in several ways. It encourages persons to accept a new behavior, reject a potential behavior, modify a current behavior, or abandon an old behavior.

**Social network and social support theory.** An interpersonal-level health theory that recognizes that social networks and the social relationships that are derived from them have powerful effects on important aspects of both physical and mental health. Social network refers to the existence of social ties. Research into how aspects of social networks influence health (positively or negatively) offers insight into the pathways that help to explain how social ties influence health. Social ties influence health through at least five primary pathways: (1) provision of social support; (2) social influence; (3) social engagement; (4) person-to-person contact; and (5) access to resources and material goods.

**Societal factors.** A cause of racial and ethnic disparities. Examples include poverty, racism, economics, health illiteracy, limited education, and educational inequality.

**Staff diversity.** A way to boost the representation of minorities in the health care workforce and a strategy for reducing health disparities.

**Staff management.** The functions of leading the staff of a program, including recruitment, training, coaching, development, day-to-day supervision, and evaluation.

**Staff members' fundraising responsibilities.** These responsibilities can include writing grant proposals, researching foundation and corporation requests for proposals, overseeing and implementing fundraising plans and strategies, and working to establish structures for effective fundraising. Collaboration with board members is a critical responsibility of development (fundraising) staff.

**Staff training.** Formal and informal education, mentoring, and coaching provided by a program to its staff in order to improve staff members' skills and service delivery, with the ultimate goal of improving the health outcomes of program participants.

**Stages of change model.** See *Transtheoretical model*.

**Stakeholders.** The people and organizations that have an interest in the health of a specific group, community, or population. Stakeholders have a legitimate interest (a stake) in what kind of health promotion program is planned and implemented.

**Standard operating procedures.** A commonly used label for program procedures that are drawn from program policies. Also see *Program procedures*.

**Standards of Practice for Health Promotion in Higher Education.** Guidelines for health promotion in the university setting. The standards espouse integration with the learning mission of higher education, collaborative practice, cultural competence, theory-based practice, evidence-based practice, and professional development and service.

**Survey questionnaires.** The most common means of gathering data for a needs assessment (for example, information about perceptions, behaviors, and issues). Questionnaires can be administered in four ways: as mail surveys, as telephone surveys, face to face, or as electronic surveys.

**Talking points.** A prepared list of issues and concepts that can be used in a variety of advocacy efforts such as meeting with a legislator, developing a public service announcement, or writing a letter to the editor. Talking points need to be succinct, on topic, and developed with a specific message in mind.

**Ten essential public health services (EPHS).** A guiding framework for the responsibilities of local public health systems, defining public health practice within local health departments and in collaboration with community partners.

**Tertiary health promotion.** The use of health promotion programs designed to improve the lives of individuals currently in treatment for a medical or health problem or individuals with chronic illness and to help them avoid further deterioration or relapses.

**Tertiary prevention.** Improving the lives of individuals currently in treatment for a medical or health problem or individuals with chronic illness.

**Theory.** A "set of interrelated concepts, definitions, and propositions that present a systematic view of events or situations by specifying relationships among variables in order to explain and predict the events or situations" (F. N. Kerlinger, *Foundations of Behavioral Research*, 3rd ed. [New York: Holt, Rinehart & Winston, 1986], p. 25).

**Theory of planned behavior.** A derivative of the theory of reasoned action, this theory postulates that people are motivated to change on the basis of their perceptions of norms, attitudes, and control over behaviors. Each of these factors can either increase or decrease a person's intent to change their behavior. Intention to change behavior, then, is thought to be directly related to behavior change.

**Theory of reasoned action.** Developed by Martin Fishbein and Icek Ajzen in 1975 to examine the relationship between attitudes and behavior, the theory of reasoned action looks at behavioral intentions rather than attitudes as the main predictors of behavior. According to this theory, attitudes toward a behavior (or more precisely, attitudes toward the expected outcome or result of a behavior) and subjective norms (the influence other people have on a person's attitudes and behavior) are the major predictors of behavioral intention.

**Transtheoretical model.** This model (also called stages of change model) is an individual-level health theory that proposes that behavior change is a process that occurs in stages and that people move through these stages in a specific sequence as they change. The stages are pre-contemplation, contemplation, preparation, action, and maintenance. People can move forward or backward (relapse) through the stages. The dimension of time—that is, each of the stages being associated with a specific time frame—is unique to the stages of change model.

**United Way.** There are more than 1,300 United Ways in the United States, and they pool their fundraising efforts. The focus of these local nonprofit organizations is identifying and resolving pressing community issues, as well as making measurable changes in the communities through partnerships with schools, government agencies, businesses, organized labor, financial institutions, community development corporations, voluntary and neighborhood associations, the faith community, and others.

**Universal preventive interventions.** These interventions target the general public or a population that has not been identified on the basis of individual risk. They are found to have mild to strong influences on different health concerns among different populations. Examples of this type of intervention include mass media campaigns via public service announcements on TV and social skills instruction provided to all K–12 students.

**Validity.** The degree to which an instrument or procedure (for example, a needs assessment survey, evaluation questionnaire, or key informant interview) accurately reflects or assesses the specific concept that the program staff, stakeholders, or participants are attempting to measure.

**Variable.** A construct (also called an indicator) that is assigned a specific property and that can be measured.

**Volunteers.** Individuals who serve an organization or cause and who do not receive compensation for services rendered. In health promotion programs, volunteers perform many tasks from direct service delivery to service on boards of directors or as program advocates. Popular in many schools are service-learning programs, in which students volunteer in community health organizations as part of their course work. Volunteers provide countless hours of services in health promotion programs through community health organizations.

**Wellness.** Physical well-being, especially when it is maintained or achieved through good diet and regular exercise.

**Wellness committee.** A group of employees from key departments or subgroups within an organization that have an interest in or commitment to workers' health and safety. Also see *Advisory board*.

**Workplaces.** One of the four major settings for health promotion programs, including any setting where people are employed—in business or industry (small, large, or multinational) as well as in government (for example, in the armed services; local, state, or federal civil service; or offices of elected officials) or in the nonprofit sector.

**World Health Organization.** The directing and coordinating authority for health within the United Nations system. It is responsible for providing leadership on global health matters, shaping the health research agenda, setting norms and standards, articulating evidence-based policy options, providing technical support to countries, and monitoring and assessing health trends.

**Youth Risk Behavior Survey.** The biannual national school-based survey conducted by the Centers for Disease Control and Prevention and state, territorial, tribal, and local surveys conducted by state, territorial, and local education and health agencies and tribal governments. The survey is part of the Youth Risk Behavior Surveillance System, which monitors priority health-risk behaviors and the prevalence of obesity and asthma among youths and young adults.

**Zone of drastic mutation.** The point after which further modification of a program to fit a target population other than the one it was designed for will compromise the program's integrity and effectiveness.